Infection Prevention Competency Review Guide 4th Edition

Association for Professionals in Infection Control and Epidemiology, Inc.

Carol M. McLay, RN, MPH, DrPH, CIC

© Copyright 2010

Association for Professionals in Infection Control and Epidemiology, Inc. (APIC)
1275 K Street, NW, Suite 1000
Washington, DC 20005-4006

All rights reserved.
No part of this publication may be reproduced, stored in a retrieval system
or transmitted, in any form or by any means, electronic, mechanical, photocopying,
recording or otherwise, without the prior written permission of the
Association for Professionals in Infection Control and Epidemiology, Inc.

Disclaimer

The *Infection Prevention Competency Review Guide (4th Edition)* was developed to assist individuals preparing to become Certified in Infection Control® (CIC) by the Certification Board for Infection Control (CBIC). The *Study Guide* is not intended to cover every aspect of the certification exam, nor does APIC have any knowledge of the contents of the exam. Rather, the *Study Guide* is intended to provide an overall review for the practice of infection prevention and control. Questions set forth in the *Study Guide* do not necessarily reflect the type of questions found in the certification exam. The outline for each topic in the *Study Guide* is not meant to contain all of the answers for the questions in the exam, nor does each outline contain all the information found on the test. It is highly recommended that the *Study Guide* not be used as the sole means of preparation for the CIC® certification exam. Further study should include the *APIC Text of Infection Control and Epidemiology*, 2009 edition.

Questions

For questions directly related to the *Infection Prevention Competency Review Guide*, contact APIC Headquarters:

Phone: (202) 789–1890
Fax: (202) 789–1899
E-mail: apicinfo@apic.org
Website: www.apic.org

For questions related to the Certification Board of Infection Control (CBIC) or the certification examination, contact CBIC directly at:

Certification Board of Infection Control and Epidemiology, Inc.

555 East Wells Street
Suite 1100
Milwaukee, WI 53202-3823
Phone: (414) 918-9796
Email info@cbic.org
Website: www.cbic.org

Description

The *Review Guide* consists of seven chapters that correspond to the areas of testing as defined by the Certification Board of Infection Control (CBIC) as well as a general chapter about taking the certification exam:

  I.   Identification of Infectious Disease Processes

  II. Surveillance and Epidemiological Investigation

  III. Preventing/Controlling the Transmission of Infectious Agents

  IV. Employee/Occupational Health

  V.   Management and Communication (Leadership)

  VI. Education and Research

  VII. The Certification Exam

Suggestions for using the *Review Guide* include individual study as well as group study. Most of the questions are referenced to the *APIC Text of Infection Control and Epidemiology*, 2009 edition. The Centers for Disease Control and Prevention (CDC) provide additional important resources and current infection prevention guidelines at: www.cdc.gov.

In addition to sample questions, a copy of the CIC® certification examination content outline has been included for more in-depth study.

Note: The *Infection Prevention Competency Review Guide* will not necessarily cover all of the material included on the certification exam.

Introduction

The *Infection Prevention Competency Review Guide (4th Edition)* has been revised to reflect the most recent national guidelines, practice recommendations and public health issues. The *APIC Text of Infection Control and Epidemiology*, 2009 edition, is also recommended for a more extensive study of the subjects covered in the *Review Guide*. For the most current information related to evidence-based practice or national guidelines, visit the CDC website (www.cdc.gov) and the APIC website (www.apic.org). The certification exam and content outline were revised based on the results of the 2009 CBIC Practice Analysis Survey. Questions included in the *Review Guide* reflect all levels of the exam questions:

1. Cognitive Level I (recall—simple recall of memory)
2. Cognitive Level II (application—simple application or interpretation of data)
3. Cognitive Level III (analysis—evaluation of data or problem solving)

The *Review Guide* is designed to fulfill the need for a formalized study tool to assist infection prevention professionals in preparing for certification in infection control.

Certification has, as its primary purpose, the increased protection of the public by providing an objective measurement of standardized current knowledge recognized and respected within and outside the field of infection prevention and control and epidemiology. Certification represents both an individual and organizational commitment to continual improvement of infection prevention and control functions and their overall contribution to healthcare and patient safety.

APIC supports certification as a mechanism for infection preventionists (IPs) to establish their mastery of specialized knowledge by taking and passing a comprehensive examination developed by APIC's independent credentialing arm, the Certification Board for Infection Control and Epidemiology (CBIC). IPs who are certified are authorized and encouraged to use the internationally recognized initials CIC after their names and in their titles.

In preparation for certification, this *Review Guide* is intended for use as a supplement to other references, pertinent journal articles and guidelines. For further study, a bibliography is included at the end of each section. It is strongly recommended that IPs use the resources listed in the bibliography in preparation for the certification exam. Individuals seeking certification are encouraged to develop a customized study plan that includes reviewing the CBIC content outline and taking a practice test (both available at www.cbic.org) to identify subjects or areas on which they most need to focus.

Carol M. McLay, RN, MPH, DrPH, CIC
Author (4th Edition)

Author 4th Edition   Carol M. McLay RN, MPH, DrPH, CIC

2010 Edition Reviewers   Kathleen M. McMullen, MPH, CIC
Kathleen Meehan Arias, MS, MT, SM, CIC
Sara Straub, RN, MPH, CIC

Contents

	Article	Page
Chapter One:	CBIC Content Outline	2
Identification of Infectious Disease Processes	I. Fundamental Principles of Infection and Immunity	3
	II. Basic Microbiology	11
	III. Clinical Microbiology	15
	IV. Laboratory Testing and Diagnostics	20
	V. Microbial Pathogenesis	21
	VI. Antimicrobial Therapy	24
	VII. Selected Infectious Diseases and Conditions	29
	Practice Questions for Chapter One	62
	References	79
Chapter Two:	CBIC Content Outline	82
Surveillance and Epidemiological Investigation	I. Epidemiology	84
	II. Statistics	88
	III. Design of Surveillance Systems	100
	IV. Collection and Compilation of Surveillance Data	104
	V. Interpretation of Surveillance Data	105
	VI. Outbreak Investigation	107
	VII. CDC Definitions of Healthcare-Associated Infections	110
	Practice Questions for Chapter Two	132
	References	161

Chapter Three:

Preventing/ Controlling the Transmission of Infectious Agents

CBIC Content Outline		164
I.	Policy Review	165
II.	Disasters and Biological Events	165
III.	Hand Hygiene	170
IV.	Cleaning, Disinfection and Sterilization	172
V.	Specific Care Settings	185
VI.	Therapeutic and Diagnostic Procedures and Devices	189
VII.	Recalls	195
VIII.	Isolation Precautions	196
IX.	Environmental Hazards	198
X.	Immunization of Patient	200
XI.	Construction and Renovation	200
XII.	Prevention of Transmission of Tuberculosis	204
XIII.	Prevention of Bloodborne Pathogens	205
XIV.	Elimination of *Clostridium difficile*	207
XV.	Prevention and Control of MDROs in Healthcare Settings	208
	Practice Questions for Chapter Three	210
	References	236

Chapter Four:

Employee/ Occupational Health

CBIC Content Outline		244
I.	Infection Prevention Objectives of an Employee/ Occupational Health Program	255
II.	Major Components of an Employee/Occupational Health Program	255
	Practice Questions for Chapter Four	266
	References	276

Chapter Five:

Management and Communication

CBIC Content Outline		286
I.	The Infection Prevention and Control Program	281
II.	Communication and Feedback	286
III.	Quality/Performance Improvement	287
	Practice Questions for Chapter Five	292
	References	308

Chapter Six:		CBIC Content Outline	312
Education and Research		Section A: Education	313
	I.	Basic Principles in Teaching and Learning	313
	II.	Educational Program Development	314
		Section B: Research	318
	I.	Critiquing Published Research Studies	318
	II.	Incorporating Research Findings into Practice	320
		Practice Questions for Chapter Six	322
		References	337
Chapter Seven:	I.	Description of the CBIC Exam	340
The Certification Exam	II.	Types of Exam Takers	342
	III.	Preparation for the Exam	345
	IV.	Exam-Taking Techniques	346
	V.	The Computerized Version of the Exam	347
	VI.	Self-Assessment Recertification Examination	349
	VII.	Contact Information	350

CHAPTER ONE

IDENTIFICATION OF INFECTIOUS DISEASE PROCESSES

CONTENTS

Article	Page
CBIC Content Outline for Identification of Infectious Disease Processes	2
Chapter One: Identification of Infectious Disease Processes	3
I. Fundamental Principles of Infection and Immunity	3
II. Basic Microbiology	11
III. Clinical Microbiology	15
IV. Laboratory Testing and Diagnostics	20
V. Microbial Pathogenesis	21
VI. Antimicrobial Therapy	24
VII. Selected Infectious Diseases and Conditions	29
Practice Questions for Chapter One	62
References	79

CBIC CONTENT OUTLINE

Identification of Infectious Disease Processes (18 Questions)

A. Differentiate among colonization, infection and contamination

B. Identify occurrences, reservoirs, incubation periods, periods of communicability, modes of transmission, signs and symptoms and susceptibility associated with the disease process

C. Interpret results of diagnostic findings/laboratory reports

D. Recognize limitations and advantages of types of tests used to diagnose infectious processes

E. Recognize epidemiologically significant organisms for immediate review and investigation

F. Differentiate among prophylactic, empiric and therapeutic uses of antimicrobials

G. Identify indications for environmental microbiological monitoring

Chapter One: Identification of Infectious Diseases Processes

I. Fundamental Principles of Infection and Immunity

A. Definitions

1. Colonization—presence of microorganisms in or on a host with growth but without tissue invasion or damage
2. Infection—entry of an infectious agent in the tissues of the host that multiplies and creates symptoms
3. Contamination—presence of microorganisms on inanimate objects (e.g., clothing, surgical instruments), on skin or in substances (e.g., water, food, milk)

B. Components of the Infectious Disease Process (Chain of Infection)

1. Causative agent
2. Reservoir of the agent
3. Portal of exit of the agent from the reservoir
4. Mode of transmission of the agent
5. Portal of entry into host
6. Susceptible host

Figure 1–1. Chain of infection. Components of the infectious disease process.

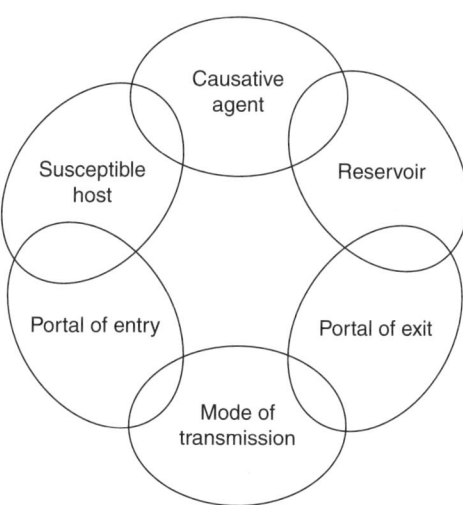

(Source: *APIC Text of Infection Control and Epidemiology*, 2009; 2–5.)

C. **Mechanisms of Microbe Pathogenicity**
   1. Virulence—measure of a microbe's ability to invade and create disease in a host, determined by:
      a. Ability to survive in the environment during transit between hosts
         (1) Blood-borne pathogens survive in blood outside of the body
         (2) Genetic characteristics to protect against drying
         (3) Carried within a vector (insect, etc.)
      b. An effective mechanism for transmission to a new host
         (1) Vectors that carry organisms also transmit them when biting, etc.
         (2) Motility of organisms that permit movement through an aqueous environment in the host to an appropriate receptor site
         (3) Airborne transmission
         (4) Fomites
      c. Ability to attach to the structure it will infect
         (1) Electrostatic charge on many bacteria permits attachment to oppositely charged cells common in humans
         (2) Specific adhesions on most bacteria favor attachment to sites of infection (e.g., protein-, polysaccharide- or foreign body–binding adhesions)
      d. Mechanism for proliferation
         (1) Secreted enzymes from pathogen that enhance spread through tissue planes
         (2) Exotoxins that kill or immobilize cellular defenses of the host
         (3) Capsules that inhibit phagocytosis or protect organisms after phagocytosis
         (4) Biofilm—slime that prevents water-soluble elements such as antibiotics and disinfectants from reaching pathogens
         (5) Digestive enzymes that dissolve nutrients essential for bacterial metabolism
      e. Invasion and dissemination
         (1) Rigid cell wall is a physical barrier
         (2) Cell surface components that inhibit phagocytosis
         (3) Ability to alter the cell surface to avoid host-created antibodies
         (4) Deterrents to intracellular killing after phagocytosis
   2. Bacterial toxins
      a. Exotoxins (enterotoxins, secreted by bacteria and proteins)
         (1) Commonly secreted by gram-positive bacteria
         (2) More susceptible to heat inactivation but variable
         (3) Neutralized by specific antibody
         (4) May possess enzymatic activity
         (5) Examples: Panton-Valentine leukocidin of methicillin-resistant *Staphylococcus aureus* (MSRA) enhances invasion by killing neutrophils and enhances rapid spread by digesting proteins; toxin A and B of *Clostridium difficile* create ulcers in the mucosa of the colon

CHAPTER ONE: IDENTIFICATION OF INFECTIOUS DISEASE PROCESSES | 5

   b. Endotoxins (complexes of bacterial proteins, lipids and polysaccharides)
      (1) Surface component of gram-negative bacteria
      (2) Not destroyed by boiling or autoclaving
      (3) Partially neutralized by antibodies
      (4) Produce physiological changes by interacting with host systems to set off cascades of responses that can induce fever, swelling, vascular leaking, pain and shock, such as the complement system
      (5) Example—cholera toxin increases secretion of fluids in the gastrointestinal (GI) tract

D. **Cellular Immune System**[1-5]
   1. Cell-mediated immunity (CMI) is the immune response induced, mediated or regulated by T lymphocytes and mononuclear phagocytes
   2. Cellular immune system interacts with humoral system via the effects of CD4 T on B lymphocytes and granulocytes
   3. Precursors of T lymphocytes originate in bone marrow, migrate to the thymus during fetal development and infancy, mature in the thymus and lead to production of T cells, which thereafter originate from spleen, lymph nodes and bone marrow
   4. Specificity of CMI depends on the presence of specific receptors on the surface of reactive T lymphocytes
   5. Cellular immune response
      a. Initially foreign substances are taken up by large phagocytic cells (called macrophages or Langerhans' cells) or B lymphocytes; initial binding occurs to immunoglobulin G (IgG) receptors on the surface of the cells
      b. Materials are engulfed by cells, where they are processed to small molecules and bound to major histocompatibility complexes (MHCs)
      c. Processing appears to depend on whether materials are within compartments called phagosomes or free in the cytoplasm of the phagocytic cell; those within phagosomes are processed to small molecules, bound to MHC and transferred to CD8 cytotoxic lymphocytes
      d. Transfer to CD4 lymphocytes of processed molecules that are bound to MHC occurs in conjunction with release of lymphokines interleukin-1 (IL-1) and interleukin-6 (IL-6)
      e. When complex binds to specific CD4 cell binding sites, cells proliferate and release other lymphokines
      f. Alterations in CMI directly compromise the ability to mount a defense against certain viral infections and can indirectly decrease antibody production
   6. T lymphocytes—descriptions and functions
      a. CD3 surface marker, present on T cells, identifies them

b. CD4 marker is on subpopulation of CD3 cells; these CD4 cells function as helper lymphocytes for:
  (1) Promotion of phagocytosis by other cells
  (2) Enhancement of activity of other T or B lymphocytes—mediated by release of lymphokines (cytokines)
  (3) Anamnestic response (long-term memory)—vaccine protection
c. CD8 cells, a subpopulation of CD3 cells, are cytotoxic and suppressor lymphocytes
  (1) Cytotoxic lymphocytes kill cells in which viruses are replicating
  (2) Suppressor CD8 cells control the intensity of T- and B-lymphocyte activity by suppressing their reproduction and metabolism
d. Natural killer (NK) cells are neither CD4 nor CD8 cells; NK cells have ability to lyse tumor cells and virus-infected cells; NK cells have CD16 and CD56 markers on their surface

7. Cytokines
  a. Interleukin-1 (IL-1)
    (1) Produced by many cell lines in the cellular immune system
    (2) Originally described as endogenous pyrogen, induces fever
    (3) Stimulates the differentiation of primitive T lymphocytes to specific T-cell lines
    (4) Increases the production of other cytokines: IL-2, INF-γ, IL-4, colony-stimulating factors, and antibody production from B cells
    (5) Increases chemotaxis of macrophages
  b. Interleukin-2 (IL-2)
    (1) Produced by CD4 cells
    (2) Growth stimulator for T cells
    (3) Enhances activity of NK cells
  c. Interleukin-4 (IL-4)
    (1) Produced by all T cells and mast cells
    (2) Stimulates growth of T and B lymphocytes, mast cells and eosinophils
  d. Interleukin-6 (IL-6)
    (1) Produced by macrophages and T and B lymphocytes
    (2) Promotes B-lymphocyte differentiation
    (3) Causes proliferation of T lymphocytes
    (4) Causes differentiation of cytotoxic T lymphocytes, macrophages and neutrophils
    (5) Induces fever
  e. INF-α and INF-β
    (1) Termed type I interferons (INFs)
    (2) Produced by circulating white blood cells (WBCs) and fibroblasts
    (3) Interfere with reproduction of viruses within infected cells

f. INF-γ
      (1) Produced by activated T lymphocytes
      (2) Inhibits virus growth
   g. Tumor necrosis factor (TNF)
      (1) Produced by macrophages
      (2) Causes involution and death of tumor cells
      (3) Causes protein catabolism in host with loss of muscle mass
   h. Lymphotoxin
      (1) Similar to TNF
      (2) Promotes inflammation
      (3) Simulates neutrophils
   i. Granulocyte macrophage colony-stimulating factor (GM-CSF)
      (1) Produced by many cell lines
      (2) Stimulates reproduction of all granulocyte and macrophage cell lines
   j. Granulocyte colony-stimulating factor (G-CSF)
      (1) Produced by many cells of the reticuloendothelial system and vascular endothelium
      (2) Stimulates reproduction of granulocyte cell lines
   k. Monocyte colony-stimulating factor (M-CSF)
      (1) Produced by many reticuloendothelial cell lines
      (2) Stimulates reproduction of monocytes

E. Humoral Immune System[6]

1. Cellular sources of humoral immunity (antibody)
   a. Precursors of B lymphocytes originate from fetal liver and bone marrow; populate the spleen and lymph nodes
   b. When B lymphocytes are stimulated by native or macrophage-processed soluble antigen, they divide and mature into antibody-producing cells called plasma cells or plasmacytes
2. Classes of immunoglobulins (antibodies)
   a. Antibody molecules contain structural sites: Fab (fragment antigen-binding), which reacts with specific antigens, and Fc (fragment, crystallizable), which distinguishes among the various classes
   b. Immunoglobulin G (IgG)
      (1) Major circulating and extravascular antibody
      (2) Protein molecule
      (3) Late-occurring immunoglobulin of an immune response and longest-lived
   c. Immunoglobulin M (IgM)
      (1) First reacting antibody or immunoglobulin to be produced to fight off infection

(2) Generally present only 6 months after initial exposure to foreign antigen; exceptions are polysaccharides and ABO blood group substances
(3) Mainly intravascular and represents the first line of defense against infection
   d. Immunoglobulin A (IgA) is the principal secretory antibody, formed by plasma cells residing in mucous membranes, present in saliva, breast milk and tissues of bladder, prostate and GI tract
   e. Immunoglobulin D (IgD) is present on the surface of lymphocytes, where it serves to determine their antigen specificity
   f. Immunoglobulin E (IgE) is the principal allergy-inducing immunoglobulin; stimulates release of large quantities of histamine and other inflammatory substances, found on mucous membranes of individuals with seasonal allergies; may aid in protection against intestinal parasites

F. Nonspecific Host Defenses[7-9]

1. Genetic constitution
   a. Caucasians and African Americans possess vigorous natural resistance to deep mycoses and to rubeola virus, whereas Asians lack resistance to both
   b. Alaskan and Hawaiian natives are naturally deficient in resistance to rubeola
2. Mechanical barriers to infection
   a. Intact skin and mucous membranes
   b. Normal skin bacterial flora depletes its environment of essential nutrients for pathogens, competes for tissue binding sites and secretes naturally occurring antibiotics and fatty acids that are lethal to pathogens
3. Physiological barriers to pathogens
   a. Fever
      (1) Centrally controlled in anterior hypothalamus
      (2) Beneficial—many organisms are inhibited by high temperatures
      (3) Harmful—febrile convulsions, worsening congestive heart failure
      (4) Whether fever is beneficial or harmful continues to be debated[10-12]
   b. Secretions
      (1) Lysozyme is a low-activity enzyme secreted by mucous membrane cells, which kills some gram-positive bacteria
      (2) Gastric acid provides major barrier to infection of the intestinal tract; artificial elevation of gastric pH by histamine antagonist or antacids allows overgrowth of bacteria in the stomach
      (3) Secreted enzymes from salivary glands, pancreas and intestinal cells partially digest invading pathogens
      (4) Motility of alimentary and urinary tracts expels invading pathogens

4. Circulating defenses in the vascular tree
   a. Natural, or cross-reactive, antibodies are antibodies that are produced without any previous infection, vaccination or other foreign exposure. Natural antibodies can activate the classical complement pathway leading to lysis of a pathogen before the adaptive immune response is activated.
   b. Fibronectin-circulating protein that binds to pathogen receptors and prevents their adherence to cells
   c. Estrogens control secretion and characteristics of mucous membrane cells
   d. Circulating neutrophils, monocytes and macrophages in the reticuloendothelial system ingest and kill many pathogens

G. **Complement System**[13,14]
   1. Consists of 11 sequentially reacting serum proteins that in their activated forms possess biological activities essential to host defense against many invading microorganisms and tumor cells
   2. Activation may be through two pathways
      a. Classical pathway
         (1) Thorough contact with IgG, IgM antibody
         (2) Components of complement system include C1q, r and s; C4; C2; C3; C5; C6; C7; C8; and C9
      b. Alternative pathway
         (1) Contact with certain microorganisms
         (2) Pathway starts with direct activation of C3, then proceeds as defined previously
   3. Genetic deficiencies have been determined to exist in some individuals

H. **Phagocytic Cell System**[15,16]
   1. Components
      a. Granulocytes (polymorphonuclear [PMN] leukocyte)
         (1) Have inclusions (granules) within the cytoplasm that are released into the surrounding location of an infection to degrade and kill pathogens
         (2) Specific staining of the inclusions differentiates the three classes:
            (a) Neutrophils—first cells to arrive at an inflammatory focus
            (b) Stages of development: myeloblast, myelocyte, metamyelocyte, nonfilamented neutrophil (bands, juveniles, stabs), mature neutrophil
            (c) "Left shift" implies abundance of immature neutrophils in peripheral blood
            (d) Basophils—no part in infection resistance, contain histamine and participate in allergic response
            (e) Eosinophils—important in hypersensitivity reactions and host defense against many parasites

(3) Stages of PMN function in host defense
   (a) Chemotaxis—migration of infection site
   (b) Opsonization—coating of microbe by antibody and complement to promote phagocytosis
   (c) Phagocytosis—attachment and engulfment with enclosure of microbe in a vacuole (phagosome)
   (d) Oxidative burst—increased oxygen consumption by neutrophil is converted to oxygen metabolites, which when released into the phagosome are microbicidal
   (e) Degranulation and killing—rupture of granules after coalescence and release into vacuole; also release of chemoattractants for PMNs and monocytes
   (f) Terms
      i. Normal WBC count: 4000–10,000 cells/mm^3
      ii. Leukocytosis: WBC count >10,000 cells/mm^3
      iii. Leukopenia: total WBC count <4000 cells/mm^3
      iv. Neutropenia: PMN or band forms WBC count <500 cells/mm^3 or absolute neutrophil count <1000 cells/mm^3 (high risk for fatal infection)
      v. Absolute neutrophil count = total WBC count × percentage of mature and immature neutrophils
b. Mononuclear phagocytes
   (1) Effector cells of inflammation, arrive after neutrophils
   (2) Major defense against intracellular pathogens
   (3) Function as antigen-presenting cells for inducing immune response and disposal of damaged or nonfunctioning host cells
   (4) Repair tissue damage and lessen cellular response that occurs during inflammation
   (5) Types:
      (a) Monocytes (circulate in peripheral blood)
      (b) Macrophage (tissue-fixed counterpart to monocytes)
         i. Kupffer's cells (liver)
         ii. Alveolar macrophages (lungs)
         iii. Histocytes (spleen)
         iv. Dendroglia (central nervous system [CNS])

II. Basic Microbiology

A. Classification Schemes

Based on the degree of genetic similarity between different species
1. Kingdom
2. Division
3. Class
4. Order
5. Family
6. Genus
7. Species

B. Microorganism Classification

1. Prokaryotes—smaller, unicellular organisms with no membrane envelope around nuclear DNA, replicate by binary fission, have plasmids and typically have a cell wall; include bacteria, cyanobacteria, rickettsiae, chlamydiae, mycoplasmas
2. Eukaryotes—larger and more complex, distinct nucleus and organelles, replicate by mitosis and meiosis, do not have cell wall (exception is fungi); includes fungi, protozoa, simple algae
3. Archaebacteria—microorganisms that grow under extreme environmental conditions

C. Bacteria (Single-Cell Prokaryotes)

1. Internal structure
    a. Small, simple, single-cell
    b. Single, long circular molecule of double-stranded DNA
    c. Ribosomes—transcribe messenger RNA into essential proteins
    d. Cell (plasma) membrane—phospholipid bilayer that has selective permeability for nutrient intake
    e. Often contain double-stranded DNA molecules called plasmids that may carry genes for activities such as antibiotic resistance, production of toxins and synthesis of enzymes; can be transferred from one bacterium to another, and genes may move from plasmid to chromosome (called transposable genetic elements or transposons)
    f. Certain bacteria (e.g., *Clostridium, Bacillus*) form endospores or spores; can survive heat, lack of water and toxic chemicals; may enter vegetative state until encountering ideal living conditions at which time they germinate and begin to reproduce
2. External structure
    a. Cell wall—rigid layer surrounding the cell membrane that provides mechanical support of the cell and protection from lysis; composed of layers of peptidoglycan (many layers in gram-positive, few layers in gram-negative)

b. Glycocalyx—substances that surround cells; if organized and attached to cell wall, it forms a capsule, which may contribute to virulence and offer protection from phagocytosis; if unorganized and loosely attached to cell wall, it forms a slime layer
c. Some bacteria also have:
(1) Flagella—filaments that confer motility, can be polar (end of cell) or peritrichous (surrounding cell)
(2) Fimbriae and pili—protein filaments aid in attachment, adherence and/or conjugation
3. Size, shape and arrangements of bacterial cells
a. Range from 0.2 to 2.0 µm in diameter, 2 to 8 µm in length
b. Basic shapes—spherical coccus, rod-shaped bacillus and spiral
4. Bacterial replication: Cellular division—rate of division varies—every 15 minutes to 12 to 24 hours
a. Cell enlarges
b. Chromosome replicates itself
c. Septation forms in cell wall
d. Daughter cells divide
5. Genetic variation
a. Plasmids—circular strands of DNA that are separate from chromosomal DNA; carry genetic information for antibiotic resistance, etc.
b. Transfer of genetic information via:
(1) Transformation—uptake of free DNA into cell (e.g., penicillin resistance genes)
(2) Transduction—DNA ferried into cell by bacteriophage (nonlethal infection by virus adds DNA that is integrated into cell chromosome)
(3) Conjugation—direct linking of two cells results in transfer of part or all of plasmid from donor to a recipient cell (e.g., gentamicin resistance)
6. Mutation is random base pair substitution in DNA caused by replication errors; has the ability to cause antibiotic resistance as well (e.g., rifampin resistance)
7. Submicroscopic bacteria
a. Mycoplasma (unicellular prokaryote lacking a cell wall)
(1) Smallest organism capable of self-replication
(2) Resistant to many antibiotics that act against a cell wall
(3) Examples: community-associated pneumonia, surgical wound infection, postpartum endometritis, urinary tract infections
b. Chlamydiae (obligate intracellular parasitic bacteria)
(1) Complex life cycle
(a) Elementary body—compact, infectious form with cell wall
(b) Reticulate body—fragile, depends on host cell for energy (adenosine triphosphate [ATP]); divides to form large inclusion in host cell

(c) Inclusion cells condense to elementary bodies, lyse cell and begin new infection cycle
            (2) Examples: ocular trachoma, genital tract infection, atypical pneumonia and psittacosis
        c. Rickettsiae (obligate intracellular parasitic bacteria)
            (1) Size—small coccobacilli contain DNA, RNA and energy-producing enzymes
            (2) Divide by binary fission
            (3) Examples: Rocky Mountain spotted fever, Q fever, epidemic typhus, rickettsialpox

D. **Fungi (Eukaryotic Organisms with Cell Walls That Lack Photosynthetic Capability)**

   1. Organisms exist as saprophytes of dead organic matter or parasites of living organisms
   2. Morphological classification
        a. Yeasts—single-celled, reproduce by budding
        b. Molds—multinucleated network of filaments
        c. Dimorphic fungi—may grow as yeast or fungi depending on conditions
   3. Cellular structure—nuclear membrane, mitochondria, endoplasmic reticulum, vacuoles and rigid polysaccharide cell wall
   4. Reproduction—yeasts bud, molds contain spores, diploid sexual phase, haploid spores form by meiosis
   5. Examples: *Candida* fungemia, *Aspergillus* necrotizing pneumonia, disseminated histoplasmosis, *Pneumocystis carinii* pneumonia (PCP)

E. **Yeasts**

   1. Single-celled, microscopic, round-to-oval organisms
   2. Range in size from 2 to 60 μm
   3. Usually form smooth, creamy colony
   4. Single nucleus with a nuclear membrane and contains organelles
   5. Usually reproduce by budding, some through fission
   6. Examples: *Candida* spp., *Cryptococcus neoformans*

F. **Molds**

   1. Consist of long, branching filaments of cells called hyphae
   2. May reproduce asexually
   3. Also may reproduce sexually or asexually by formation of spores
   4. Examples: *Aspergillus* spp., *Rhizopus*

G. Virus (Smallest Infectious Agent—DNA or RNA in a Protein Coat)

1. Can replicate only in cells of other living organisms
2. Viral life cycle within the cell
   a. Attachment—virion attaches to receptor site on host cell
   b. Penetration—virion enters host cell via endocytosis
   c. Replication—viral DNA or RNA direct host cell to begin synthesis of viral components
   d. Maturation—assembly of progeny genomes and capsids into daughter virions
   e. Release—lysis of cell, releasing daughter virions
3. Grouped into families based on
   a. Genome type
   b. Number of strands in genome
   c. Presence of absence of an envelope

H. Prions (Infectious Agent Composed of Protein)

1. Can replicate only in cells of living organisms
2. Affect the brain or neural tissue; are untreatable and universally fatal
3. Examples: Creutzfeldt-Jakob disease, mad cow disease in cattle

I. Parasites

1. Any organism living within or on another living creature and deriving advantage from doing so while causing disadvantage to the host
   a. Ectoparasites
      (1) Infestations are fairly common in the community
      (2) Can be spread in a healthcare facility
      (3) Examples: scabies, bedbugs, lice
   b. Protozoa
      (1) Unicellular, free-living eukaryotic organisms
      (2) Most are not pathogenic to humans; not typically related to healthcare facilities but have important public health considerations
      (3) Examples: *Leishmania, Toxoplasma, Giardia*
   c. Helminths
      (1) Parasitic worms
      (2) Examples: roundworms, tapeworms and flatworms

III. Clinical Microbiology

A. Diagnostic Bacteriology

Goal is to classify pathogenic bacteria to determine origin or predict response to antibacterial therapy

B. Techniques Used in the Observation, Cultivation and Identification of Microorganisms

1. Light microscopy
   a. Bright-field microscopy—oil immersion lens results in $1000\times$ magnification; scanning lens is $40\times$ magnification
   b. Dark-field microscopy—bright objects appear on dark background; used for motile spirochetes (such as treponemes); used on fresh material that cannot be stained
   c. Phase-contrast microscopy—cellular elements of different densities appear to stand out from the background—used in viral isolation in living tissue
   d. Fluorescent microscopy—uses ultraviolet (UV) light on naturally fluorescent substances, coupled with direct or indirect fluorescent antibody (DFA or IFA) for rapid diagnosis
   e. Confocal microscopy—specimens are stained with fluorochromes and will emit light; laser is used to illuminate the specimen; may be used with computer to develop 3-dimensional images
2. Electron microscopy—mainly used for viruses and large molecules; uses electron-emitting tungsten filament, which is focused on specially prepared microscope; images are viewed on a computer—less often used because of cost
   a. Transmission electron microscopy—uses a finely focused beam
   b. Scanning electron microscopy—allows for 3-dimensional view
3. Specimen preparation
   a. Direct examination—must be performed as soon as possible; may require the specimen to be diluted with saline; most often used for fungi and parasites
   b. Fixation—heat or chemicals used to kill the organisms and attach them to the slide
   c. Simple stains—stains all bacteria equally to outline shape (coccus, bacillus, spiral), size or arrangement (single, diplo, chains, clusters); wet mounts generally use methylene blue, crystal violet, malachite green and safranin
   d. Differential stains—use two or more stains to stain certain bacteria different colors
      (1) Gram stains—use crystal violet (primary dye), iodine (mordant), acid-alcohol (decolorizer) and safranin (counterstaining dye); gram-positive cells are purple, gram-negative are red
      (2) Acid-fast stains—Kinyoun (cold), Ziehl Neelsen (hot) for *Mycobacteria*, modified for *Nocardia*

(3) Calcofluor white—rapid screen for fungal elements or pneumocysts
(4) Immunofluorescent staining—dye converts UV light into visible light coupled with antibody directed against a specific genus or species; if antibody binds with organism it appears to glow against a dark background (*Chlamydia, Legionella*)
(5) Trichrome stain—differentiates the internal structures of cysts, trophozoites or other forms of parasites; useful for examination of stool samples

C. Identification of Bacteria
1. Physical conditions required for the growth of bacteria
   a. Nutrition (media)
   b. Temperature (ideal for most bacteria—35°C)
   c. Atmospheric conditions—aerobic (must have oxygen), obligate anaerobes (grow without oxygen, killed or inhibited in presence of oxygen), facultative anaerobes (can grow with or without presence of oxygen), and microaerophilic (require 2% to 10% oxygen and may require increased carbon dioxide)
2. Growth media types—choice depends on requirements of bacteria, site being cultured and need for bacterial inhibition
   a. Nutrient agar (blood agar)—general purpose, supports growth of wide variety of bacteria
   b. Enrichment media—chocolate agar, charcoal yeast; for hard-to-grow (fastidious) bacteria
   c. Selective media—MacConkey inhibits gram-positive bacteria; Sabouraud inhibits bacteria to allow fungal growth; Thayer-Martin includes antibiotics to inhibit normal flora
   d. Differential media—promotes specific organisms but inhibits others
3. Additional testing for bacterial characteristics
   a. Stain characteristics—e.g., gram-positive vs. gram-negative
   b. Morphological features—coccus, bacillus, etc.
   c. Oxygen utilization—aerobe vs. anaerobe vs. facultative anaerobes
   d. Classification by enzymatic tests and sugar fermentations
   e. Catalase test—differentiates streptococci (–) from staphylococci (+)
   f. Coagulase test—differentiates *S. aureus* (+) from other *Staphylococcus* sp. (–)
   g. Hemolysis on blood agar—color classifies *Streptococcus*
      (1) Alpha (green)—*S. viridans, S. pneumoniae*
      (2) Beta (clear)—*S. pyogenes, S. agalactiae*
      (3) Gamma (no hemolysis)—*S. bovis*
   h. Optochin inhibition, Bile esculin and Lancefield grouping are additional tests to differentiate *Streptococcus* sp.

D. **Antimicrobial Susceptibility Testing**
   1. Determine correct antimicrobial therapy
   2. Determine adequate amount of appropriate antimicrobial
   3. Determine exact organism (in outbreak or cases of multiple transmission)
   4. Methods
      a. Disk diffusion—Kirby Bauer (paper disks impregnated with antimicrobial then placed on agar with growth of organism) measure zone of inhibition around disk. Measured as susceptible, intermediate or resistant
      b. Broth dilution—determines MIC (minimum inhibitory concentration)—may be manual or automated (Vitek® or WalkAway®)
      c. E Test—impregnated plastic strip placed on agar plate; read for MIC (used to confirm a case of vancomycin-resistant enterococci [VRE])
      d. Beta-lactamase detection—presence of enzyme that causes specific antimicrobials to be resisted (penicillins)
      e. Disk Approximation Test—shows inducible clindamycin resistance
      f. Miscellaneous tests:
         (1) Synergy test—determines inhibitory ability of combinations of antibiotics
         (2) Hodge test—detect presence of extended-spectrum beta-lactamases (ESBL) resistance in gram-negative organisms
         (3) Minimal bacteriocidal concentration (MBC)—determine minimal concentration of antibiotic needed to kill organism

E. **Identification of Fungi**
   1. Some fungi can be identified directly from a clinical specimen (e.g., skin scraping)
   2. Some yeasts grow on routine agars (e.g., *Candida* spp.)
   3. Germ-tube and sugar assimilation tests are used for yeast
   4. If cultures are done, specimens need to be incubated for several weeks at room temperature; identification then based on colony appearance and microscopic examination
   5. Direct antigen detection methods (e.g., latex agglutination) may be used
   6. Serologic test methods can be used to identify coccidioidomycosis, histoplasmosis and *Aspergillus* spp.

F. **Identification of Viruses**
   1. Direct detection methods
      a. Electron microscopy
      b. Enzyme-linked immunosorbent assay (ELISA) for viruses such as respiratory syncytial virus (RSV), hepatitis B surface antibody and rotavirus

c. Latex agglutination for viruses such as RSV and rotavirus
   d. DNA probes for viruses such as cytomegalovirus (CMV)
   e. Polymerase chain reaction (PCR) for DNA detection for viruses such as human immunodeficiency virus (HIV) types 1 and 2
   f. Optical immunoassay (OIA), an antibody antigen–based test for detection of influenza viruses A and B from respiratory specimens
   g. Light microscopy of cell scrapings
 2. Antibody assay for serum
   a. Determine presence or absence of immunoglobulins; limitations include cross-reactions to other antibodies, dependence on immune system function; paired sera sometimes needed for diagnosis
 3. Viral culture—specialized media containing antibacterial and antifungal agents, cultured on mammalian host cells (detection of growth changes in host cells)

G. Identification of Parasites

1. Microscopy—direct or concentrated examination based on morphological appearance (protozoa or helminths)
2. Serological methods used by reference laboratories when direct examination of tissue is difficult or unrevealing

H. Identification of Mycobacteria

1. Requires special culture techniques
2. Must kill commensal bacteria first
3. Planted on special media, incubated 4 to 6 weeks
4. Rapid techniques include BACTEC method, PCR, DNA probes

I. Identification of Mycoplasma

1. Fastidious growth requirements; culture rarely attempted
2. Serological tests generally used to diagnose infection

J. Identification of Chlamydiae

1. Requires tissue culture, not attempted in most laboratories
2. Direct-detection methods include direct florescent staining and ELISA technique

K. Identification of Rickettsiae and Other Tick-Borne Microbes

1. Serological studies used to detect specific infections
2. ELISA best diagnostic test

L. Microbiological Environmental Sampling

1. Generally not recommended because it is costly, requires special laboratory procedures, there is no standard for comparison and may result in the implementation of unnecessary procedures or treatment
2. Routine environmental monitoring—routine microbiological sampling for quality assurance purposes should be limited to:
    a. Biological monitoring of sterilization processes (see Chapter 3)
    b. Monthly cultures and endotoxin testing of water and dialysate in hemodialysis units
    c. Short-term evaluation of the impact of infection prevention measure or changes in infection prevention protocols (e.g., evaluating new cleaning procedures and/or products, or water culturing after *Legionella* abatement)[17]
3. Special environmental monitoring—use when epidemiological investigation suggests a source or reservoir exists
    a. May monitor personnel, medical devices, air, water, food or surfaces
    b. Quantitative methods should be used to determine the amount of burden

M. Specimen Collection and Transport

1. Specimens should be collected aseptically, placed in sterile container
2. Some specimens may be placed directly on culture media (e.g., blood cultures, genital cultures)
3. Special handling techniques may be necessary for some specimens (e.g., anaerobic culture)
4. Prompt delivery essential
5. If transport delayed, some specimens may be refrigerated (e.g., urine, stool, sputum); others should be maintained at room temperature (e.g., genital, eye, spinal fluid)

N. Techniques Used to Type Organisms During Outbreak Investigation

1. Laboratory can assist in the identification of an outbreak by
    a. Confirming identity of organism
    b. Recognizing organism clusters
    c. Detecting unusual organisms and/or antimicrobial susceptibility patterns
    d. Can retrieve/review archival data to determine background rates and determine if outbreak situation exists
    e. Can save organism isolates and assist in testing to determine if organisms same or related
2. Phenotypic techniques
    a. Colony morphology
    b. Biotyping—patterns of metabolic activities

   c. Antimicrobial susceptibility testing
   d. Serotyping
   e. Bacteriophage and bacteriocin typing
   f. Electrophoretic protein typing and immunoblotting
  3. Genotypic techniques
   a. Plasmid analysis
   b. Restriction endonuclease analysis
   c. Restriction fragment length polymorphisms (RFLPs) and ribotyping
   d. Pulse field gel electrophoresis (PFGE): chromosomal DNA
   e. PCR typing systems

IV. Laboratory Testing and Diagnostics

A. Direct Examination

1. Gram stain
2. Histology/cytology
   a. Gross and microscopic evaluation of a specimen or tissue
   b. Special fixing or staining techniques may be used
   c. Useful for diagnosing infections with agents that are difficult to culture (e.g., actinomycosis, *Chlamydia*, CMV, genital herpes)
3. Wet mount
   a. Microscopic examination of fresh specimens (e.g., sputum for fungal elements, stool, for larvae, worms; cerebral fluid for *Cryptococcus neoformans*)

B. Detection of the Antigen/Antibody Reaction

1. Antigen detection
2. Antibody detection

C. Molecular Diagnostic Testing

1. Target amplification methods
2. Probe amplification methods
3. Signal amplification methods

D. Test for Infectious Process

1. Body fluid analysis
2. Cerebrospinal analysis
3. Cold agglutinins
4. C-reactive protein

5. Complete blood count
6. Complete blood count; absolute neutrophil count
7. Fecal leukocytes
8. Lymphocyte subset
9. Sedimentation rate
10. Toxin production testing
11. Weil-Felix agglutinin
12. Urinalysis

V. Microbial Pathogenesis

A. Terms

1. Normal flora—bacteria commonly found on healthy human body surfaces
2. Colonization— the presence of a microorganism in the absence of symptoms or deep tissue invasion (these may be normal flora or pathogenic organisms)
3. Asymptomatic infection—viable organisms are present in a body site without causing any obvious symptoms (latent tuberculosis)
4. Opportunistic infections—infections with organisms that cause disease primarily in immunodeficient hosts (e.g., *C. neoformans, L. pneumophila, M. avium*)
5. Pathogenic organism—infection can be caused by any organism if it is introduced into a normally sterile area/tissue; causes tissue damage

B. Sources of Microorganisms

1. Exogenous—outside the host
   a. Other humans
   b. Food
   c. Contaminated water
   d. Vector-borne
   e. Animals
   f. Air from environment
   g. Direct contact
2. Endogenous—from host's own flora (pneumonia, urinary tract infection, wound infections)
3. The host may become colonized with this organism then proceed to active infection condition

Table 1–1. Organisms by Site—Normal Flora and Pathogens

Site	Normal Flora	Pathogens
Respiratory tract	Alpha *Streptococcus, Staphylococcus aureus,* Coagulase-negative *Staphylococcus, Neisseria, Haemophilus, Moraxella, Corynebacterium, Micrococcus, Candida,* mixed anaerobes	*Streptococcus pyogenes, Arcanobacterium, Chlamydia pneumoniae, Neisseria gonorrhoeae, Corynebacterium diphtheriae, Mycoplasma pneumoniae, Candida, Staphylococcus aureus, Streptococcus pneumoniae, Haemophilus influenzae, Moraxella catarrhalis,* enteric gram-negative rods, *Pseudomonas, Legionella, Microbacterium tuberculosis, Bordetella pertussis, Chlamydia trachomatis, Chlamydia psittaci,* mixed anaerobes, *Histoplasma, Blastomyces, Coccidioides, Cryptococcus*
Genitourinary tract	*Corynebacterium, Lactobacillus, Staphylococcus,* nonpathogenic *Neisseria,* enteric rods, *Gardnerella, Enterococcus, Mycoplasma, Ureaplasma, Propionibacterium, Candida,* mixed anaerobes	*N. gonorrhoeae, Haemophilus ducreyi, C. trachomatis, Mycoplasma, Ureaplasma, Actinomyces, Bacteroides, Fusobacterium, Clostridium, Candida,* enteric gram-negative rods, *Pseudomonas, Enterococcus, Staphylococcus saprophyticus, S. aureus, M. tuberculosis, Corynebacterium urealyticum, Candida*
Gastrointestinal tract	*Lactobacillus, Enterococcus,* enteric rods, *Corynebacterium, Streptococcus, Staphylococcus, Propionibacterium, Candida,* mixed anaerobes	*Helicobacter pylori, Campylobacter, Salmonella, Shigella, Vibrio cholerae, S. aureus, Bacillus cereus, Yersinia, Escherichia coli, Blastomyces*
Skin, ear, eye	*Corynebacterium, Staphylococcus, Micrococcus,* nonpathogenic *Neisseria, Propionibacterium, Peptostreptococcus, Candida, Mucor, Absidia*	*S. pneumoniae, H. influenzae, M. catarrhalis, Pseudomonas, Aspergillus, Candida, S. aureus,* coagulase negative *Staphylococcus, H. influenzae* subsp. *aegypticus, N. gonorrhoeae, M. catarrhalis, Bacillus, Chlamydia trachomatis*
Bone and joint		*S. aureus,* coagulase-negative *Staphylococcus, N. gonorrhoeae, Streptococcus, H. influenzae,* enteric gram-negative rods, *Pseudomonas, Mycobacterium, Sporothrix, Coccidioides, Candida*
Blood		*S. aureus,* coagulase-negative *Staphylococcus, S. pneumoniae, Enterococcus,* enteric gram-negative rods, *Pseudomonas, H. influenzae, Candida, Bacteroides*
Central nervous system		*S. pneumoniae, H. influenzae, Neisseria meningitidis, Streptococcus agalactiae,* coagulase-negative *Staphylococcus, S. aureus, Listeria, Escherichia coli, M. tuberculosis, Nocardia, Candida, Cryptococcus*

(Source: Adapted from APIC Text of Infection Control and Epidemiology, 2005 and APIC Ready Reference to Microbes, 2002.)

Table 1-2. Common Pathogens by Site

Type of Infection	Common Pathogens
Skin, subcutaneous tissue	*Staphylococcus aureus, Streptococcus pyogenes, Candida*, dermatophytes, coagulase-negative *Staphylococcus, Pseudomonas, Clostridium*
Sinusitis	*Streptococcus pneumoniae, Haemophilus influenzae, S. pyogenes, S. aureus,* gram-negative bacilli, *Mucorales*
Pharyngitis	Respiratory viruses, *S. pyogenes, Candida albicans, Neisseria gonorrhoeae, Corynebacterium diphtheriae*
Bronchitis	Respiratory viruses (especially respiratory syncytial virus [RSV]) among pediatrics), *S. pneumoniae, H. influenzae, Bordetella pertussis*
Pneumonia (community acquired)	Respiratory viruses (e.g., influenza, RSV, hantavirus, *S. pneumoniae, H. influenzae, Mycoplasma pneumoniae, Chlamydia pneumoniae, Mycobacterium tuberculosis, S. aureus*, gram-negative bacilli, *Legionella pneumophila, Pneumocystis carinii*
Empyema	*Anaerobes*, oral streptococci, *S. aureus, S. pyogenes, H. influenzae*
Nosocomial pneumonia	*Pseudomonas, Enterobacteriaceae, S. aureus, Legionella, S. pneumoniae*
Endocarditis	*Streptococcus viridans, S. aureus, Enterococcus, Haemophilus, Staphylococcus epidermidis, Candida*
Gastroenteritis	*Salmonella, Shigella, Campylobacter*, invasive *Escherichia coli*, viruses, *Giardia, Yersinia, Vibrio*
Peritonitis, abdominal	*Bacteroides*, anaerobic cocci, Enterobacteriaceae, *Enterococcus*, abscess *S. aureus, Candida*
Urinary tract infection	*E. coli, Klebsiella, Proteus, Enterococcus, Pseudomonas, Staphylococcus saprophyticus, Candida*
Pelvic inflammatory	*Chlamydia trachomatis, Gonococcus, Bacteroides*, Enterobacteriaceae disease
Osteomyelitis	*S. aureus, Salmonella, Pseudomonas, Staphylococcus. Agalactiae*

Table 1-2. Common Pathogens by Site *(Continued)*

Type of Infection	Common Pathogens
Septic arthritis	S. aureus, N. gonorrhoeae, S. pneumoniae, S. pyogenes, Pasteurella multocida
Meningitis	H. influenzae, Neisseria meningitidis, S. pneumoniae, S. agalactiae, M. tuberculosis
Septicemia	S. aureus, S. pneumoniae, E. coli, Klebsiella, Salmonella, Candida, Clostridium, Listeria
Device-associated infections	Coagulase-negative Staphylococcus, Corynebacterium, gram-negative bacilli, infection Candida, or any organism listed under septicemia

(Source: *APIC Text of Infection Control and Epidemiology,* 2009.)

VI. Antimicrobial Therapy

Seeks to suppress or kill microorganisms with minimal toxicity and/or side effects to the patient

A. Antimicrobial Mechanisms

1. Antibacterials—interfere with cell wall biosyntheses, inhibit bacterial ribosomes, interfere with DNA replication or RNA transcription or inhibit metabolic pathways
   a. Beta-lactam drugs possess bactericidal activity by inhibiting cell wall synthesis (i.e., penicillin, cephalosporins, monobactams, carbapenems)
   b. Fluoroquinolones inhibit bacterial enzymes important in DNA replication (i.e., ciprofloxacin)
   c. Macrolides inhibit protein synthesis; mostly bacteriostatic, therefore used for less serious infection (i.e., azithromycin)
   d. Aminoglycosides act at the site of bacterial ribosomes; used for combination therapy for serious or multidrug-resistant infection (i.e., gentamicin)
2. Antifungals—alter permeability of fungal membrane, inhibit membrane biosyntheses or inhibit DNA synthesis
3. Antivirals—inhibit formation of DNA precursors, inhibit DNA polymerase, inhibit HIV reverse transcription, interfere with viral uncoating or confer viral resistance on uninfected cells

B. **Definitions**
1. Prophylactic—antimicrobial given to prevent infection (before infection develops) when there has been potential exposure to infection or when situation will involve potential risk for infection such as certain surgeries
2. Empiric—antimicrobial therapy (usually broad spectrum) initiated when no information about causative pathogen is known, patient is sufficiently ill to warrant treatment before culture and sensitivity tests are available, or clinical site of infection may give an indication of likely pathogen (culture may or may not be done)
3. Therapeutic (pathogen directed)—antimicrobial therapy initiated because infecting agent is known, susceptibility tests have been done and appropriate antimicrobial and dosage are known

C. **Interpretation of In Vitro Susceptibility Test Result**
1. Disk diffusion test results are expressed qualitatively
   a. Susceptible (S)—drug is probably effective at standard dose
   b. Intermediate (I)—relationship between MIC and achievable body fluid level should be used to help select the most effective route and dosage; may be referred to as moderate or moderately susceptible
   c. Resistant (R)—drug is probably not effective in the blood by systemic administration at nontoxic dosages
2. Agar and broth diffusion test results are usually expressed quantitatively as the MIC—the minimum concentration of drug required to inhibit the organism in vitro; this allows more refined consideration of the choice, route and dosage of antimicrobial based on the specific strain, site infected, penetration of various antibiotics into the infected site and projected pharmacokinetics in the particular patient

D. **Factors That Affect Outcome in Antimicrobial Therapy**
1. Prompt institution of an appropriate antimicrobial
2. The "bug factor" related to the virulence and susceptibility of the infecting organism
3. The "drug factor" related to the activity of the antimicrobial at a particular site of infection
4. The "host factor" related to the underlying condition and immunocompetence of the patient
5. The "site factor" related to the fact that infections at certain body sites (e.g., meninges, heart valves) are inherently more difficult to treat[18]
6. Problems with antibiotic administration
   a. Timeliness of administration
   b. Storage

c. Deterioration of antibiotic
d. Poor patient compliance
e. Absorption failure after intramuscular or oral administration

E. Host Factors That Require Reduction of Antimicrobial Dosage
1. Renal failure requires dosage reduction of antimicrobials that are excreted by the kidney
2. Liver failure requires dosage reduction of antimicrobials that are excreted by the liver

F. Antimicrobial Resistance
1. Mechanisms of antimicrobial resistance
   a. Alteration of drug-receptor/target sites (methicillin resistance in *Staphylococcus aureus*)[19]
   b. Drug inactivation—occurs when a bacterium produces an enzyme that can destroy or inactivate the antimicrobial (e.g., bacteria may produce beta-lactamase enzymes that destroy penicillins and cephalosporins[20]
   c. Decreased drug permeability or efflux (imipenem resistance in *Pseudomonas aeruginosa*)[21]
   d. Bypass of a metabolic pathway (resistance to trimethoprim-sulfamethoxazole [TMP-SMX])
2. Transmission
   a. Point mutations usually occur in the chromosome and are passed on only to daughter cells via cell division
   b. Mobile genetic elements (resistance factors [R factors]) can promote transmission of genes between strains
      (1) Plasmid—extrachromosomal circular DNA that can replicate itself
      (2) Transposon—small piece of DNA that can move from plasmid to plasmid or from chromosome to plasmid; mechanism allows bacteria to assemble new plasmids

G. Antimicrobial Use and Selective Pressure
Strong evidence in the literature supports an association between antibiotic use and resistance in hospitals. To reduce selective pressure:
1. Perform surveillance of antimicrobial resistance annually (antibiogram) to show which antimicrobials are overused or misused
2. Monitor the number of patients with new infection or colonization from problem organisms (e.g., MRSA, *C. difficile*)
3. Perform antimicrobial audits (e.g., costs, how used, appropriate dose) to identify problem areas

4. Interventions when inappropriate use is encountered
   a. Computer-assisted drug protocols
   b. Restrictions on certain drugs (i.e., exclusion from formulary, requirement for approval before use, and antibiotic cycling)
   c. Didactic instruction and institutional antimicrobial guidelines for prescribers

H. Antibiogram

Simplifies multiple patients' antimicrobial sensitivity information at an institution into a single number for pathogens of interest
   1. Provides information on what antimicrobial classes are most used and potentially misused
   2. Helps to monitor trends merging in drug resistance at each facility
   3. Should be published at least annually

I. Measures to control resistant organisms

   1. Antibiotic stewardship
   2. Surveillance
   3. Antibiograms
   4. Appropriate use of vaccines
   5. Appropriate isolation precautions
   6. Hand hygiene

Index for Selected Infectious Diseases

A. Anthrax
B. Arthropod-Borne Viral Diseases
C. Aspergillosis
D. Botulism
E. Brucellosis
F. Candidiasis
G. Cat-Scratch Disease
H. Chickenpox/Herpes Zoster
I. Cholera
J. Conjunctivitis/Keratitis
K. Creutzfeldt-Jakob Disease/Kuru
L. Cryptosporidiosis
M. Dengue
N. Diphtheria
O. Ebola-Marburg Viral Diseases
P. Ehrlichiosis
Q. Erythema Infectiosum
R. Foodborne Diseases
S. Hantaviral Diseases
   1. Hemorrhagic Fever with Renal Syndrome
   2. Pulmonary Syndrome
T. Hepatitis, Viral
   1. Hepatitis A
   2. Hepatitis B
   3. Hepatitis C
   4. Hepatitis D—delta hepatitis
   5. Hepatitis E
U. Histoplasmosis
V. Human Immunodeficiency Virus (HIV) Acquired Immune Deficiency Syndrome (AIDS)
W. Influenza (Avian, H1N1, Pandemic, Seasonal Swine)
X. Kawasaki Syndrome
Y. Lassa Fever
Z. Legionellosis
AA. Leprosy
BB. Leptospirosis
CC. Lyme Disease
DD. Malaria
EE. Measles
FF. Meningitis
   1. Bacterial Meningitis
   2. Viral Meningitis
   3. Chronic Meningitis
   4. Shunt-Associated or Epidural-Associated Meningitis
   5. Brain Abscess
   6. Prevention
GG. Mononucleosis
HH. Mumps
II. Pediculosis and Phthiriasis
JJ. Pertussis
KK. Plague
LL. Poliomyelitis
MM. Psittacosis
NN. Rabies
OO. Rocky Mountain Spotted Fever
PP. RSV
QQ. Rubella
RR. Severe Acute Respiratory Syndrome (SARS)
SS. Scabies
TT. Sexually Transmitted Diseases
   1. Gonorrhea
   2. Syphilis
   3. Herpes Simplex
   4. Chlamydia
   5. Warts
UU. Tetanus
VV. Tuberculosis
WW. Tularemia
XX. Typhoid Fever
YY. Typhus Fever
ZZ. West Nile Virus
AAA. Yellow Fever
BBB. Yersiniosis

VII. Selected Infectious Diseases and Conditions

A. Anthrax

1. Etiology—*Bacillus anthracis*
2. Identification—acute bacterial disease usually affecting the skin; may rarely involve oropharynx, lower respiratory tract, meningitis, intestinal tract, mediastinal widening, sepsis, shock and death within 3 to 5 days
3. Diagnostic testing—laboratory confirmation is made by demonstration of the causative organism in blood, lesions or discharges by direct polychrome methylene blue–stained smears or by culture; serological studies for titer rise in paired sera can be carried out only by specialized laboratories
4. Incubation period—hours to 7 days, most within 48 hours
5. Isolation Precautions—Contact Precautions with all drainage, secretions, and body fluids; inhalation of anthrax spores results in risky industrial processes, such as tanning of hides or wool or bone processing, where aerosols of *B. anthracis* spores are present. Accidental infection has occurred in laboratory settings. Transmission from person to person is rare, but spores from contaminated soil can remain infective for decades
6. Treatment—immunization and treatment with penicillin, ciprofloxacin, tetracycline, erythromycin or chloramphenicol
7. Case fatality—5% to 20%

B. Arthropod-Borne Viral Diseases—Arboviral Diseases

1. Etiology—over 100 different arboviruses—best known:
   a. *Togaviridae* (e.g., eastern equine encephalomyelitis, Mucambo, Venezuelan equine encephalomyelitis; western equine encephalomyelitis)
   b. *Flaviviridae* (e.g., dengue, St. Louis encephalitis, West Nile, yellow fever)
   c. *Bunyaviridae* (e.g., Anopheles A group, group C, Bunyamwera group, Bwamba group, California group [California encephalitis], Guama group, Mapputta group, Simbu group, Phlebovirus [sand fly fever group], Nairovirus)
   d. *Reoviridae* (e.g., Changuinola group, Kemerovo group, Colorado Tick fever)
   e. *Rhabdoviridae* (e.g., Vesicular stomatitis group, LeDantec group)
   f. *Orthomyxoviridae* (e.g., Dhori, Thogoto)
2. Pathogenesis—viruses are maintained in zoonotic cycles; humans are usually an unimportant host in maintaining the cycle; infections in humans are incidental and are acquired most frequently during blood feeding by an infected arthropod vector. In only a few cases can humans serve as the principal source of virus amplification and vector infection, such as dengue and yellow fever. Most viruses are transmitted by mosquitoes; the rest are transmitted by ticks, sand flies or biting midges

3. Identification—fever, rash, encephalitis, arthritis and, rarely, hemorrhagic fever, which involves extensive hemorrhagic involvement, external or internal, associated with capillary leakage, shock, liver damage (hepatitic damage most severe in yellow fever) and high case-fatality rates
4. Diagnostic testing—diagnosis by clinical picture and serological titers for IgM and IgG, complement fixation (CF), haemagglutination inhibition (HI), fluorescent antibody (FA) or ELISA. Viruses may cross-react within a virus group
5. Incubation period—most are 3 to 15 days, but range depends on specific virus
6. Isolation precautions—Contact Precautions except for dengue fever or yellow fever; special care should be used with all blood and body fluids for hemorrhagic fevers in the hospital setting; avoid splash or aerosol spray of contaminated fluids; use mosquito screening
7. Case fatality rates—dengue hemorrhagic fever or shock syndrome if untreated or mistreated—40% to 50%; yellow fever—20% to 50% fatality in jaundiced cases—overall fatality rate below 5%; other arboviral diseases—range 0.3% to 60%, with Japanese encephalitis, Murray Valley fever and eastern equine encephalomyelitis among the highest
8. Control—for dengue fever or yellow fever: vector control, immunization for yellow fever (for contacts of both viruses), animal quarantine; for other arboviral diseases: immunize animals but no human immunizations available in United States for contacts
9. Treatment—supportive treatment: for most arboviral diseases there is no specific treatment; intravenous ribavirin and convalescent plasma have been used for viral hemorrhagic fevers; fresh plasma, fibrinogen and platelet concentration used to treat severe hemorrhage; INF approved for treatment of West Nile—see also page 60, West Nile virus

C. Aspergillosis

1. Etiology—*Aspergillus fumigatus, A. flavus, A. niger*
2. Identification—allergy to aspergillus results in bronchial damage and intermittent bronchial plugging; clumps of hyphae may form within bronchi, or a large mass of hyphae may fill a previously existing cavity (fungus ball or aspergilloma); invasive aspergillosis in immunocompromised patients with dissemination to the brain, kidneys, or other organs is often fatal; invasion of blood vessels with thrombosis and infarction, cardiac prosthetic valve vegetation, otomycosis, invasion of paranasal sinuses
3. Diagnostic testing—intradermal or scratch tests resulting in wheal/flare responses; episodes of bronchial plugging, eosinophilia, serum-precipitating antibodies against *Aspergillus*, elevated serum concentration of IgE, transient pulmonary infiltrates, endobronchial culture, culture of sputum or plugs of expectorated hyphae, serum

precipitins to antigens of *Aspergillus* spp., and fungus balls in the lungs may be diagnosed by chest radiograph
4. Incubation period—few days to weeks
5. Isolation precautions—no special precautions
6. Treatment—corticosteroid suppression therapy, surgical resection, amphotericin B (Fungizone), itraconazole (for slowly progressing cases) and discontinuation or reduction of immunosuppressive therapy

D. Botulism
1. Etiology—caused by toxins produced by *Clostridium botulinum*
2. Types
    a. Foodborne botulism—severe intoxication resulting from ingesting food contaminated by preformed toxin
    b. Wound botulism—wound contaminated by the organism in anaerobic conditions
    c. Infant botulism—most common; caused by ingestion and toxin production in the intestine by organism; affects infants under 1 year of age
3. Identification—acute bilateral cranial nerve impairment, descending weakness or paralysis; visual difficulty (blurred or double vision), dysphagia, dry mouth; flaccid paralysis in a paradoxically alert person; vomiting, constipation, diarrhea; fever if complicating infection occurs; **infant symptoms**—lethargy, listlessness, poor feeding, ptosis, difficulty swallowing, loss of head control, hypotonia, "floppy baby," respiratory insufficiency, arrest; may be related to 5% of cases of sudden infant death syndrome (SIDS)
4. Diagnostic testing—for botulinum toxin in stool, serum and/or gastric secretions or wound culture
5. Incubation period—12 to 36 hours, up to several days
6. Isolation precautions—no special isolation: handwashing, Standard Precautions
7. Treatment—IV 2 vials of trivalent botulinum antitoxin (from Centers for Disease Control and Prevention [CDC]), respiratory support, wound debridement, and appropriate antibiotics (e.g., penicillin); **infant treatment**—botulinum antitoxin (an equine product) is NOT used because of hazard of anaphylaxis; antibiotics do not improve course of the disease; aminoglycosides may worsen by causing a synergistic neuromuscular blockade; respiratory assistance
8. Case fatality rates—foodborne, 5% to 10%; infant, <1% and may be responsible for 5% of SIDS cases

E. Brucellosis—Undulant Fever, Malta Fever, Mediterranean Fever
1. Etiology—*Brucella abortus, B. melitensis, B. suis, B. canis*
2. Identification—fever, headache, weakness, profuse sweating, chills, arthralgia depression, weight loss and generalized aching; localized suppurative infections of

organs, including the liver and spleen; chronic localized infections may occur, may last months or years if not adequately treated; osteoarticular complications in 20% to 60% of cases; sacroiliitis, most common joint affected; genitourinary involvement in 2% to 20%, with orchitis and epididymitis common
3. Diagnostic testing—serological tests on blood, bone marrow, tissues, discharge
4. Incubation period—5 to 60 days, 1 to 2 months common
5. Isolation precautions—Contact Precautions with drainage and secretions
6. Treatment—rifampin, streptomycin and doxycycline for 6 weeks; tetracycline (avoid in children), TMP-SMX effective but relapses common (30%); relapses occur in 5%, should be retreated with original regimen; arthritis may occur in recurrent cases
7. Case fatality—untreated cases <2% usually from endocarditis from *B. melitensis*

F. Candidiasis—Moniliasis, Thrush

1. Etiology—*Candida albicans, C. tropicalis, C. glabrata*
2. Identification—mycosis usually confined to superficial layers of skin or mucous membranes, oral thrush, intertrigo, vulvovaginitis, paronychia or onychomycosis; ulcers or pseudomembranes in esophagus, stomach, or intestine; hematogenous dissemination (usually in neutropenic persons) arises from GI or IV catheters; may produce lesions in kidney, spleen, lungs, liver, eye, meninges, brain, cardiac valves or prosthetic cardiac valves
3. Diagnostic testing—microscopy: pseudohyphae and/or yeast cells; culture confirmation
4. Incubation period—2 to 5 days
5. Isolation precautions—no special precautions, Standard Precautions
6. Treatment—treat underlying causes, topical nystatin, miconazole, clotrimazole, ketoconazole, fluconazole (oral troches or suspension, IV), butoconazole, terconazole, tioconazole, amphotericin B, 5-fluorocytosine

G. Cat-Scratch Disease (CSD)—Cat-Scratch Fever, Benign Lymphoreticulosis

1. Etiology—*Bartonella henselae*, (*B. quintana* causes similar disease in immunocompromised); *Afipia felis* felt to play minor role in CSD
2. Identification—bacterial disease characterized by malaise, granulomatous lymphadenitis, fever, red papular lesion; regional lymph node involvement within 2 weeks; papule can be found at inoculation site in 50% to 90% of cases; Parinaud oculoglandular syndrome after inoculation of the eye and encephalopathy, optic neuritis can occur; prolonged high fever accompanied by osteolytic lesions, hepatic, splenic granulomata; bacteremia, peliosis hepatica and bacillary angiomatosis seen in immunocompromised; can be confused with tularemia, brucellosis, tuberculosis, plague and pasteurellosis

3. Diagnostic testing—serologic titer of antibody to *Bartonella* is considered positive at >1:64 by IFA assay
4. Incubation period—3 to 14 days from inoculation to primary lesion and 5 to 50 days from inoculation to lymphadenopathy
5. Isolation precautions—no special precautions
6. Treatment—ciprofloxacin, TMP-SMX, rifampin, gentamicin, erythromycin or doxycycline

H. Chickenpox/Herpes Zoster—Varicella/Shingles

1. Etiology—human herpesvirus 3 (varicella-zoster [VZ] virus, member of Herpesvirus group
2. Identification—sudden onset of slight fever, skin eruptions that are maculopapular for hours, vesicular for 3 to 4 days, then granular scab; vesicles are monolocular and collapse on puncture (smallpox lesions are multilocular and noncollapsing vesicles); lesions appear on scalp, axilla, mucous membranes of mouth and upper respiratory tract and conjunctiva; occur in areas of irritation; may be unnoticed because small in number; infection may be mild or severe
3. Diagnostic testing—serum antibodies, viral DNA by PCR, examination by electron microscope
4. Incubation period—2 to 3 weeks, average 13 to 17 days
5. Isolation precautions—chickenpox: Airborne Precautions with negative pressure ventilation and Contact Precautions; zoster: Standard Precautions unless disseminated zoster (then Airborne and Contact Precautions); maintain isolation for at least 5 days after eruption first appears or until vesicles become dry; personnel who have not had chickenpox should avoid contact
6. Treatment—susceptible contacts may be given varicella-zoster immunoglobulin (VZIG) within 96 hours of exposure; vidarabine and acyclovir are effective in treating VZ infections; acyclovir and famciclovir shorten the duration and symptoms of zoster
7. Case fatality—chickenpox: overall rate is 2/100,000, but in adults it is 30/100,000; cause of death in infants is sepsis or encephalitis; in adults, primary viral pneumonia; children with leukemia, 5% to 10% mortality; neonates of mothers who develop chickenpox 5 days before birth to 10 days after birth are at risk for generalized chickenpox, with fatality rate of up to 30%

I. Cholera

1. Etiology—*Vibrio cholerae* serogroup 01 or 0139
2. Identification—sudden onset, profuse, painless watery stools, vomiting, dehydration, acidosis, circulatory collapse, hypoglycemia in children and renal failure

3. Diagnostic testing—dark-field microscopy: "shooting stars"; antitoxic/vibriocidal antibodies; stool culture
4. Incubation period—few hours to 5 days; mean, 2 to 3 days
5. Isolation precautions—Contact Precautions
6. Treatment—prophylaxis: tetracycline, doxycycline, furazolidone or TMP-SMX; adequate rapid hydration, electrolyte replacement, tetracycline, TMP-SMX, sulfamethoxazole, trimethoprim or erythromycin
7. Case fatality—untreated 50% within hours; treated <1%

J. Conjunctivitis/Keratitis—Pink Eye, Keratoconjunctivitis
1. Etiology
    a. Bacterial—*Haemophilus influenzae, Streptococcus pneumoniae, Moraxella* spp., *Neisseria meningitidis, Corynebacterium diphtheriae, Pseudomonas aeruginosa, Streptococcus viridans*
    b. Viral—adenovirus types 5, 8, 19 and 37
2. Identification
    a. Bacterial—lacrimation, irritation, hyperemia of the palpebral and bulbar conjunctivae of one or both eyes, edema of lids and mucopurulent discharge; severe cases may have ecchymoses of bulbar conjunctiva and marginal infiltration of the cornea with photophobia
    b. Viral—sudden onset of eye pain, photophobia, blurred vision, low-grade fever, headache, malaise, tender preauricular lymphadenopathy; keratitis may leave discrete subepithelial opacities that may interfere with vision for a few weeks and rarely may leave scarring of cornea
3. Diagnostic testing—bacterial diagnosed by smear and culture of drainage; viral diagnosed by FA staining of corneal scrapings or by immunoelectron microscopy (IEM), viral antigen may be detected by ELISA
4. Incubation period—bacterial: 24 to 72 hours; viral: 5 to 12 days
5. Isolation precautions—Contact Precautions for acute viral conjunctivitis
6. Treatment—bacterial: ophthalmic ointments or drops containing polymyxin B, neomycin or trimethoprim, ampicillin, chloramphenicol, TMP-SMX, rifampin; viral: no treatment during the acute phase but may use corticosteroids for residual opacities

K. Creutzfeldt-Jakob Disease—Kuru, Spongiform Encephalopathy
1. Etiology—caused by a self-replicating protein particle called a prion
2. Identification—confusion, progressive dementia, variable ataxia, (99% of patients are older than 35 years), myoclonic jerks appear; routine cerebrospinal fluid (CSF) laboratory studies are normal and there is no fever; disease progresses rapidly,

death occurs within 3 to 12 months, mean 7 months; two main types: sporadic and familial. New variant CJD may be result of bovine-to-human transmission of bovine spongiform encephalopathy by ingestion of contaminated meat
3. Diagnostic testing—diagnosis by clinical symptoms, periodic high-voltage complexes on electroencephalogram (EEG) and histopathological findings (abnormal amyloid protein in biopsied brain tissue) CSF fluid testing for 14–3–3 protein, PrPsc from brain tissue, or analysis of DNA from blood or brain
4. Incubation period—15 months to 30 years; those with CNS tissue exposure <10 years
5. Isolation precautions—Standard Precautions; great care should be taken with tissues, EEG electrodes and surgical instruments contaminated tissue. See Chapter 3 for specific instructions for decontamination and sterilization of instruments and equipment
6. Treatment—none
7. Case fatality—all die within 3 to 12 months

L. Cryptosporidiosis

1. Etiology—*Cryptosporidium parvum*
2. Identification—a parasitic infection that affects the epithelial cells of the GI, biliary, and respiratory tracts; diarrhea, anorexia, vomiting, cramping, abdominal pain, general malaise, fever that usually lasts <30 days; immunocompromised may not be able to get over the infection, which can contribute to death
3. Diagnostic testing—diagnosis by identification of oocysts in fecal smears; ELISA assays, fluorescein-tagged monoclonal antibody testing is helpful
4. Incubation period—1 to 12 days with mean of 7 days
5. Isolation precautions—Standard Precautions: restrict infected persons from food handling or patient care
6. Treatment—rehydration; immunosuppressive drugs should be stopped or reduced

M. Dengue and Dengue Hemorrhagic Fever/Shock Syndrome

1. Etiology—flaviviruses serotypes 1, 2, 3 and 4
2. Identification—acute febrile viral disease, sudden onset, fever for 3 to 5 days, intense headache, myalgia, arthralgia, retro-orbital pain, anorexia, GI disturbances and rash; hemorrhagic fever, also vascular permeability, hypovolemia, abnormal blood clotting, severe restlessness, facial pallor, diaphoresis, circumoral cyanosis, hypotension, shock is usually the principal pathophysiologic symptom; petechiae, easy bruisability, epistaxis, bleeding at venipuncture sites, GI hemorrhage, liver enlargement, liver necrosis, effusions in the thorax or abdomen, thrombocytopenia, hemoconcentration, accumulation of fluids in serosal cavities

3. Diagnostic testing—low serum albumin, elevated transaminases, prolonged prothrombin time, low levels of C3 complement protein
4. Incubation period—3 to 14 days, commonly 5 to 7 days
5. Isolation precautions—Standard Precautions: special care to prevent splash or spray of blood/body fluids
6. Treatment—supportive oxygen therapy, rapid replacement with fluid and electrolyte solutions, plasma expanders, blood transfusions, heparin, fresh plasma, fibrinogen and platelet concentrate
7. Case fatality—untreated or mistreated 40% to 50%, with adequate fluid replacement 1% to 2%

N. Diphtheria

1. Etiology—*Corynebacterium diphtheriae*
2. Identification—acute bacterial disease involving tonsils, pharynx, larynx, nose, occasionally conjunctivae or genitalia; characterized by lesions marked by patches of grayish membrane with a surrounding inflammation; throat is moderately sore; lymph node swelling and edema of the neck; laryngeal diphtheria is serious in infants and young children; lesions of cutaneous diphtheria may resemble impetigo; after 2 to 6 weeks, cranial and peripheral motor and sensory nerve palsies, and myocarditis
3. Diagnostic testing—Diphtheria: presumptive: asymmetrical, grayish-white membrane of pharyngeal area; confirmed by bacteriologic examination of lesions
4. Incubation period—usually 2 to 5 days
5. Isolation precautions—Droplet Isolation for pharyngeal diphtheria; Contact Precautions for cutaneous diphtheria until 2 negative cultures (24 hours apart) from nose and throat after cessation of antimicrobial therapy
6. Treatment—antitoxin after testing to ensure not allergic, erythromycin, procaine penicillin G; prophylactic treatment of carriers: benzathine penicillin G or erythromycin
7. Case facility—5% to 10% for noncutaneous

O. Ebola—Marburg Viral Disease

1. Etiology—*Filoviridae* virions, Marburg virus and Ebola virus (Zaire, Ivory Coast, Sudan, and Reston strains)
2. Identification—severe acute viral illness, sudden onset of fever, malaise, myalgia and headache; followed by pharyngitis, vomiting, diarrhea; then finally hemorrhagic diathesis, hepatic damage, renal failure and then CNS involvement, terminal shock with multiorgan dysfunction
3. Diagnostic testing—diagnosis by ELISA antigen detection in the blood, use of an IFA test to detect virus antigen in liver cells; virus may be seen by electron microscope in liver secretions

4. Incubation period—3 to 9 days with Marburg and 2 to 21 days with Ebola
   5. Isolation precautions—Contact Precautions with special care to prevent all splashes and sprays of blood or body fluids
   6. Treatment—supportive, adequate fluid replacement, ribavirin should be started within the first 6 days
   7. Case fatality—combined fatality rate is 70% for types except Ebola Reston (affects monkeys only with symptomatic disease)

P. **Ehrlichiosis**
   1. Etiology—*Ehrlichia sennetsu, E. chaffeensis* (majority of human cases), member of *Rickettsia* genus, *E. phagocytophila* (causes human granulocytic ehrlichiosis [HGE])
   2. Identification—Sennetsu fever (in Japan): sudden-onset fever, chills, malaise, headache, muscle and joint pain, sore throat, sleeplessness, generalized lymphadenopathy; human ehrlichiosis: mild to severe disease; fever, headache, anorexia, nausea, myalgia and vomiting; leukopenia, thrombocytopenia
   3. Diagnostic testing—elevated liver function tests; development of antibodies to *Ehrlichia chaffeensis* in the IF test
   4. Incubation period—14 days for Sennetsu fever; 7 to 21 days for American ehrlichiosis
   5. Isolation precautions—Standard Precautions, no special precautions
   6. Treatment—tetracycline; chloramphenicol for pregnant women or children under age 8
   7. Case fatality—fatal cases have not been reported

Q. **Erythema Infectiosum—Fifth Disease**
   1. Etiology—human parvovirus B19 belonging to the family *Parvoviridae*
   2. Identification—erythematous eruption, usually mild, nonfebrile, "slapped-face" appearance (communicability greatest before onset of rash), lace-like rash on trunk and extremities, which may recur for 1 to 3 weeks with exposure to sunlight or warmth; arthralgias lasting days to months may occur, >25% are asymptomatic; anemic patients may develop transient aplastic crisis, intrauterine infection has resulted in hydrops fetalis and fetal death in 10% of pregnancies; immunocompromised persons may develop chronic anemia
   3. Diagnostic testing—diagnosis by IgM antibodies for parvovirus B19, rise in IgG antibodies, B19 antigen and DNA can be detected in acute stage, and nucleic acid hybridization techniques for autopsy tissues from infected fetuses
   4. Incubation period—4 to 20 days
   5. Isolation precautions—transient aplastic crisis should be on Droplet Precautions; children should be excluded from school while feverish (most infectious before rash)
   6. Treatment—immunocompromised persons with chronic anemia can be treated with intravenous immunoglobulin (IGIV)

R. Foodborne Diseases—Food Poisoning, Foodborne Infections

1. Etiology
   a. Bacteria: *Salmonella typhimurium, S. enteritidis, S. schottmülleri, S. hirschfeldii* (200 more serotypes in the United States); *Shigella dysenteriae, S. sonnei, S. flexneri, S. boydii; Campylobacter jejuni, C. coli, C. fetus; Vibrio parahaemolyticus, V. vulnificus; Clostridium perfringens, C. welchii,* C. botulinum (infection produced by toxins); *Brucella abortus, B. suis, B. canis, B. melitensis; S. aureus* (toxin); *Bacillus cereus* (toxin); *Escherichia coli* (toxin); *Listeria monocytogenes*
   b. Viruses: hepatitis A, rotaviruses in the *Reoviridae* family, Norwalk-like viruses in the *Caliciviridae* family
   c. Parasites: *Giardia lamblia, G. intestinalis; Toxocara canis, T. cati* (toxocariasis); *Toxoplasma gondii* (toxoplasmosis); *Trichinella spiralis* (trichinellosis/trichinosis); *Taenia solium, saginata*
2. Identification—depends on the specific causative agent, most cause nausea, vomiting, diarrhea, fever, dehydration, hypotension, sepsis; laboratory diagnosis frequently involves smears and culturing for bacteria, serology for viruses, and microscopy for parasite identification; clinical symptoms vary with illness but may enable diagnosis, such as a 2-hour onset of vomiting may indicate *S. aureus* or *Bacillus cereus*
3. Diagnostic testing—foodborne diseases: quantitative stool cultures; enterotoxin testing; phage typing; in outbreaks/semi-quantitative food cultures
4. Incubation period—depends on specific causative agent:

S. aureus	30 minutes to 8 hours, average 2 to 4 hours
B. cereus	1 to 6 hours vomiting; 6 to 24 hours diarrhea
Salmonella	6 to 72 hours; average 12 to 36 hours
Shigella	12 to 96 hours; average 1 to 3 days
Shigella dysenteriae	to 1 week
Campylobacter	1 to 10 days; average 2 to 5 days
Clostridium perfringens	6 to 24 hours; average 10 to 12 hours
Vibrio	12 to 24 hours
Rotavirus	24 to 72 hours
Norovirus	24 to 48 hours
Norwalk-like viruses	24 to 48 hours
Hepatitis A	15 to 50 days; average 25 to 30 days
Trichinellosis/trichinosis	5 to 45 days; average 8 to 15 days
Toxoplasmosis	10 to 23 days
Giardiasis	3 to 25 days; average 7 to 10 days

5. Isolation precautions—Contact Precautions, Standard Precautions

6. Treatment—fluid replacement, electrolyte replacement, parasites may be treated with metronidazole, quinacrine, furazolidone, mebendazole (trichinellosis), pyrimethamine with sulfadiazine and folinic acid (for severe toxoplasmosis), or spiramycin for pregnant women; severe cases of salmonellosis or shigellosis: ciprofloxacin, ampicillin, amoxicillin, TMP-SMX, or chloramphenicol; *E. coli* diarrhea treatment with TMP-SMX is controversial and may precipitate hemolytic-uremic syndrome

S. Hantaviral Diseases—Hemorrhagic Fever with Renal Syndrome and Pulmonary Syndrome

1. Etiology—hantavirus of the *Bunyaviridae* family; pulmonary syndrome is usually Sin Nombre virus (southwest United States) or the Black Creek Canal virus (Florida)
2. Identification—hemorrhagic fever: abrupt onset of fever, lower back pain, malaise, anorexia, nausea, vomiting, facial flushing, petechiae, conjunctival injection, hypotension, oliguria, renal involvement, hemorrhage; pulmonary syndrome: abrupt onset, respiratory distress and hypotension; progresses to severe respiratory failure and cardiogenic shock
3. Diagnostic testing—hemorrhagic fever: diagnosis by detection of IgM antibodies using ELISA or IFA, presence of proteinuria, leukocytosis, thrombocytopenia and elevated blood urea nitrogen; pulmonary syndrome: diagnosis by IgM antibodies using ELISA or western blot techniques, PCR analysis of autopsy or biopsy tissues
4. Incubation period—hemorrhagic: 2 to 60 days, average 2 to 4 weeks; pulmonary: suspected to be 2 to 6 weeks but may occur in days
5. Isolation Precautions—Standard Precautions; transmission occurs through aerosol transmission from rodent excreta
6. Treatment—support for shock and renal failure, prevent overhydration, ribavirin IV given early may benefit hemorrhagic fever
7. Case fatality—hemorrhagic: 5%; pulmonary: 40% to 50%

T. Hepatitis, Viral[22]

1. Hepatitis A
   a. Etiology—hepatitis A virus (HAV); single-stranded RNA virus (picornavirus)
   b. Identification—jaundice, fatigue, abdominal pain, loss of appetite, nausea, diarrhea; symptoms last <2 months (rare cases as long as 6 months) with complete recovery, no chronic infection
   c. Incubation period: 15 to 50 days
   d. Diagnostic testing—anti-HAV IgM is the antibody that appears during the acute illness and declines over 6 to 12 months; anti-HAV IgG rises later than IgM but persists indefinitely and is believed to be the neutralizing, protective antibody responsible for lifelong immunity after natural infection

e. Incidence—25,000 new infections/year in the United States
f. Prevalence—29% of Americans show evidence of past infection
g. Transmission—fecal-oral; food/waterborne outbreaks; blood-borne (rare)
h. Prevention—hepatitis A vaccine (HAVRIX); immune globulin
i. Isolation precautions—Standard Precautions
j. Risk groups—household/sexual contacts; international travelers; persons living on American Indian reservations/Alaska native villages; persons in outbreak areas such as day care centers, men who have sex with men, injecting drug users

2. Hepatitis B
   a. Etiology—hepatitis B virus (HBV); double-shelled particle, member of hepa-DNA viruses
   b. Identification—jaundice, fatigue, abdominal pain, loss of appetite, nausea, vomiting
   c. Diagnostic testing—HBsAg (hepatitis B surface antigen) is an outer surface component of HBV that serves as a marker for ongoing infection. It is found in the serum 1 to 2 months after exposure. Persistence of this antigen beyond 6 months will indicate chronic infection. Hepatitis B core antibody IgM (Anti-HBc IgM) is the first antibody detected and usually appears at the same time as symptoms begin. It can persist for 3 to 12 months in self-limited cases. Anti-HBc IgG persists for life and serves as a marker for previous natural HBV infection
   d. Incidence—43,000 new infections/year in United States
   e. Prevalence—4.3% to 5.6% of Americans show chronic infection (800,000 to 1.4 million Americans); 3000 deaths each year result from cirrhosis and liver cancer
   f. Incubation period: 45 to 180 days
   g. Transmission—blood-borne, sexual, perinatal
   h. Prevention—hepatitis B vaccine; screening done of pregnant women and treatment of infants born to infected women; routine vaccination of infants and 11- to 12-year-olds; vaccination of high-risk groups; screening of blood/organ/tissue donors
   i. Isolation precautions—Standard Precautions
   j. Risk groups—injecting drug users; sexually active heterosexuals; men who have sex with men; infants/children of immigrants from disease-endemic areas; low socioeconomic level; sexual/household contacts of infected persons; infants born to infected mothers; healthcare workers; hemodialysis patients

3. Hepatitis C
   a. Etiology—hepatitis C virus (HCV); single-stranded RNA virus (flavivirus)
   b. Identification: jaundice, fatigue, abdominal pain, loss of appetite, nausea/vomiting; 70% are asymptomatic
   c. Diagnostic testing—antibody to HCV (Anti-HCV) can be detected between 4 and 24 weeks after onset of hepatitis but may not be present for up to a year after

d. Incidence—17,000 new infections in the United States per year
   e. Prevalence—1.3% to 1.9% of Americans have been infected with HCV; 2.7 to 3.9 million are chronically infected
   f. Incubation period: 2 weeks to 6 months
   g. Transmission—blood-borne, sexual (less efficient than HBV), perinatal
   h. Prevention—screening of blood/organ/tissue donors; counseling to reduce/modify high-risk practices
   i. Isolation Precautions—Standard Precautions
   j. Treatment—INF-α2b, may be combined with ribavirin; effective in 10% to 40% of persons; high rates of side effects seen; relapse also seen with retreatment beneficial
   k. Risk groups—injecting drug users; hemodialysis patients; healthcare workers; sexual contacts; persons with multiple sex partners; recipients of transfusions before July 1992; recipients of clotting factors made before 1987; infants born to infected women
4. Hepatitis D—delta hepatitis
   a. Etiology—hepatitis D virus (HDV) occurs as a coinfection with HBV or as a superinfection of persons with chronic HBV infection; small defective RNA virus that resembles plant satellite viruses
   b. Identification—same as with HBV; persons with HBV/HDV coinfection may have more severe acute disease and higher risk for fulminant hepatitis and chronic liver (70% to 80%)
   c. Diagnostic testing—detection of HDV antibody by radioimmunoassay (RIA) or electroimmunoassay (EIA); positive IgM titer; reverse transcription PCR (RT-PCR) detects viremia
   d. Incidence—25% to 50% of fulminant hepatitis suspected to be from hepatitis D
   e. Prevalence—very low in the United States, worldwide, highest rates in populations at high risk for HBV infection; Russia, Romania, southern Italy (20% to 60%); moderate risk in northern Italy, Spain, Turkey, and Egypt (10% to 50%); also seen in Africa and South America; in hemophiliacs, drug addicts and those in frequent contact with blood; severe epidemics in tropical South America (Brazil, Venezuela and Colombia), Central African Republic and among drug addicts in Worcester, Massachusetts
   f. Incubation period: 2 to 8 weeks
   g. Transmission—same as with HBV, but sexual transmission of HDV is less efficient than for HBV
   h. Prevention—prevent hepatitis B through vaccine and modification of high-risk behaviors; no products exist to prevent HDV superinfection in persons with chronic HBV infection
   i. Isolation precautions—Standard Precautions

j. Risk groups—same as for hepatitis B
k. Case fatality—in outbreaks, disease has been severe, with rapid progression to fulminant hepatitis and fatality rates of 10% to 20%

5. Hepatitis E
   a. Etiology—a nonenveloped particle of the Calicivirus family
   b. Identification—clinical illness similar to hepatitis A; brief prodromal illness characterized by anorexia, nausea, vomiting and abdominal pain followed by an icteric phase; usually a benign, self-limiting disease except mortality rates of 10% to 20% seen in pregnancy; no evidence of chronic infection
   c. Diagnostic testing—tests for hepatitis E virus (HEV) and anti-HEV antibody are not yet widely available, but immunoassays, Western blot assays, PCR tests and immunofluorescent antibody blocking assays are available in research laboratories
   d. Incidence/prevalence—only seen in the United States as an imported disease; primarily seen in India, Asia, Africa and Central and South America
   e. Transmission—fecal/oral transmission, predominantly waterborne-associated outbreaks
   f. Incubation period—15 to 64 days
   g. Prevention—no available vaccine; water treatment and sanitation will reduce HEV infection in endemic areas
   h. Isolation precautions—Standard Precautions

U. Histoplasmosis

1. Etiology—*Histoplasma capsulatum* var. *capsulatum* (American), *Histoplasma capsulatum* var. *duboisii* (African)
2. Identification—*H. capsulatum*: Systemic mycosis with primary lesion usually in lungs, five clinical forms:
   a. Asymptomatic with hypersensitivity to histoplasmin
   b. Acute benign respiratory illness, fever, chills, myalgia, chest pains, nonproductive cough, scattered calcifications in lungs, hilar lymph nodes and spleen
   c. Acute disseminated histoplasmosis with fever, GI symptoms, bone marrow, hepatosplenomegaly, lymphadenopathy; most frequent in immunocompromised individuals, usually fatal
   d. Chronic disseminated disease with low-grade fever, weight loss, weakness, hepatosplenomegaly, mild hematological abnormalities, focal disease (e.g., meningitis), progression over 10 to 11 months, usually fatal
   e. Chronic pulmonary, resembles tuberculosis with cavitation
3. Diagnostic testing—diagnosis confirmed by culture or smear using Giemsa or Wright stains, serological tests can cross-react with other mycoses
4. Incubation period—3 to 17 days, average 10 days

5. Isolation precautions—Standard Precautions
6. Treatment—ketoconazole, itraconazole, amphotericin B for disseminated histoplasmosis

V. **Human Immunodeficiency Virus (HIV)/Acquired Immune Deficiency Syndrome (AIDS)**[23]
   1. Etiology—HIV is a double-stranded RNA virus; viral genomic RNA is copied into a DNA provirus by the viral enzyme reverse transcriptase
   2. Identification—acute retroviral syndrome (1 to 4 weeks after exposure)—fever, malaise, lethargy, anorexia, nausea, myalgias, headaches, sore throat, diarrhea and generalized lymphadenopathy; followed by latent period where patient remains asymptomatic; followed by active disease evidenced by damage to the immune system with development of infections (pneumonia most common)—bacterial, viral, fungal or parasitic and cancers or lymphoma
   3. Diagnostic testing—enzyme-linked immunosorbent assay (ELISA) and SUDS HIV-1 test measure antibody responses to HIV antigens; usually positive within 3 weeks to 6 months after exposure (average of 25 days). In rare cases, antibodies might not appear until 6 months after exposure. False-positive results after flu vaccines or associated with lupus have been seen. In low-risk populations, a positive test has a higher predictive positive result. Western blot testing (detects antibody-bound HIV protein) is confirmatory if 2 of 3 bands of significance are positive (anti-gp 160/120, anti-gp41 and anti-p24). Test results are listed as indeterminate if positive bands other than these are detected. If positive results are seen at least 2 weeks after an indeterminate finding, seroconversion is likely. IFA can be used to differentiate HIV-1 from HIV-2 infection or resolve an indeterminate Western blot result. Polymerase chain reaction (PCR) can detect either HIV-1 proviral DNA in peripheral or HIV-1 RNA in serum. Virus cultures have been largely replaced by PCR except in research laboratories. CD4 (T helper) measurements give indicators about HIV-infected person's immunity
   4. Incidence/prevalence—Approximately 56,300 new HIV infections occur in the United States each year. The CDC estimates that more than 1 million people are living with HIV in the United States, 21% of which are undiagnosed. More than 18,000 people with AIDS still die each year in the U.S.
      a. Men who have sex with men (MSM) account for more than half (53%) of all new HIV infections in the United States each year, as well as nearly half (48%) of people living with HIV
      b. Individuals infected through heterosexual contact account for 31% of annual new HIV infections and 28% of people living with HIV
      c. As a group, women account for 27% of annual new HIV infections and 25% of those living with HIV

d. Injection drug users represent 12% of annual new HIV infections and 19% of those living with HIV
   (CDC: HIV/AIDS Update);
5. Transmission—blood-borne, sexual, perinatal
6. Incubation period—1 to 3 months
7. Prevention—screening of blood/organ/tissue donors, counseling to reduce or modify high-risk behaviors, screening of all pregnant women, with treatment of infants born to HIV-positive mothers; vaccines are currently in development
8. Isolation precautions—Standard Precautions
9. Treatment
   a. Nucleoside reverse transcriptase inhibitors: zidovudine (AZT), didanosine (ddI), zalcitabine (ddC), stavudine (d4T), lamivudine (3TC)
   b. Nonnucleoside RT inhibitors: delavirdine, efavirenz, nevirapine
   c. Protease inhibitors: saquinavir, amprenavir, lopinavir + ritonavir, indinavir, ritonavir, nelfinavir
   d. Nucleotides: tenofovir DF
   e. Immune system modulators: interleukin-2 (IL-2)

W. Influenza (Avian, H1N1, Pandemic, Seasonal, Swine)

1. Etiology—influenza types: A, B or C; subtypes: H1N1, H2N2 and H3N2; subtypes are classified by the antigenic properties of the surface glycoproteins, the hemagglutinin (H) and the neuraminidase (N); strains of the virus are described by the geographic site of isolation, the culture number and the year of isolation (e.g., A/Beijing/32/92(H3N2); antigenic shift of type A viruses occurs at irregular intervals, vaccine is reformulated annually (avian flu—H5N1 [type A strain] from poultry)
2. Identification—sudden onset, fever, headache, sore throat, cough, prostration, myalgia (avian flu has an aggressive clinical course with rapid deterioration, multiorgan failure and high fatality [4 to 13 days]. Most cases have been bird to human transmission)
3. Diagnostic testing—diagnosis by clinical symptoms, nasopharyngeal swab with FA test, ELISA or serological response between acute and convalescent sera (avian flu—rapid antigen immunofluorescence assay or enzyme immunoassay, viral culture, or PCR)
4. Incubation period—1 to 3 days (avian: up to 10 days)
5. Isolation precautions—Droplet Precautions (control measures for avian flu include proper identification and disposal of sick and exposed birds, quarantining and disinfecting of poultry farms, and immediate screening and medical care for any suspected humans with H5N1 flu)

6. Treatment*—for influenza A: amantadine, rimantadine; for influenza A or B: anamivir, oseltamivir; vaccine is the most effective preventive method
7. Case fatality—average of 36,000 deaths each year from flu-associated illness
   ***Note**—because of changing resistance patterns, check CDC website for latest treatment recommendations

X. Kawasaki Syndrome—Kawasaki Disease

1. Etiology—unknown
2. Identification—criteria for diagnosis based on fever lasting more than 5 days, exclusion of other causes and at least four of the following:
   a. Bilateral conjunctival injection
   b. Injected or fissured lips, injected pharynx or "strawberry tongue," periungual desquamation
   c. Rash
   d. Cervical lymphadenopathy >1.5 cm; coronary artery aneurysms or ectasia resulting from coronary arteritis occur in 15% to 25% reduces to 8% with appropriate therapy
3. Diagnostic testing—no diagnostic test for Kawasaki syndrome but elevated erythrocyte sedimentation rate (ESR), C-reactive protein, and platelet counts >450,000 common
4. Incubation period—unknown
5. Isolation precautions—Standard Precautions
6. Treatment—high-dose IVIG can reduce fever, inflammatory signs and aneurysm formation; high-dose aspirin during the acute phase, then low dose for 2 months
7. Case fatality—0.1% to 1%

Y. Lassa Fever

1. Etiology—Lassa virus, an arenavirus, related to lymphocytic choriomeningitis, Machupo, Junin, Guanarito and Sabia viruses
2. Identification—acute viral illness, onset gradual with malaise, fever, headache, sore throat, cough, nausea, vomiting, diarrhea, myalgia, chest and abdominal pain, inflammation and exudation of the pharynx and conjunctivae; in severe cases: hypotension, shock, pleural effusion, hemorrhage, seizures, encephalopathy and edema of the face and neck; transient alopecia and ataxia may occur in convalescence, eighth cranial nerve deafness occurs in 25%, with half recovering after 1 to 3 months
3. Diagnostic testing—diagnosis by albuminuria and hemoconcentration are present, early lymphopenia then late neutrophilia, platelet count depression, platelet function normal

4. Incubation period—6 to 21 days
   5. Isolation precautions—Droplet/Contact Precautions for duration of acute phase; males should not have unprotected sex until semen is free of virus, usually 3 months. Use Airborne Precautions when the air may be contaminated with rodent excretions
   6. Treatment—ribavirin
   7. Case fatality—in pregnancy, fetal loss is >80%, fatality rate is 15% in hospitalized patients

Z. Legionellosis—Legionnaires' Disease and Pontiac Fever

   1. Etiology—*Legionella pneumophila, L. micdadei, L. bozemanii, L. longbeachae* and *L. dumoffii* (35 species with 45 serogroups)
   2. Identification—anorexia, malaise, myalgia, headache, rapidly rising fever with chills (102° to 105°F), nonproductive cough, abdominal pain and diarrhea; chest radiograph may show patchy or focal areas of consolidation that may progress to respiratory failure
   3. Diagnostic testing—isolation of organism on special media, direct IF stain, detection of antigens in urine by RIA, or 4-fold rise in IFA titer between acute and convalescent serum
   4. Incubation period—Legionnaires' disease: 2 to 10 days, average 5 to 6 days, Pontiac fever: 5 to 66 hours, average 24 to 48 hours
   5. Isolation precautions—Standard Precautions
   6. Treatment—erythromycin, clarithromycin, azithromycin, fluoroquinolones with rifampin used as an adjunct
   7. Case fatality—39%

AA. Leprosy—Hansen's Disease

   1. Etiology—*Mycobacterium leprae*
   2. Identification
      a. Lepromatous leprosy—nodules, papules, macules and diffuse infiltrations, usually bilaterally symmetrical; involvement of nasal mucosa with crusting, breathing difficulty, epistaxis, ocular involvement with iritis and keratitis
      b. Tuberculoid leprosy—skin lesions few, asymmetrical; peripheral nerve involvement severe
   3. Diagnostic testing—diagnosis by skin and nerve function examination, acid-fast smear and culture of skin scrapings or biopsy tissues
   4. Incubation period—9 months to 20 years, average 4 years for tuberculoid and 8 for lepromatous; rarely seen in children under age 3
   5. Isolation precautions—Standard Precautions for tuberculoid, Contact Precautions for lepromatous

6. Treatment—rifampin, dapsone and clofazimine combination therapy for 2 years; Bacille Calmette Guérin (BCG), dapsone, or acedapsone has been shown to prevent infections in 50% of cases

BB. Leptospirosis—Well Disease, Canicola Fever, Hemorrhagic Jaundice
   1. Etiology—leptospires are member of the order Spirochaetales, 23 serogroups, common serogroups are *L. icterohaemorrhagiae, L. canicola, L. autumnalis, L. hebdomadis, L. australis, L. pomona, L. interrogans* and *L. hardjo*
   2. Identification—sudden onset fever, headache, chills, severe myalgia, conjunctival suffusion, meningitis, rash, hemolytic anemia, jaundice, mental confusion/depression, myocarditis, and pulmonary involvement with or without hemoptysis
   3. Diagnostic testing—diagnosis is confirmed by rising titer in microscopic agglutination test; isolation of leptospires from blood; first 7 days of CSF (days 4 to 70) and urine after day 10
   4. Incubation period—4 to 19 days, average 10 days
   5. Isolation precautions—Standard Precautions with special care to prevent splash or spray of body fluids, person-to-person transmission rare
   6. Treatment—penicillin, cephalosporins, lincomycin, erythromycin, doxycycline, penicillin G, amoxicillin
   7. Case fatality—low but 20% in cases with jaundice or kidney damage

CC. Lyme Disease
   1. Etiology—*Borrelia burgdorferi*
   2. Identification—red macule or papule that expands into an annular shape called erythema migrans, must be 5 cm for case definition; malaise, fatigue, fever, headache, stiff neck, myalgia, migratory arthralgias and/or lymphadenopathy lasting weeks
   3. Diagnostic testing—serology by IFA, ELISA and immunoblotting techniques, cross-reacting seen with syphilis, relapsing fever, leptospirosis, HIV, Rocky Mountain spotted fever, mononucleosis, lupus, or rheumatoid arthritis, skin biopsy, PCR
   4. Incubation period—3 to 32 days after exposure to tick
   5. Isolation precautions—Standard Precautions
   6. Treatment—doxycycline, amoxicillin, cefuroxime, erythromycin, ceftriaxone

DD. Malaria
   1. Etiology—*Plasmodium P. vivax, P. malariae, P. falciparum,* or *P. ovale*
   2. Identification—fever, chills, sweats, cough, diarrhea, respiratory distress, headache, icterus, coagulation defects, shock, renal and liver failure, encephalopathy, pulmonary and cerebral edema, coma and death

3. Diagnostic testing—microscopy of blood, DNA probe, antibody detection by IFA
4. Incubation period—*P. falciparum, P. vivax* or *P. ovale* is 7 to 14 days, *P. malariae* is 7 to 30 days; with some strains of *P. vivax* incubation period may be up to 8 to 10 months, with infection by blood transfusion usually 2 months
5. Isolation precautions—Standard Precautions and patients should be in mosquito-proof areas from dusk to dawn
6. Treatment—chloroquine, mefloquine, halofantrine, quinine dihydrochloride or gluconate
7. Case fatality—<10%

EE. Measles—Rubeola, Red Measles

1. Etiology—measles virus of genus *Morbillivirus* of the family Paramyxoviridae
2. Identification—prodromal fever, conjunctivitis, coryza, cough, and Koplik spots on buccal mucosa, red blotchy rash on third to seventh day, beginning on face; becomes generalized and occasionally ends in brawny desquamation, leukopenia, otitis media, pneumonia, laryngotracheobronchitis, diarrhea and encephalitis
3. Diagnostic testing—detection of measles specific IgM antibodies present 3 to 4 days after rash onset; significant rise in antibody between acute and convalescent sera
4. Incubation period—7 to 18 days, average 10 days
5. Isolation precautions—Airborne Precautions in hospital setting through fourth day of rash
6. Treatment—immunization of contacts with live virus vaccine within 72 hours, immunoglobulin (IG) may be used within 6 days; specific treatment: none
7. Case fatality—3% to 5% globally, 10% to 30% in some areas

FF. Meningitis

1. Meningitis, bacterial
    a. Identification: sudden-onset fever, intense headache, nausea/vomiting, convulsions, stiff neck, irritability, bulging fontanel in infants, and frequently petechial rash with pink macules; delirium and coma
    b. Diagnostic testing
        (1) Cerebrospinal fluid (CSF) should be examined for: blood cells, leukocyte differential cell count, protein and sugar (with simultaneous blood glucose level), Gram stain, culture and bactogens (latex agglutination for pneumococcus, meningococcus or *H. influenzae*)
        (2) Blood cultures are positive in 30% to 60% of cases
        (3) Additional testing: limulus lysate (detects endotoxin from gram-negative bacilli) and lactic acid level (elevated in bacterial)

c. Isolation precautions—Droplet Precautions (wear a mask when within 3 feet of the patient) or Airborne Precautions; usually maintained for 24 hours after patient is on appropriate antimicrobial therapy (evidence of improved clinical condition)
d. Treatment
   (1) Pneumococcal or meningococcal: penicillin, cefotaxime, ceftriaxone or chloramphenicol plus TMP-SMX
   (2) *H. influenzae:* ampicillin plus ceftriaxone or cefotaxime
   (3) Gram-negative rods: cefotaxime or ceftriaxone combined with aminoglycoside
   (4) Group B streptococcus: penicillin
   (5) *L. monocytogenes:* penicillin or ampicillin
   (6) Dexamethasone given before the antibiotic in infants and children (younger than 7 years of age) reduces morbidity and mortality
e. Specific types of bacterial meningitis
   (1) Pneumococcus *(Streptococcus pneumoniae)*
      (a) One-fourth of all cases; most common cause of adult meningitis; affects all ages
      (b) Usually associated with focus infection: otitis media, mastoiditis, basilar skull fracture or pneumonia
      (c) Mortality of treated cases 25%
      (d) Convulsions, hemiparesis and hearing loss are infrequent sequelae
   (2) Meningococcus *(Neisseria meningitidis)*
      (a) One-fourth of all cases; affects infants, children and young adults primarily
      (b) Usually not associated with a predisposing factor
      (c) Most cases are caused by serogroups A and C (epidemic cases) and B and Y (sporadic cases)
      (d) Epidemic disease usually occurs in closed populations such as military recruit camps, college dormitories, etc.
      (e) Mortality of treated cases is 5% to 10%
      (f) Risk for development in patients with meningococcemia
      (g) Intimate exposure to case should be treated prophylactically
         (i) Ciprofloxacin 500 mg PO, single dose to nonpregnant adults
         (ii) Rifampin 600 mg PO twice a day for 2 days (adults); children over 1 month old, 10 mg/kg; or <1-month old, 5 mg/kg
         (iii) ceftriaxone 250 mg IM in single dose may be given to pregnant adults; 125 mg IM to children under 15 years of age
   (3) *Haemophilus influenzae*
      (a) Accounts for 10% to 15% of all cases
      (b) Usually associated with preexisting infection such as otitis media or pharyngitis

- (c) Mortality in treated cases: 5%
- (d) Neurological sequelae include mental retardation, deafness occurs in up to 50% of surviving patients
- (e) Close contacts, usually family only, are treated prophylactically for exposure
- (f) Rates have significantly declined since advent of Hib vaccine
- (4) *Listeria monocytogenes*
  - (a) Occurs primarily in immunosuppressed patients, renal transplant recipients, neonates and elderly
  - (b) Source is usually endogenous but clusters have been reported
2. Meningitis, viral
   a. Usually occurs in July, August and September
   b. Most often seen in patients <40 years of age
   c. Same signs and symptoms as bacterial meningitis but usually no mental impairment
   d. Etiology
      (1) Enteroviruses such as echovirus and coxsackievirus account for more than 50% of cases
      (2) Other causes: adenovirus, lymphocytic choriomeningitis virus, herpesvirus, cytomegalovirus and Epstein-Barr virus
      (3) Encephalitis viruses—St. Louis, California, and western equine encephalitis
      (4) Clinical features may be clue to origin or cause, such as rash with varicella-zoster infection or oral herpes infection
      (5) Standard Precautions are adequate
   e. Recovery usual without sequelae
   f. Diagnostic testing
      (1) Viral cultures of CSF
      (2) Cultures from rectal swab, stool or pharyngeal tissue may be positive in 50% of cases but do not establish cause
      (3) Antibody titers to virus—must show 4-fold rise in titer to confirm diagnosis
   g. Treatment—acyclovir may be of value for herpes; no specific treatment for other types of viral
3. Chronic meningitis—persistent or progressive for over 4 weeks
   a. Most commonly caused by *Mycobacterium tuberculosis* or fungi (*Cryptococcus neoformans*, *Histoplasma capsulatum*, and *Coccidioides immitis*)
   b. Isolation precautions—follow Standard Precautions
   c. Frequently seen in immunocompromised individuals
   d. Diagnostic testing
      (1) India ink preparation of CSF—positive in 50% of cases caused by *Cryptococcus neoformans*

(2) Acid-fast stain and culture for mycobacteria
(3) Fungal cultures
(4) Screen for cryptococcal antigen in CSF and blood
   e. Treatment
      (1) Coccidioidal: amphotericin B
      (2) Cryptococcal: amphotericin B plus flucytosine, for HIV-infected add fluconazole
      (3) *Histoplasma*: amphotericin B, in HIV-infected itraconazole
      (4) Tuberculous: isoniazid, rifampin, ethambutol and pyrazinamide with or without dexamethasone
4. Shunt-associated or epidural-associated meningitis
   a. Up to one third of patients with ventriculoatrial or ventriculoperitoneal shunts develop meningitis
   b. Usual organisms include: coagulase-negative *Staphylococcus*, *S. aureus*, gram-negative rods and enterococci
   c. Isolation precautions—follow Standard Precautions
   d. Diagnostic testing—same as for bacterial meningitis
   e. Treatment—antibiotics as indicated for bacterial meningitis with removal of shunt or epidural catheter critical to recovery
5. Brain abscess
   a. Etiology—*Streptococcus, Bacteroides, Enterobacter* commonly found; *S. aureus* and fungi are less frequent
   b. Pathogenesis—usually spread from infection site such as sinusitis or otitis, or from head trauma
   c. Identification—headache, fever, focal neurological deficit, mental status changes, nausea/vomiting, seizures, nuchal rigidity and papilledema
   d. Diagnostic testing—should not undergo lumbar puncture because of risk for brainstem herniation; brain scan (with technetium 99), computerized axial tomography (CAT) scan, and magnetic resonance imaging (MRI) are sensitive and noninvasive
   e. Treatment—aspiration, open surgical drainage or surgical excision necessary for cure along with appropriate antibiotic as indicated by focus of infection:
      (1) Otogenic or cryptogenic: penicillin G, metronidazole, cefotaxime or ceftriaxone
      (2) Paranasal sinus: penicillin G and metronidazole
      (3) Traumatic: nafcillin or vancomycin in penicillin-allergic patient and metronidazole
6. Prevention
   a. Bacterial infections—vaccines are now available for prevention of meningococcus, pneumococcus, *H. influenzae*
   b. Viral infections—vaccines for measles, polio, mumps, rabies

c. Fungal—immunocompromised persons may be treated with fluconazole or itraconazole
d. Tuberculosis—antitubercular drugs to prevent active disease

GG. Mononucleosis—Epstein-Barr Disease

1. Etiology—Epstein-Barr virus, human (gamma) herpesvirus
2. Identification—acute viral syndrome, fever, sore throat, lymphadenopathy, splenomegaly; 50% recovery can take weeks, but person may take weeks to regain former energy level; jaundice in about 4%
3. Diagnostic testing—95% will have abnormal liver function tests, lymphocytosis >50%, IFA test for IgM and IgA antibody specific for viral capsid antigen or antibody
4. Incubation period—4 to 6 weeks
5. Isolation precautions—Standard Precautions
6. Treatment—none except steroids for extreme cases

HH. Mumps—Infectious Parotitis

1. Etiology—mumps virus, family Paramyxoviridae, genus *Rubulavirus*
2. Identification—fever, swelling and tenderness of one or more salivary glands, usually parotid and sometimes sublingual or submaxillary glands, orchitis occurs in 20% to 30% of postpubertal males and oophoritis in 5% of postpubertal females, CNS may be involved (rare) with aseptic meningitis or encephalitis, pancreatitis occurs in 4%, neuritis, arthritis, mastitis, nephritis, thyroiditis or pericarditis may cause spontaneous abortion in first trimester
3. Diagnostic testing—diagnosis by serological tests (CF, HI, EIA and neutralization)
4. Incubation period—12 to 25 days, average 18 days
5. Isolation precautions—Droplet Precautions from 9 days past onset of swelling
6. Treatment—none

II. Pediculosis and Phthiriasis—Head Lice, Body Lice, Crab Lice

1. Etiology—*Pediculus humanus capitis, humanus corporis, Phthirus pubis*
2. Identification—infestation with head lice, body lice or crab lice in genital area; adult lice, nymphs and nits (egg cases); species involved in outbreaks of typhus, trench fever and louse-borne relapsing fever
3. Diagnostic testing—infested hair is fluorescent under UV light
4. Incubation period—eggs of lice hatch in 7 to 10 days, nymphal stages last about 7 to 13 days, egg-to-egg cycle averages 3 weeks
5. Isolation precautions—Contact Precautions

6. Treatment—1% permethrin, pyrethrins synergized with piperonyl butoxide, carbaryl, benzyl benzoate, gamma benzene hexachloride (lindane not recommended for infants, young children, pregnant or lactating women or persons with low seizure threshold); retreatment may be necessary after 7 to 10 days; environment cleaning necessary

JJ. Pertussis—Parapertussis—Whooping Cough

1. Etiology—*Bordetella pertussis* or *B. parapertussis*
2. Identification—insidious onset of irritating cough, which becomes paroxysmal within 1 to 2 weeks, lasts for 1 to 2 months or longer; cough has characteristic crowing or high-pitched inspiratory whoop; vomiting; parapertussis is similar to pertussis but milder
3. Diagnostic testing—diagnosis by nasopharyngeal culture, direct FA staining
4. Incubation period—6 to 20 days
5. Isolation precautions—droplet isolation for at least 5 days when on appropriate antibiotic
6. Treatment—erythromycin
7. Case fatality—<1% in infants younger than 6 months in the United States; in countries not administering immunizations it is among the highest causes of death among infants and young children

KK. Plague—Pestis

1. Etiology—*Yersinia pestis*
2. Identification—fever, chills, malaise, myalgia, nausea, prostration, sore throat, headache, lymphadenitis, septicemia, meningitis, endotoxic shock, disseminated intravascular coagulation, pneumonia
3. Diagnostic testing—diagnosis by bipolar staining, FA test, antigen capture ELISA, confirmation by culture or 4-fold rise in antibody titer
4. Incubation period—1 to 7 days, for primary plague pneumonia 2 to 4 days
5. Isolation precautions—(pneumonic plague) Droplet Precautions for 72 hours after appropriate antibiotic has been given; remove clothing that will probably be infested with fleas, use insecticides
6. Treatment—streptomycin, gentamicin, tetracyclines or chloramphenicol
7. Case fatality—untreated 50% to 60% mortality

LL. Poliomyelitis

1. Etiology—poliovirus (genus *Enterovirus*) types 1, 2 and 3
2. Identification—acute onset of flaccid paralysis, fever, malaise, headache, nausea, vomiting, severe muscle pain, stiffness of the neck and back with and without flaccid

paralysis, paralysis is asymmetrical, maximum extent is reached in 3 to 4 days, paralysis of the muscles of respiration or swallowing is life-threatening; may improve but paralysis seen after 60 days is permanent
3. Diagnostic testing—diagnosis by isolation of virus from stool specimen, CSF or oropharyngeal secretions, 4-fold rise in antibody levels
4. Incubation period—3 to 35 days, average 7 to 14 days
5. Isolation precautions—Contact Precautions
6. Treatment—none, but illness is preventable by vaccines

MM. Psittacosis—Parrot Fever, Avian Chlamydiosis

1. Etiology—*Chlamydia psittaci*
2. Identification—fever, headache, rash, myalgia, chills, respiratory infection, cough, pleuritic chest pain, splenomegaly, encephalitis, myocarditis, thrombophlebitis
3. Diagnostic testing—diagnosis by isolation of organism from sputum, blood or postmortem tissues
4. Incubation period—1 to 4 weeks
5. Isolation precautions—Standard Precautions
6. Treatment—tetracycline, erythromycin

NN. Rabies—Hydrophobia

1. Etiology—Rabies virus, a rhabdovirus of genus *Lyssavirus*
2. Identification—viral encephalomyelitis, onset by sense of apprehension, headache, fever, malaise, sensory changes, excitability, aerophobia, progresses to paresis or paralysis, spasm of swallowing muscles, fear of water (hydrophobia), delirium, convulsions, death is often caused by respiratory paralysis
3. Diagnostic testing—diagnosis by specific FA staining of brain tissue
4. Incubation period—9 days to 7 years, usually 3 to 8 weeks
5. Isolation precautions—Contact Precautions
6. Treatment—intensive supportive medical care

OO. Rocky Mountain Spotted Fever

1. Etiology—*Rickettsia rickettsii*
2. Identification—sudden onset of fever, malaise, deep muscle pain, severe headache, chills, conjunctival infection (50%) maculopapular rash on extremities including the palms and soles of feet, petechiae and hemorrhages
3. Diagnostic testing—diagnosis by serological response to specific antigens
4. Incubation period—3 to 14 days
5. Isolation precautions—Standard Precautions

CHAPTER ONE: IDENTIFICATION OF INFECTIOUS DISEASE PROCESSES | 55

6. Treatment—tetracycline, chloramphenicol
7. Case fatality—13% to 25%

PP. RSV (Respiratory Syncytial Virus)

1. Etiology—respiratory syncytial virus
2. Identification—bronchiolitis and pneumonia in infants and children under 1 year of age, begins with fever, runny nose, cough and/or wheezing (2% may require hospitalization), elderly and immunocompromised persons may also suffer
3. Diagnostic testing—virus isolation, viral antigens, viral RNA or rise in serum antibodies
4. Incubation period—1 to 10 days
5. Isolation precautions—Contact Precautions (can only live a few hours on environmental surfaces) but can be spread by droplet
6. Treatment—for mild disease no treatment, children with severe disease may require oxygen, ribavirin aerosol, RSV-IGIV and anti-RSV–humanized murine monoclonal antibody (may be used in an outbreak).

QQ. Rubella—German Measles

1. Etiology—rubella virus in family *Togaviridae*, genus *Rubivirus*
2. Identification—diffuse, punctate, maculopapular rash that resembles measles, low-grade fever, headache, malaise, mild coryza, conjunctivitis, postauricular, occipital and posterior cervical lymphadenopathy, arthralgia, arthritis, encephalitis
3. Diagnostic testing—thrombocytopenia, 4-fold rise in specific antibody titer between acute and convalescent-phase serum specimens by ELISA, HAI, passive HA or LA or rubella-specific IgM
4. Incubation period—14 to 23 days, average of 16 to 18 days
5. Isolation precautions—Droplet Precautions for 7 days after rash development
6. Treatment—none

RR. Severe Acute Respiratory Syndrome (SARS)

1. Etiology—SARS-associated coronavirus (SARS-CoV)
2. Identification—high fever (>100.4°F), headache, body aches, mild respiratory symptoms at outset, diarrhea; after 2 to 7 days; dry cough then pneumonia
3. Diagnostic testing—reverse transcription PCR (RT-PCR) test on blood, stool and nasal secretions, antibodies in serum and/or viral culture
4. Incubation period—up to 10 days
5. Isolation precautions—Droplet and Contact Precautions (CDC states some cases may have been spread by airborne and other ways not presently known).

6. Treatment—same treatment as for any serious community-acquired atypical pneumonia, CDC states various antiviral drugs are being studied.
   (Last known cases April 2004 in China)

SS. Scabies

1. Etiology—*Sarcoptes scabiei*
2. Identification—parasitic disease of the skin caused by a mite whose penetration causes papules, vesicles or tiny linear burrows, intense itching may cause scaling, vesiculation and crusting
3. Diagnostic testing—diagnosis by skin scraping or biopsy for microscopy
4. Incubation period—2 to 6 weeks, persons who have previously been infested 1 to 4 days after re-exposure
5. Isolation precautions—Contact Precautions for 24 hours after treatment
6. Treatment—permethrin, 1% gamma benzene hexachloride (contraindicated in young children, pregnant women or persons susceptible to seizures) crotamiton, tetramethylthiuram monosulfide, benzyl benzoate

TT. Sexually Transmitted Diseases (Gonorrhea, Syphilis, Herpes, Chlamydia, and Venereal Warts [Condyloma Acuminatum])

1. Etiology—*Neisseria gonorrhoeae, Treponema pallidum*, herpes simplex virus in the family Herpesviridae, *Chlamydia trachomatis*, human papillomavirus of the papovavirus group of DNA viruses
2. Identification
   a. Gonorrhea
      (1) Males—purulent discharge from penis; females: urethritis, cervicitis (may be mild), endometritis, salpingitis, pelvic peritonitis causing risk for infertility and ectopic pregnancy, can cause conjunctivitis in newborn and blindness if not treated; septicemia occurs in 0.5% to 1% with arthritis, skin lesions and rarely endocarditis and meningitis (which can cause death)
      (2) Diagnostic testing—diagnosis by Gram stain and culture, antigen detection testing
   b. Syphilis—if untreated
      (1) Chancre (painless ulcer), followed by painless lymph node; secondary eruption: symmetrical maculopapular rash involving palms and soles with lymphadenopathy, then latent for weeks to years followed by recurrence of lesions of skin and mucous membranes; lesions in aorta; gummas may occur in the skin viscera, bone and mucosal surfaces; CNS damage; neurosyphilis may occur in conjunction with HIV infection, which proceeds to CNS symptoms, may result in death

(2) Diagnostic testing—diagnosis by rapid plasma reagin (RPR), Venereal Research Laboratory (VDRL), fluorescent treponemal antibody absorbed (FTA-Abs), microhemagglutination assay for antibody to *T. pallidum* (MHA-TP), or *T. pallidum* hemagglutinating antibody (TPHA)
  c. Herpes simplex 2
    (1) Blisters or lesions on cervix and vulva of women, recurrent episodes may occur in the perineal skin, legs and buttocks; in men lesions appear on the glans penis, prepuce, anus or rectum of those engaging in anal sex; other sites may be involved, such as the mouth, depending on sexual practices; aseptic meningitis or radiculitis
    (2) Diagnostic testing—diagnosis by tissue scrapings or biopsy, direct FA tests or isolation of the virus from oral or genital lesions, PCR of spinal fluid or DNA analysis
  d. Chlamydia
    (1) Males—urethritis, mucopurulent discharge of scanty or moderate quantity, urethral itching, burning on urination, 25% of males may be asymptomatic, epididymitis, infertility, Reiter syndrome, proctitis; females: mucopurulent endocervical discharge with edema, erythema, endocervical bleeding, salpingitis, infertility, ectopic pregnancy, or chronic pelvic pain, perihepatitis, proctitis; pregnancy: premature rupture of preterm delivery, conjunctival and pneumonia infection of newborn
    (2) Diagnostic testing—diagnosis by direct IF test with monoclonal antibody of swab material, EIA, DNA probe, PCR, or cell culture
  e. Warts—hyperkeratotic, rough-textured, painless papule, may be cauliflower-like, fleshy growth
3. Incubation period—gonorrhea 2 to 7 days; syphilis 10 days to 3 months, average 3 weeks; herpes 2 to 12 days; chlamydia few hours to 5 days; warts 1 to 20 months, average 2 to 3 months
4. Isolation precautions—Standard Precautions
5. Treatment
  a. Gonorrhea—gonorrhea, syphilis, herpes, chlamydia, and venereal warts (condyloma acuminatum) ceftriaxone, ciprofloxacin, ofloxacin, cefixime or spectinomycin
  b. Syphilis—gonorrhea, syphilis, herpes, chlamydia and venereal warts (condyloma acuminatum); long-acting penicillin G, doxycycline, tetracycline
  c. Herpes—gonorrhea, syphilis, herpes, chlamydia and venereal warts (condyloma acuminatum) trifluridine, adenine arabinoside (vidarabine), acyclovir
  d. Chlamydia—gonorrhea, syphilis, herpes, chlamydia, and venereal warts (condyloma acuminatum) doxycycline, tetracycline, erythromycin, azithromycin

e. Warts—gonorrhea, syphilis, herpes, chlamydia and venereal warts (condyloma acuminatum); liquid nitrogen to freeze and remove; podophyllin in tincture of benzoin, trichloroacetic acid or 5-fluorouracil for widespread lesions; INF-α2b; surgical removal; laser therapy; cesarean section may be required for extensive genital warts

UU. Tetanus—Lockjaw

1. Etiology—*Clostridium tetani*
2. Identification—exotoxin of the tetanus bacillus, anaerobic, painful muscular contractions, primarily of masseter and neck muscles and then trunk muscles; abdominal rigidity, generalized spasms, stimulated by sensory, opisthotonus, facial expression "risus sardonicus"
3. Diagnostic testing—diagnosis by clinical symptoms
4. Incubation period—1 day to several months, average 3 to 21 days
5. Isolation precautions—Standard Precautions
6. Treatment—tetanus immune globulin (TIG) IM, tetanus antitoxin IV; IV metronidazole

VV. Tuberculosis[24]

1. Etiology—*Mycobacterium tuberculosis* an acid-fast bacterium
2. Identification—cough/congestion-sputum may be bloody, weakness or fatigue, weight loss, chills, fever, night sweats, chest pain
3. Diagnostic testing—acid-fast sputum analysis (smear and culture) or bronchial lavage specimen, PCR, DNA probe; chest radiographs help describe extent of infection or differentiate between infection and disease; tuberculin skin testing (TST) shows presence of tuberculosis (TB) infection/disease if person's immune system is competent, anergy testing done for mumps, histoplasmosis, etc.; TST may be slightly positive for atypical mycobacterial infections such as *M. avium-intracellulare*; QuantiFERON-TB blood test can be used for determining TB infection. INF-γ release assays (IGRA) provide rapid testing within 24 to 48 hours, not affected by BCG status, immunosuppression status
4. Incidence/prevalence: 12,904 new cases of TB disease in the United States in 2008
5. Transmission—airborne by inhalation of droplet nuclei
6. Prevention/isolation—adequate airborne isolation procedures for any patient suspected of having TB (negative pressure isolation rooms, N95 respirators, etc.), direct observed therapy for all new cases, adequate treatment of all new cases of TB infection where appropriate
7. Treatment—isoniazid (INH), rifampin (RIF), pyrazinamide (PZA), ethambutol (EMB), and streptomycin; treatment for TB disease will last 6 to 12 months unless HIV positive, then may last 18 months; culture must be tested for drug sensitivity as soon

as growth is present to rule out drug resistance and aid in selection of antitubercular drugs

WW. Tularemia—Rabbit Fever, Deer Fly Fever

1. Etiology—*Francisella tularensis*, gram-negative, coccobacillus
2. Identification—tick bite: swelling of regional lymph nodes, ulcerations, from nodes; ingestion of organism: pharyngitis, abdominal, pain, diarrhea, vomiting; inhalation of organisms: pneumonia, septicemia; conjunctivitis with lymphadenitis
3. Diagnostic testing—diagnosis by rise in serum antibody titers, cross-reactions occur with *Brucella* species, FA testing of drainage from ulcers, lymph node aspirates, biopsy of lymph nodes often induces septicemia, culture on cysteine-glucose blood agar but due to the caution that must be used in the laboratory, most are diagnosed serologically
4. Incubation period—1 to 14 days, average 3 to 5 days
5. Isolation precautions—Contact Precautions when lesions present
6. Treatment—streptomycin or gentamicin

XX. Typhoid Fever—Paratyphoid Fever

1. Etiology—*Salmonella typhi* (paratyphoid) group strains I to VI
2. Identification—typhoid fever: sustained fever, severe headache, malaise, anorexia, bradycardia, splenomegaly, rose spots on the trunk in 25% of light-skinned persons, nonproductive cough, constipation, ulceration of Peyer patches in the ileum producing intestinal hemorrhage or perforation, cerebral dysfunction; paratyphoid: same symptoms but milder
3. Diagnostic testing—diagnosis by culture of organisms from blood, urine, feces or bone marrow, 4-fold rise in titers, monoclonal antibody testing
4. Incubation period—3 days to 3 months, average 1 to 3 weeks; paratyphoid is 1 to 10 days
5. Isolation precautions—exclude typhoid carriers from handling food; Contact Precautions until 3 negative stool cultures not earlier than 1 month after onset
6. Treatment—chloramphenicol, amoxicillin, TMP-SMX, quinolones, cephalosporins, supportive care
7. Case fatality—typhoid fever untreated 10%, reduced to <1% with appropriate antibiotic treatment early; paratyphoid is much lower

YY. Typhus Fever—Louse-borne Typhus Fever, Murine Typhus Fever

1. Etiology—*Rickettsia prowazekii, R. typhi*
2. Identification—sudden onset of headache, chills, prostration, fever, general pains, macular eruption on the upper trunk then spreads to entire body on fifth to sixth day, but not on palms, soles or face; severe toxemia

3. Diagnostic testing—diagnosis by IF test most commonly but may not discriminate between louse-borne and murine, EIA, CF with group-specific or washed type-specific rickettsial antigens and toxin-neutralization test, antibody testing usually positive in second week
4. Incubation period—1 to 2 weeks, commonly 12 days
5. Isolation precautions—Standard Precautions after delousing patient
6. Treatment—tetracycline, chloramphenicol, doxycycline

ZZ. West Nile Virus—West Nile Encephalitis or Meningitis, West Nile Fever

1. Etiology—West Nile virus
2. Identification—80% of infections are asymptomatic; 20% develop West Nile fever characterized by fever, myalgia, rash (maculopapular or morbilliform rash involving the neck, trunk, arms or legs), lymphadenopathy, eye pain, nausea/vomiting, anorexia and malaise; a small percentage develop West Nile meningitis, encephalitis, or poliomyelitis, which may be characterized by fever, weakness, GI symptoms, change in mental status, severe muscle weakness, flaccid paralysis, neurological presentations: ataxia and extrapyramidal signs, cranial nerve abnormalities, myelitis, optic neuritis, polyradiculitis, seizures
3. Diagnostic testing—diagnosis by serum or CSF collected 8 days after illness onset for IgM antibody (MAC-ELISA). Patients with related flaviviruses or vaccinated against may have positive WNV MAC-ELISA results
4. Incubation period—3 to 14 days
5. Isolation precautions—Standard Precautions
6. Treatment—ribavirin in high doses and INF-α2b; corticosteroids, antiseizure, or osmotic agents in the management of WNV encephalitis

AAA. Yellow Fever

1. Etiology—yellow fever virus, genus *Flavivirus*, family Flaviviridae
2. Identification—sudden-onset fever, chills, headache, backache, generalized muscle pain, prostration, nausea and vomiting, slow and weak pulse (Faget sign), jaundice, albuminuria, anuria, hemorrhagic symptoms: epistaxis, gingival bleeding, hematemesis, melena, liver and renal failure
3. Diagnostic testing—diagnosis by viral antigen in the blood by ELISA, viral genome in blood and liver tissue by PCR or hybridization probes, specific IgM in early sera
4. Incubation period—3 to 6 days
5. Isolation precautions—Standard Precautions, protect patient from mosquitoes
6. Treatment—none
7. Case fatality—20% to 50% of jaundiced cases are fatal, overall case-fatality rate is <5%

BBB. Yersiniosis
1. Etiology—*Yersinia pseudotuberculosis, Y. enterocolitica*
2. Identification—acute febrile diarrhea, enterocolitis, acute mesenteric lymphadenitis mimicking appendicitis, erythema nodosum, postinfectious arthritis and systemic infection, bloody diarrhea seen 10% to 30%, joint pain in 50% of adults
3. Diagnostic testing—diagnosis by stool culture, agglutination test, or by ELISA
4. Incubation period—3 to 7 days
5. Isolation precautions—Contact Precautions
6. Treatment—aminoglycosides, TMP-SMX, ciprofloxacin, tetracyclines

Practice Questions for Chapter One

Chapter One:

Identification of Infectious Disease Processes Questions

1. A urine specimen collected from an indwelling urinary catheter was sent to the laboratory for culture and sensitivity. Culture results reported a colony count of 50,000 cc/mL of *Escherichia coli*. Sensitivity testing reported resistance to cephalosporin and sensitivity to ciprofloxacin. This organism is an example of:
   a. Methicillin resistance
   b. Aminoglycoside resistance
   c. Extended-spectrum beta-lactam resistance
   d. Quinolone resistance

2. The validity of a culture report is dependent on the quality of the specimen sent. To determine if an expectorated specimen was sputum and not saliva, the Gram stain should show:
   a. Fewer than 10 epithelial cells per low-power field
   b. More than 10 epithelial cells per low-power field and moderate to abundant polys
   c. More than 10 epithelial cells per low-power field and abundant *Pseudomonas aeruginosa* in pure culture
   d. Many WBCs and organisms on low-power field

3. To increase recovery of AFB from expectorated or induced sputum, specimens should be collected:
   a. Once a week for 3 consecutive weeks
   b. Every day for 1 week
   c. First morning specimen for 3 consecutive days
   d. Three specimens 1 hour apart on the same day

4. A patient has a nasal swab positive for MRSA. This is an example of:
   a. Normal flora
   b. Colonization
   c. Asymptomatic infection
   d. Symptomatic infection

Questions 5–6

5. A 27-year-old man is admitted with symptoms suggestive of meningitis. The patient has a history of head trauma from a motor vehicle collision. The laboratory calls to report that a gram-positive organism is noted in the CSF. What is your next action?
   a. Have the charge nurse compile a list of exposed staff
   b. Notify the employee health nurse that several employees will need prophylaxis
   c. Tell the staff that no one should be treated until the culture report is final
   d. Ensure that employees understand which organisms are treated and which are not

6. The type of isolation or precautions to be followed when providing direct care to this patient would be:
   a. Droplet Precautions
   b. Airborne isolation
   c. Standard Precautions
   d. Respiratory etiquette

7. Which of the following is not a mechanical barrier to infection?
   a. Intact skin
   b. Mucous membranes
   c. Secretions
   d. Normal bacterial flora

8. Patients with cell-mediated immunity dysfunction are susceptible to infections attributed to pathogenic intracellular bacteria. Examples of these organisms include:
   (1) *Salmonella typhi*
   (2) *Bacteroides fragilis*
   (3) *Listeria monocytogenes*
   (4) *Staphylococcus aureus*
      a. 2, 3
      b. 1, 3
      c. 1, 2
      d. 3, 4

9. What is the name for a substance that prevents water-soluble elements such as antibiotics and disinfectants from reaching pathogens?
   a. Cell wall
   b. Biofilm
   c. Sludge
   d. Biocarbon

10. A gram-negative bacterium responsible for chronic antral gastritis and a major factor in peptic ulcer disease is:
    a. H. pyogenes
    b. S. typhi
    c. C. difficile
    d. H. pylori

11. The spirochete *Borrelia burgdorferi* is the agent responsible for:
    a. Legionnaires' disease
    b. Lyme disease
    c. Aseptic meningitis
    d. Syphilis

12. Higher morbidity rates in chronic HBV carriers are associated with a co-infection of:
    a. Enteric NANB hepatitis
    b. Hepatitis D
    c. Hepatitis C
    d. Hepatitis E

13. Gram stains classify an organism as gram-positive or gram-negative. The determinant factors for Gram stains are cell wall components of:
    a. Peptidoglycans
    b. Lipids
    c. Polysaccharides
    d. Mycolic acids

14. Microorganisms are grown on culture media made of an agar base. Additives to media vary according to growth requirements of organisms and/or the desire to select out a specific organism. Fastidious organisms require _____media, and _____media is used to inhibit normal commensals.
    (1) Differential
    (2) Enrichment
    (3) Selective
    (4) Nutrient broth
    (5) Synthetic sheep blood agar
        a. 1, 3
        b. 2, 3
        c. 3, 4
        d. 5, 1

15. An example of an obligate intracellular parasitic bacterium would be an organism responsible for:
    (1) Hepatitis
    (2) Q fever
    (3) Malaria
    (4) Epidemic typhus
        a. 2, 3
        b. 2, 4
        c. 3, 4
        d. 1, 2

Questions 16–17

16. You are notified by the microbiology laboratory that three patients on the oncology ward have cultures positive for *Aspergillus fumigatus*. Chart review confirms that the cultures are responsible for invasive disease. Two specimens are bronchial lavages and the third a sinus cavity. All three cultures were taken on the same day. Your FIRST course of action is:
    (1) Notify the head nurse and medical director of the unit
    (2) Set up a meeting with engineering staff to discuss air handling
    (3) Ask the microbiology laboratory to do a retrospective review of *Aspergillus* cultures
    (4) Notify the administration personnel of fungal infection outbreak
        a. 1, 3
        b. 1, 2
        c. 3, 4
        d. 1, 4

17. Review of microbiology logs revealed four additional patients with positive *Aspergillus* cultures within the past 6 months. Chart review of the four determined that the patients were from different units and medical services and the cultures represented community-associated colonization. Based on this information, you:
    a. Decide no follow-up is necessary because oncology patients are at high risk for *Aspergillus* infection
    b. Look for a common factor in all seven patients
    c. Look for a common factor among the three oncology patients only
    d. Continue investigating all seven patients by doing phone interviews

18. While touring the oncology unit and the outside perimeter of the hospital, you notice active road construction one block from the hospital. The oncology unit is at the street level, facing the construction. Assuming this to be the source of the *Aspergillus*, you determine factors allowing *Aspergillus* spores to enter the building, including:
    (1) Staff props outside doors open when they go out to smoke
    (2) Pigeons roost on the unit's windowsills
    (3) The air intake system on the roof faces the construction
    (4) The unit's utility room has an open window
    a. 1, 3
    b. 2, 4
    c. 1, 4
    d. None, the construction is too far away to be a factor

19. A meeting was called with the head nurse, medical director, and vice president of engineering. Proposed interventions included adding an alarm to sound when the outside door was open for longer than 30 seconds, placing a positive-airflow vent over the doorway, and locking the utility room window. To determine whether these measures were effective, you will:
    a. Monitor every patient on the unit for the next 6 months
    b. Have the microbiology laboratory notify you immediately in the event of another positive culture
    c. Tour the unit daily to ensure the engineering controls are in place
    d. Consider the problem solved and move on to other issues

20. Microorganisms that can only live and grow in the presence of oxygen are:
    a. Anaerobes
    b. Pathogens
    c. Aerobes
    d. Molds

21. Of the following viruses, which is the most common healthcare-associated pathogen in pediatric wards?
    a. Respiratory syncytial virus
    b. Adenovirus
    c. Herpes simplex virus
    d. Cytomegalovirus

22. Five cases of prosthetic valve endocarditis caused by *Staphylococcus epidermidis* are observed in one hospital. Of the following available methods, which is BEST for determining whether all five isolates were derived from a single source?
    A. Serotyping
    B. Restriction fragment length polymorphism analysis
    C. Antimicrobial susceptibility testing
    D. Bacteriophage typing

23. Which of the following statements is TRUE regarding bacterial spores?
    a. They are resistant to antibiotics.
    b. They allow the bacteria to multiply in adverse conditions.
    c. They are usually formed by gram-negative bacteria.
    d. They can be identified with Gram stains.

Questions 24–28 A 10-year-old boy is admitted to the hospital with a 3-day history of fever, abdominal pain, diarrhea, and vomiting. He and his family have just returned from a week-long camping expedition in the mountains that included trips to the seashore.

24. A stool culture is reported with many lactose-negative colonies. The most probable causing organism is:
    a. *Providencia alcalifaciens*
    b. *Providencia stuartii*
    c. *Yersinia enterocolitica*
    d. *Providencia rettgeri*

25. Which of the following organisms can grow in the small bowel and cause diarrhea in children and traveler's diarrhea through the production of enterotoxins?
    a. *Yersinia enterocolitica*
    b. *Escherichia coli*
    c. *Salmonella typhi*
    d. *Shigella dysenteriae*

26. Which disease requires a very small inoculum of organisms to cause diseases?
    a. Dysentery *(Shigella)*
    b. *Salmonella*
    c. *Campylobacter*
    d. *Giardia*

27. A liquid stool specimen is collected from the patient (the 10-year-old boy) at 9 pm. The physician has ordered a culture, ova and parasites. The specimen is refrigerated until 9 am the following day, when the physician calls and requests the laboratory to look for amebic trophozoites. The best course of action is:
    a. Request a fresh specimen
    b. Perform a concentration on the original stool specimen
    c. Perform a trichrome stain on the original specimen
    d. Perform a saline wet mount on the original specimen

28. Which organism found in food poisoning causes the most rapid onset of symptoms?
    a. *Salmonella enteritidis*
    b. *Shigella sonnei*
    c. *Staphylococcus aureus*
    d. *Escherichia coli*

29. The IP referred a new nurse in the labor and delivery suite to the occupational health department to be tested for immunity to rubella. The laboratory would test for the presence of:
    a. Opsonin
    b. Antigen
    c. Antibody
    d. Agglutinin

30. The IP is teaching nurses how to assess infection risks in patients. Depletion of what cell type provides the BEST indication of susceptibility to most bacterial infections?
    a. Monocyte
    b. Eosinophil
    c. Neutrophil
    d. Lymphocyte

31. The IP is reviewing the chart of a patient with a sputum culture positive for pathogens. Which of the following findings indicates that the specimen had been properly collected from a patient with possible bacterial pneumonia?
    a. Numerous neutrophils and few if any epithelial cells
    b. Presence of blood
    c. Many epithelial cells and few neutrophils
    d. Variety of both gram-positive and gram-negative bacteria

32. The IP has been seeing an increased number of positive surgical site cultures from patients who are not infected. The IP suspects that the cultures may have been improperly collected. While discussing the problem with the unit nurse manager, the IP reviews the proper technique for collecting wound cultures. Wound swabs for cultures should be obtained from the:
    a. Skin surface adjacent to the wound
    b. Purulent material from the dressing
    c. Wound surface before cleaning
    d. Drainage after cleaning wound surface

33. The IP is asked to review with a group of staff nurses how to interpret antibiotic susceptibility tests. The susceptibility test that allows a determination of the least amount of antibiotic per milliliter that impedes the growth of an organism is known as a:
    a. Minimum inhibitory concentration
    b. Kirby-Bauer disc method
    c. Minimum bactericidal concentration
    d. Serum-cidal level

34. When reviewing microbiology laboratory data looking for isolates of methicillin- resistant *Staphylococcus aureus* (MRSA), the laboratory does not use methicillin for susceptibility testing. Which of the following antimicrobial agents is the MOST similar to methicillin and is most commonly used in susceptibility testing?
    a. Carbenicillin
    b. Oxacillin
    c. Gentamicin
    d. Amikacin

35. A child with chickenpox has been admitted to your facility. Which of the following is FALSE?
    a. The child should be placed on airborne and contact precautions with an N95 respirator
    b. Personnel who have not had chickenpox should avoid contact with this patient
    c. The vesicles are monolocular and collapse on puncture
    d. The incubation period is 2 to 3 weeks, with an average of 13 to 17 days

36. Antivirals act in all but which of the following methods?
    a. Inhibition of formation of DNA precursors
    b. Interference with viral uncoating
    c. Conference of viral resistance on uninfected cells
    d. Inhibition of cell wall synthesis

37. Your patient has a low absolute neutrophil count. Of the following choices, which is true of your patients?
    i. They are especially susceptible to disease
    ii. You can determine the absolute neutrophil count by multiplying the total WBC count by the percentage of mature and immature neutrophils
    iii. The patient's WBC count is between 4000 and 10,000
    iv. The patient's complement system will only be activated through the alternative pathway
    a. i
    b. i and ii
    c. iii
    d. d. i, ii and iv

38. A 14-year-old boy from rural Maryland was seen in the emergency room with fever, fatigue, chills, headache and a large annular lesion on his left thigh which the patient described as burning and itching. What is the most probable vector of this child's illness?
    A. Tick
    B. Mosquito
    C. Flea
    D. Louse

39. A sputum specimen is obtained and sent to the microbiology laboratory. The most valid indication for setting the specimen up for culture is:
    a. The Gram stain contained many epithelial cells
    b. The specimen was collected in the early morning
    c. The Gram stain contained polymorphonucleocytes
    d. The patient rinsed or gargled before giving the specimen

40. Which immune marker represents past exposure to disease?
    a. IgG
    b. IgE
    c. IgM
    d. IgA

41. A patient presents to the ER with profuse diarrhea. The patient has never traveled outside of the United States and has not had recent healthcare or antibiotic exposure. What is the most likely agent causing the diarrhea?
    a. *Vibrio cholerae*
    b. *Clostridium difficile*
    c. *Cryptosporidium parvum*
    d. Lassa fever

42. Three cases of cramping abdominal pain and diarrhea are reported to you through the emergency department within a 24-hour period. All persons are from the same community, and onset was within 12 to 36 hours of a picnic they all attended. Which foodborne illness do you suspect?
    a. *Salmonella*
    b. Hepatitis A
    c. *Staphylococcus aureus*
    d. *Clostridium perfringens*

43. When reviewing the Gram stain of a person with a wound infection, you see gram-positive organisms in clusters. Which organism would this most likely represent?
    a. *Streptococcus*
    b. *Enterococcus*
    c. Diphtheroids
    d. *Staphylococcus*

44. Which organism would commonly be found in tap water?
    a. *Salmonella*
    b. *Legionella*
    c. *Staphylococcus*
    d. *Candida*

45. You receive a call from a young man who thinks he was exposed to HIV. His baseline HIV test (ELISA) was negative. At what time period after exposure would we be most likely to detect HIV antibodies?
    a. 6 months
    b. 1 to 3 months
    c. 12 months
    d. 3 weeks

46. The isolation of a diphtheroid or *Corynebacterium*-like organism from a clinical specimen may or may not be significant. One feature that increases the likelihood of significance is:
    a. Isolation from a blood culture of a patient with a fever
    b. Isolation in the presence of a shunt or prosthetic valve
    c. Isolation from an abdominal surgical wound infection
    d. Sensitivity of the organism to vancomycin

47. The causative organism of Creutzfeldt-Jakob disease is a:
    a. Helminth
    b. Rickettsia
    c. Spirochete
    d. Prion

48. Which of the following organisms would be the most likely cause of a viral conjunctivitis in a physical therapist who performs home care?
    a. Echovirus
    b. Adenovirus
    c. Enterovirus
    d. Herpes simplex virus

49. Anaerobic cultures should be used for any of the following sites EXCEPT:
    a. Blood
    b. Transtracheal aspirate
    c. Spinal fluid
    d. Pressure ulcer

50. Greater than 80% lymphocytes in a CSF specimen, with no organisms seen, usually is indicative of meningitis caused by:
    a. Mycobacteria
    b. Fungi
    c. Bacteria
    d. Viruses

51. You examine an employee complaining about a sore throat. A culture is done. The organism most likely to be found on the culture is:
    a. *Streptococcus pyogenes*
    b. *Staphylococcus aureus*
    c. *Streptococcus viridans*
    d. *Corynebacterium diphtheriae*

52. According to the Centers for Disease Control and Prevention *Infection Control Guidelines*, routine microbiological sampling is indicated for which of the following?
    a. Respiratory therapy equipment
    b. Dialysis fluid
    c. Sterile disposable equipment
    d. Operating room surfaces

Questions 53–57 Herpes simplex virus (HSV) keratitis is suspected in an oncology patient. The patient has been hospitalized in a semi-private room for the previous 10 days. Aerobic eye cultures are negative to date. The roommate is a patient with newly diagnosed acute leukemia receiving chemotherapy.

53. Eye drainage is sent for viral studies. These studies may include:
    a. Direct immunofluorescence
    b. Gram stain
    c. Latex agglutination
    d. Complement fixation

54. A single serum sample is sent for ELISA antibody testing. The following titers are reported: HSV titer 1:128; CMV titer <1:8; EBV titer <1:8. These results indicate:
    a. Immunity to HSV
    b. Confirmation of acute HSV infection
    c. Presumptive identification of HSV infection
    d. Immunity to CMV and EBV

55. The patient's roommate has talked with his physician about prophylactic treatment. The physician will probably recommend that:
    a. The patient be moved to another room, but no treatment is indicated
    b. The patient remain in this room, and no treatment is indicated
    c. The patient remain in this room and receive treatment with acyclovir
    d. The patient be moved to another room and receive treatment with acyclovir

56. A pre-admission serum sample from the patient is recovered. ELISA antibody testing for HSV is done on the paired sera. Reported titers are: previous 1:8; current 1:128. The results indicate:
    a. Acute HSV infection
    b. Indeterminate infection
    c. Chronic infection
    d. Immunity to HSV

57. A nurse rotated to the oncology unit for one shift on the day before the patient's onset of keratitis. She passed oral medications to the patient. On the day following that shift, she noted a painful, fluid-filled vesicle on her right index finger. Viral cultures were positive for HSV. Which statement is most likely?
   a. The employee acquired HSV from this patient
   b. The employee acquired HSV from a different source
   c. The employee transmitted infection to this patient
   d. The employee's infection is probably HSV type II, and the patient's infection HSV type I, so the events are unrelated.

Questions 58–60

58. An emaciated homeless person is admitted with suspicion of TB. He has an upper lobe cavitary lesion and a positive PPD skin test measuring 10 mm. He is placed on Airborne Precautions with negative pressure. Laboratory reports indicate three positive AFB smears. This result indicates:
   a. Confirmed diagnosis of tuberculosis
   b. Presumptive mycobacterial infection
   c. Presumptive diagnosis of tuberculosis
   d. No conclusion is possible from this report

59. All of the following are CDC recommendations for TB treatment EXCEPT:
   a. Start all TB patients on 4-drug regimen
   b. Perform susceptibility testing on all isolates
   c. Start TB patient on 6-drug regimen in geographic areas with reported drug-resistant outbreaks
   d. Consider direct observed therapy (DOT) for noncompliant patients only

60. After 6 weeks, initial sputum cultures grow *Mycobacterium avium-intracellulare*. Possible reasons for a positive tuberculin skin test include all EXCEPT:
   a. Prior exposure to *M. tuberculosis*
   b. Prior BCG vaccination
   c. Cross-reactivity to skin test antigens
   d. The patient is only colonized

CHAPTER ONE: IDENTIFICATION OF INFECTIOUS DISEASE PROCESSES

Questions 61–75   A young child with an elevated temperature and respiratory symptoms is admitted to your pediatric unit.

61. Which of the following precautions will you take?
    a. Cohort with children having similar symptoms
    b. Place with clean medical patient
    c. Place in a private room in isolation
    d. Use Standard Precautions with no special placement

62. In the admitting assessment, the following symptoms were noted: elevated temperature, bronchiolitis, lethargy, and irritability. Which infectious process should be considered as the likely cause?
    a. *Legionella*
    b. Respiratory syncytial virus
    c. *Mycoplasma pneumoniae*
    d. *Haemophilus influenzae* infection

63. Control measures include all BUT which of the following?
    a. Contact Precautions
    b. Restricting healthcare workers with active respiratory illness
    c. Vaccination
    d. Strict handwashing

64. Diagnosis of this illness can be confirmed by all BUT the following:
    a. Viral isolation from nasopharyngeal secretions
    b. Rapid diagnostic procedures such as ELISA or complement fixation
    c. Serological testing of acute and convalescent serum
    d. Skin test

65. Which one of the following viral diseases has the shortest incubation period?
    a. Rubella
    b. Influenza
    c. Hepatitis A
    d. Hepatitis B

66. All of the following are tick-borne diseases associated with fever EXCEPT:
    a. Lyme disease
    b. Ehrlichiosis
    c. Tularemia
    d. Parvovirus

67. The PRIMARY reason for the emergence of multidrug-resistant TB is:
    a. Increase in the homeless population
    b. Inadequate or incomplete treatment of those infected with TB
    c. Increase in the numbers of HIV-infected persons
    d. Decrease in the effectiveness of antitubercular drugs

68. One example of pneumonia generally acquired from an environmental source is:
    a. *Legionella*
    b. Pneumococcal
    c. Influenza
    d. Varicella

69. You are caring for a patient who is extremely immunocompromised. While reviewing the laboratory data for this patient, you discover he has had a sputum examination for AFB, which is smear positive. The physician is aware but states isolation is not necessary. What is a possible reason that the patient does not need isolation?
    a. His past AFB cultures have always been negative
    b. His PPD skin test is negative
    c. He only has lower lobe infiltrates on his chest radiograph
    d. His regular sputum culture is growing *Nocardia* spp

70. A 38-year-old woman being treated for breast cancer has a WBC count of 2.3. This is an improvement over the counts seen during the past 2 weeks. Her physician has been aggressive in treating every potential infection she has had. She is currently on an antibiotic for a bloodstream infection from *Staphylococcus epidermidis*. She now has a fever of 100.4°F. What action should be taken?
    a. Her intravenous sites should be inspected frequently
    b. None because she may have neutropenic fever and no real infection
    c. More blood cultures because she may be developing fungal septicemia
    d. Antibiotics stopped because she may have a "drug fever"

71. All of the following are changes in activity of the T cells or B cells, which affect immunity associated with the elderly, EXCEPT:
    a. Delayed hypersensitivity
    b. Defense against foreign antigens
    c. Increased serum levels of IgG and IgA
    d. Shortened T-cell life in post-mature state

72. A patient has been admitted with a diagnosis of suspected West Nile fever. The doctor has not ordered any isolation precautions. What precautions should be used with this patient?
    a. Standard Precautions
    b. Airborne Precautions
    c. Contact Precautions
    d. No precautions

73. What descriptive characteristic of bacteria are you looking for when you check an anaerobic culture?
    a. Antibiotic resistance
    b. Sugar fermentation
    c. Cell morphology
    d. Oxygen utilization

74. A diagnosis of cryptococcal meningitis is suspected. What additional testing should be done to confirm this?
    a. Gram stain of CSF
    b. Anaerobic culture of CSF
    c. India ink examination of CSF
    d. Aerobic culture of CSF

75. All of the following have a vaccine that may prevent the disease EXCEPT:
    a. Hepatitis A
    b. Hepatitis B
    c. Hepatitis C
    d. Hepatitis D

Answers for Practice Questions Chapter One

1.	c	26.	a	51.	a		
2.	a	27.	a	52.	b		
3.	c	28.	c	53.	a		
4.	b	29.	c	54.	c		
5.	d	30.	c	55.	b		
6.	c	31.	a	56.	a		
7.	c	32.	d	57.	b		
8.	d	33.	a	58.	b		
9.	b	34.	b	59.	d		
10.	d	35.	a	60.	d		
11.	b	36.	d	61.	a		
12.	b	37.	b	62.	b		
13.	a	38.	a	63.	c		
14.	b	39.	c	64.	d		
15.	b	40.	a	65.	b		
16.	a	41.	c	66.	d		
17.	c	42.	a	67.	b		
18.	c	43.	d	68.	a		
19.	b	44.	b	69.	d		
20.	c	45.	b	70.	c		
21.	a	46.	b	71.	d		
22.	b	47.	d	72.	a		
23.	a	48.	b	73.	d		
24.	c	49.	d	74.	c		
25.	b	50.	a	75.	c		

References

1. Johnson RM, Brown EJ. Cell-mediated immunity in host defense against infectious diseases. In: Mandell GL, Bennett JE, Dolan R, eds. *Principles and Practice of Infectious Diseases*. 5th ed. New York: Churchill Livingstone; 2000:112–145.

2. Tosi MF, Cates KL. Immunologic and phagocytic responses to infection. In: Feigin RD, Cherry TD, eds. *Textbook of Pediatric Infectious Diseases*. 3rd ed. Philadelphia: WB Saunders; 1998:14–54.

3. Romani L, Pucetti P, Bistoni F. Interleukin-12 in infectious diseases. *Clin Microbiol Rev* 1997;10(4):611–636.

4. Yoshikai Y, Nishimura H. The role of interleukin-15 in mounting an immune response against microbial infections. *Microbes Infect* 2000;2(4):381–389.

5. Markham RB. Cell-mediated immunity. In: Gorbach SL, Bartlett JG, Blacklow HR, eds. *Infectious Diseases*. 2nd ed. Philadelphia: WB Saunders; 1998:66–81.

6. Heinzel FP. Antibodies. In: Mandell GL, Bennett JE, Dolan R, eds. *Principles and Practice of Infectious Diseases*. 5th ed. New York: Churchill Livingstone; 2000:45–66.

7. Tramont EC, Hoover DL. Innate (general or nonspecific) host defense mechanisms. In: Mandell GL, Bennett JE, Dolan R, eds. *Principles and Practice of Infectious Diseases*. 5th ed. New York: Churchill Livingstone; 2000:31–38.

8. Smith AL. Indigenous flora. In: Feigin RD, Cherry TD, eds. *Textbook of Pediatric Infectious Diseases*. 3rd ed. Philadelphia: WB Saunders; 1998:95–98.

9. Lorin MI. Fever. pathogenesis and treatment. In: Feigin RD, Cherry TD, eds. Textbook of Pediatric *Infectious Diseases*. 3rd ed. Philadelphia: WB Saunders; 1998:130–134.

10. Lorin MI. Fever. pathogenesis and treatment. In Feigin RD, Cherry TD, eds. Textbook of pediatric infectious diseases. 3rd ed. Philadelphia: WB Saunders; 1998:130–134.

11. Kazuhiro K, Hiroshi N, Atsuko H, et al. Association of human herpesvirus 6 infection of the central nervous system with recurrence of febrile convulsions. *J Infect Dis* 1993;167:1197–1200.

12. Kluger MJ. Fever revisited. *Pediatrics* 1992;90:846–850.

13. Densen P. Complement. In: Mandell GL, Bennett JE, Dolan R, eds. *Principles and Practice of Infectious Diseases*. 5th ed. New York: Churchill Livingstone; 2000:67–88.

14. Winkelstein JA. The complement system. In: Gorbach SL, Bartlett JG, Blacklow HR, eds. *Infectious Diseases*. 2nd ed. Philadelphia: WB Saunders; 1998:35–40.

15. Nauseef WM, Clark RA. Granulocytic phagocytes. In: Mandell GL, Bennett JE, Dolan R, eds. *Principles and Practice of Infectious Diseases*. 5th ed. New York: Churchill Livingstone; 2000:89–111.

16. Klempner MS, Malech HL. Phagocytes: normal and abnormal neutrophil host defenses. In: Gorbach SL, Bartlett JG, Blacklow HR, eds. *Infectious Diseases*. 2nd ed. Philadelphia: WB Saunders; 1998:41–65.

17. Centers for Disease Control and Prevention, Healthcare Infection Control Practices Advisory Committee (HICPAC). Guidelines for environmental infection control in healthcare facilities. *MMWR* 2003;52(RR-10):1–44.

18. Moellering RC, Eliopoulos GM. Principles of anti-infective therapy. In: Mandell GL. *Douglas and Bennett's Principles and Practice of Infectious Disease*. Philadelphia, PA: Churchill Livingstone; 2005:242–253.

19. Siegel JD, Rhinehart E, Jackson M, et al. The Healthcare Infection Control Practices Advisory Committee. Management of Multidrug-Resistant Organisms in Healthcare Settings, 2006. Available online at: www.cdc.gov/hicpac/mdro/mdro_0.html.

20. Davies J. Inactivation of antibiotics and the dissemination of resistance genes. *Science* 1994;264:375–382.

21. Nikaido H. Prevention of drug access to bacterial targets: permeability barriers and active efflux. *Science* 1995;264:382–388.

22. Centers for Disease Control and Prevention. Viral Hepatitis. Available at http://www.cdc.gov/hepatitis/index.htm. Accessed November 2, 2010.

23. Centers for Disease Control and Prevention. Diagnoses of HIV infection and AIDS in the United States and Dependent Areas, 2008. HIV Surveillance Report, Volume 20. Available at http://www.cdc.gov/hiv/surveillance/resources/reports/2008report/index.htm. Accessed November 2, 2010.

24. American Thoracic Society. ATS/CDC/IDSA Statement: Treatment of Tuberculosis, 2003. Report found at http://www.thoracic.org/statements/. Accessed on November 9, 2010.

CHAPTER TWO

SURVEILLANCE AND EPIDEMIOLOGICAL INVESTIGATION

CONTENTS

Article	Page
CBIC Content Outline for Surveillance and Epidemiological Investigation	82
Chapter Two: Surveillance and Epidemiological Investigation	84
I. Epidemiology	84
II. Statistics	88
III. Design of Surveillance Systems	100
IV. Collection and Compilation of Surveillance Data	104
V. Interpretation of Surveillance Data	105
VI. Outbreak Investigation	107
VII. CDC Definitions of Healthcare-Associated Infections	110
Practice Questions for Chapter Two	132
References	161

CBIC CONTENT OUTLINE

Surveillance and Epidemiological Investigation (38 Questions)

A. Design of Surveillance Systems

1. Develop a surveillance plan based on the population served, services provided and regulatory or other requirements
2. Evaluate periodically the effectiveness of the surveillance plan and modify as necessary
3. Identify appropriate critical/significant laboratory results and implement a notification system
4. Determine data needed to calculate specific rates
5. Integrate surveillance activities within healthcare settings (e.g., ambulatory, home health, long-term care, acute care)
6. Establish mechanisms for identifying those with communicable diseases requiring follow-up and/or isolation

B. Collection and Compilation of Surveillance Data

1. Use standardized definitions for the identification of outcomes and processes
2. Use a systematic approach to record surveillance data
3. Determine numerators, denominators and constants for calculations of rates for outcomes and processes
4. Organize and manage data in preparation for analysis
5. Determine the incidence or prevalence of infections
6. Calculate specific infection rates (e.g., provider-specific, unit-specific, device-specific, procedure-specific)
7. Calculate risk stratified rates
8. Incorporate post-discharge surveillance findings into calculation of rates

C. Interpretation of Surveillance Data

1. Generate, analyze and validate surveillance data
2. Use basic statistical techniques to describe data (e.g., mean, standard deviation, rates, ratios, proportions)
3. Recognize statistical significance of surveillance data
4. Monitor and interpret antibiotic resistance patterns
5. Recognize the need for an epidemiological study to investigate a problem (e.g., case control, cohort studies)

6. Compare surveillance results to published data or other benchmarks
7. Prepare and report findings of surveillance or epidemiological investigation to customers, using analyzed data, tables, graphs or charts, as appropriate
8. Develop and implement corrective action plans based on surveillance findings

D. Outbreak Investigation
1. Verify existence of outbreak
2. Collaborate with appropriate persons to establish the case definition, period of investigation and case-finding methods
2. Define the problem using time, place, person and risk factors
3. Formulate hypothesis on source and mode of transmission
5. Implement and evaluate control measures, including ongoing surveillance
6. Prepare and disseminate reports

Chapter Two: Surveillance and Epidemiological Investigation

I. Epidemiology

A. Definition

1. Study of the distribution and determinants of health conditions or events in a specified population and the application of this study to the control of health problems
2. Purpose is to aid in understanding the cause of disease by knowing distribution, natural history and determinants in terms of person, place and time
3. It is both a body of knowledge and a method of study

B. Epidemiological Triangle

Model of disease including host, agent and environment

Figure 2-1.   Epidemiological triangle model of disease causation

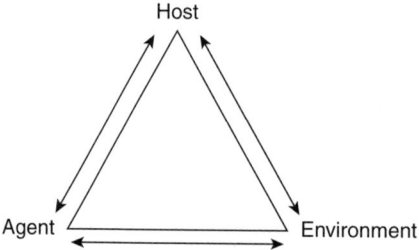

(Source: *APIC Text of Infection Control and Epidemiology*, 2009; 2–1.)

C. Association and Causation

1. Association—as one variable changes, there is a concomitant or resultant change in the quantity or quality of another variable
2. Artifactual association—a false association that can be due to chance or bias in study method
3. Indirect association—mixing of effects among exposure, disease and a third factor (e.g., confounding variable) that is associated with the exposure and independently affects the outcome
4. Causal association—when evidence indicates that one factor is clearly shown to increase the probability of the occurrence of a disease; reduction of this factor decreases the frequency of disease

a. Causality—these criteria for causality use epidemiology to determine whether a factor is causal for a given disease
    (1) Strength of association—the incidence of disease should be higher in those who are exposed to the factor under consideration
    (2) Consistency—the association should be observed in numerous studies
    (3) Specificity—refers to an association between one factor and one disease
    (4) Temporality—exposure to the causal factor must precede onset of disease
    (5) Biological gradient—dose-response relationship between increased exposure to the factor and increased likelihood of disease
    (6) Biological plausibility—should be plausible in light of current knowledge
    (7) Coherence—the association should be in accordance with other factors known about the history of the disease
    (8) Experiment—associations derived from experiments
    (9) Analogy—if similar associations have been shown to be causal, by analogy the association is more likely to be causal
b. Statistics do not prove causality; they can merely suggest that an association exists
c. Useful Terms
    (1) Incidence—number of new cases of disease in a given time period
    (2) Prevalence—number of cases, events or conditions occurring in a population
    (3) Endemic—usual presence of a disease or condition in a specific population or geographic area
    (4) Epidemic—the occurrence of more cases of a disease than expected in a given area or among a specific group of persons during a specific time period; synonym of an outbreak
    (5) Outbreak—synonymous with epidemic
    (6) Pandemic—an epidemic spread over a wide geographic area, across countries or continents
    (7) Reservoir—place where an infectious agent can survive, but may not multiply
    (8) Fomite—inanimate object on which organisms may exist for some period of time
    (9) Herd immunity—resistance of a group to invasion and spread of an infection (based on the immunity of a high proportion of members of the group)
    (10) Risk—probability or likelihood of an event occurring
    (11) Risk factor—a characteristic, behavior or experience that increases the likelihood of developing a negative health status

D. **Epidemiological Study Design**
   1. Useful terms
      a. Quantitative research—research based on traditional scientific methods, which generates numerical data and usually seeks to establish causal relationships between two or more variables, using statistical methods to test the strength and significance of the relationships.
      b. Qualitative research—research that seeks to provide understanding of human experience, perceptions, motivations, intentions, and behaviors based on description and observation and utilizing a naturalistic interpretative approach to a subject and its contextual setting.[1]
   2. Two main types of epidemiological studies (quantitative research)
      a. Observational studies—investigator does not intervene or control exposures or risk factors for study subjects
         (1) Descriptive studies—characterize a population by occurrence of an outcome by time, place or person; includes case reports and case series (e.g., describes series of patients with a disorder including characteristics and outcomes)
         (2) Analytic studies—compare individuals with and without an outcome with the presence of one or more risk factors
            (a) Cross-sectional study (prevalence, correlation or survey study)—outcome and risk factors reviewed in a population group at one point in time; outcomes measured (incidence rates cannot be determined)
            (b) Case-control study (case referent, case comparison, or retrospective study)—population of individuals with and without an outcome of interest studied for exposure to one or more risk factors; studies are quicker, less expensive and easier
            (c) Cohort study (prospective or longitudinal study)—start with sample of individuals with and without exposure to a potential risk factor who are followed for incidence of the outcome in each group; can be done retrospectively; less patient selection bias; stronger evidence of causal association
      b. Experimental studies
         Investigator controls certain factors or treatments that may influence disease process or study outcome
         (1) Clinical trials—investigator assigns interventions to one or more experimental (treated) groups and to a control (untreated) group; usually random assignment to the group to prevent selection bias; groups are compared for the outcome of interest; may be double-blinded (neither investigator nor participants knows who is assigned to which group); considered the gold standard for study design to determine causal relationships; drawback is

expense and difficulty of studies; random assignment may not guarantee that groups will be similar in characteristics
    (2) Community trials—similar to clinical trials but intervention is applied on a community-wide instead of individual basis; not as desirable as clinical trials; difficult to establish intervention was implemented to each individual; large and expensive

3. Qualitative research
Exploratory, descriptive and/or used for theory verification; persons are studied as a whole, not independent of their environment, rather than as a part of an experience; typically contain detailed, in-depth descriptions of people, events and situations
  a. Purposes
    (1) Gain detailed information about a topic
    (2) Develop understanding of a person's perception of a phenomenon
    (3) Capture the human experience associated with an event
    (4) Identify the influence of cultural roles and norms for behavior
    (5) Identify the variables and relationships of variables
    (6) Develop theories/hypotheses that can be used for future research
    (7) Develop theories/hypotheses that describe the phenomenon being studied
    (8) Obtain additional information about a phenomenon when what is known about it is biased, inconsistent or outmoded
    (9) Confirm what is theorized
  b. Types of qualitative research
    (1) Phenomenology—study of a phenomenon
    (2) Grounded theory—data studied, coded, compared until themes emerge; relationships between themes used to develop hypotheses and theory
    (3) Ethnography—studies a person's environment and culture
    (4) Hermeneutics
    (5) Heuristics
    (6) Symbolic interactionism
    (7) Chaos theory
  c. Data-gathering techniques
    (1) Focus groups
    (2) Participant observation
    (3) Interviews
    (4) Field notes
    (5) Tape recording/transcription
  d. Analysis—data studied by these methods to reduce researcher biases:
    (1) Notations in margins
    (2) Brackets of feelings, biases, beliefs
    (3) Classify data in themes and describe relationships

(4) Look for patterns and structure
(5) Verify findings by experts or participants

II. Statistics

A. Definition

1. A tool to aid in organizing and summarizing data, communicate findings clearly and meaningfully and make inferences about data

B. Role of Statistics in Hospital Epidemiology

1. To analyze data and prepare reports for healthcare facility
   a. Calculation of infection rates
   b. Frequency distributions displayed as tables, graphs or charts
   c. Numeric summaries that describe characteristics of the population being studied
2. To obtain knowledge about hospital epidemiology for the healthcare facility
3. To investigate clusters of infections and describe the outbreak
4. To perform research studies within your own facility

C. Descriptive Statistics—Provide Numerical Information about Variables

1. Scales of measurement
   a. Nominal scale—simplest level of measurement; use of categories to classify observations into mutually exclusive groups or classes; no ordering among the classifications
   b. Ordinal scale—observations are ranked so that each category is distinct; definite relationship to each other category
   c. Interval scale—ordinal data with the exact difference between any two observations on the scale is knows (if the 0 point is arbitrary, called absolute interval data)
   e. Equal-interval scales—distance between adjacent scores are equal and consistent
   f. Ratio scale data—measurements that have a true zero point, such as distance
2. Rate—an expression of the frequency with which an event occurs in a defined population per unit of time
   a. Rules:
      (1) Persons in the denominator must reflect the same population as in the numerator
      (2) Counts in the numerator and denominator should cover the same time period
      (3) Persons in the denominator should have been at risk for the event
   b. Incidence rate—a measure of the frequency with which an event occurs in a population over a defined time period; the numerator is the number of new cases

occurring during the defined time period and the denominator is the population at risk; formula = (number of new cases ÷ population at risk) × constant
  (1) Attack rate—type of incidence rate used to measure the frequency of new cases of a disease or condition in a specific population during a given time period; formula = (number of new cases ÷ population at risk) × 100
  (2) Incidence density—type of incidence rate that incorporates time into the denominator; formula = (number of new cases ÷ exposure time [e.g., device days]) × constant
 c. Prevalence rate—proportion of persons in a population with a particular disease at a specific point in time or period of time; related to the duration of disease; the numerator is the number of existing cases of disease, regardless of date of onset; denominator is the population at risk; formula = (number of existing cases ÷ population at risk) × 100
 d. Mortality rate—measure of the frequency of death in a defined population during a specified time; formula = (number of deaths ÷ population at risk) × 100
  (1) Crude mortality refers to all causes of death, cause-specific mortality is the rate of mortality from a certain cause
 e. Stratification and standardization—stratification is the grouping together of patients at similar risk for an event (e.g., acquiring a surgical site infection [SSI]). The standardization method used most often in healthcare-associated infection (HAI) surveillance is indirect standardization, which is a means of risk adjustment in which the raw rate of an event is divided by the average risk for the occurrence of the event
3. Measures of association
 a. Definition—quantify the magnitude of the effect of risk factors on disease risk; requires data to be put into 2×2 table format, based on disease and risk factor presence/absence

Table 2-1. Notation for a 2 x 2 Table

	Disease	No Disease	Total
Factor present	a	b	a + b
Factor absent	c	d	c + d
Totals	a + c	b + d	n

(Source: *APIC Text of Infection Control and Epidemiology*, 2005).

b. Relative ratio (risk ratio)—probability of developing a disease if the risk factor is present, divided by the probability of developing disease if the risk factor is not present; formula = (a ÷ [a + b]) ÷ (c ÷ [c + d])
c. Odds ratio—closely related to relative risk; probability of having a particular risk factor if a disease is present, divided by the probability of having the risk factor if disease is not present; formula = (a × d) ÷ (c × b)

4. Testing for reliability
   a. Definition—whether what is intended to be measured is, in fact, measured; often used to describe diagnostic tests; set up the 2×2 table as shown earlier, with "test" (diagnostic or otherwise) in place of the risk factor
   b. Sensitivity—percentage of persons with true positive results when a test is applied to persons known to have a disease; formula = a ÷ (a + c) × 100
   c. Specificity—percentage of persons with true negative results when the test is applied to persons without the disease; formula = d ÷ (b + d) × 100
      (1) Relationship between sensitivity and specificity usually inversely related
   d. Positive predictive value—percentage of tests that are positive when the disease is present; formula = a ÷ (a + b) × 100
   e. Negative predictive value—percentage of tests that are negative when the disease is not present; formula = d ÷ (c + d) × 100

5. Bivariate relationships
   a. Correlation—used to calculate the direction and magnitude of a relationship between two variables; values range between +1 and −1; the closer r is to ±1, the stronger is the relationship
   b. Regression—assesses the influence of one or more variables on another
   c. Confound variables—can suggest a false relationship between variables or can hide a relationship that exists; requires multivariate analysis (powerful statistical method that can describe simultaneously the effect of exposure and effect of other factors that may be confounding or modifying the effect of the exposure)

6. Measures of central tendency—describe the center of a distribution of data
   a. Mean—mathematical average of the values in a set of data; inaccurate if there are outliers in the data set
   b. Median—value or point in a series that divides the ranked values into two equal groups; good measure for ordinal data or for numeric data when the distribution is skewed
   c. Mode—value in a set of data that occurs most frequently; most useful for describing qualitative data; used for nominal data and bimodal distributions

7. Measures of dispersion (variability)
   a. Range—difference between the smallest and largest values in a sample
   b. Deviation—actual distance between an individual measurement in a data set and the mean value for the set
   c. Standard deviation—reflects the variability in values around the mean; mathematically it is obtained by taking all the deviations from the mean, squaring them, and then dividing their sum by the total number of observations minus one and, finally, taking the square root of this number
   d. Variance—the square of the standard deviation of the measurements; useful indicator of variability, but standard deviation is more commonly used
   e. Standard error of the mean—standard deviation adjusted for by the sample size
8. Frequency distribution
   a. Normal distribution—when the values on both sides of the mean are even (bell-shaped)

Figure 2–2. A normal distribution showing the percentage of values found in various ranges about the mean

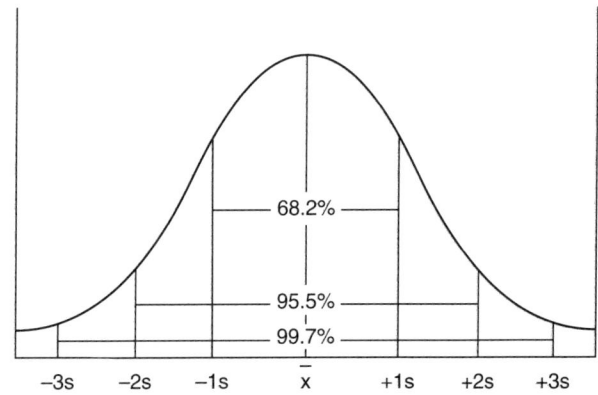

(Source: *APIC Text of Infection Control and Epidemiology*, 2002; 19–4.)

   b. Skewness—asymmetrical distribution

Figure 2–3. Negative skew (left) and positive skew (right)

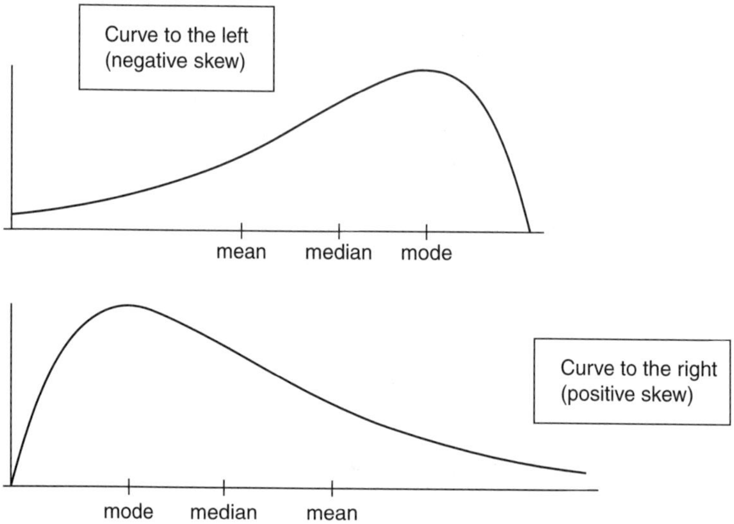

Curve to the left (negative skew)

mean   median   mode

Curve to the right (positive skew)

mode   median   mean

(Source: *APIC Text of Infection Control and Epidemiology*, 2009: 5–7.)

    c. Kurtosis—how flat or peaked a curve is

Figure 2–4. General forms of kurtosis

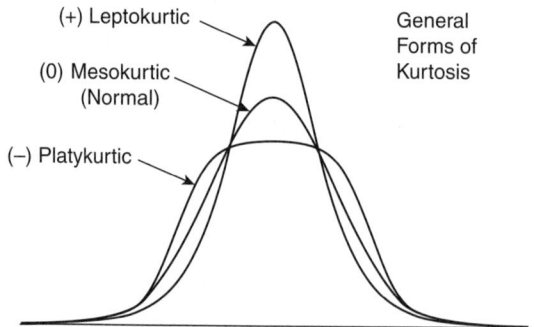

(+) Leptokurtic
(0) Mesokurtic (Normal)
(−) Platykurtic

General Forms of Kurtosis

(Source: *APIC Text of Infection Control and Epidemiology*, 2009: 5–8.)

D. **Inferential Statistics—Make an Assumption about a Population Based on a Sample of That Population**
   1. Terms
      a. Population—the total number of persons in a specified place or group
      b. Sample—group of observations selected from the population to represent the whole
   2. Hypothesis testing—estimates the likelihood (probability) that a result did not occur by chance
      a. Alternate hypothesis—states the expectation to be tested
      b. Null hypothesis—classically written as Ho; opposite of the alternate hypothesis; it is stated to be rejected; hypothesis testing will either accept or reject the null hypothesis; statement can be rejected
      c. Directionality of hypothesis
         (1) One-tailed tests—direction is specified in advance (SSI rate for doctor A is higher than doctor B)
         (2) Two-tailed tests—direction is not specific, difference in either direction is possible (SSI rates of doctor A and doctor B are different)
      d. Type I (a) error—the probability of rejecting a true null hypothesis; indicates the significance level, or p value, usually set at 0.05
      e. Type II (b) error—the probability of not rejecting a false null hypothesis; heavily influenced by sample size
         (1) Control—keeping the alpha level very small will decrease the risk for committing a type I error; no control over type II error except determination of sample size
         (2) Type I and II errors are inversely related; decreasing the risk for committing a type I error increases the risk of committing a type II error; impossible to control both simultaneously
   1. Types of inferential statistics
      a. Parametric—assume normal distribution, continuous-interval scale
         (1) z test to examine two means (sample size >30)
         (2) t test to examine two means (sample size <30)
         (3) Mann-Whitney U test when <5 in any box of a 2×2 table
      b. Nonparametric—no assumption of distribution, discrete, nominal, ordinal and interval data
         (1) Chi-square to measure observed versus expected frequency in two different groups (Fisher's exact test used when <5 in any cell of a 2×2 table)
   2. Test statistic—numeric measure, computed from a set of sample measurements, which quantifies the magnitude of discrepancy between the hypothesized population

parameter and the statistic computed from the sample; can be converted to a probability value using special tables
3. P value—the probability, given that the null hypothesis is true, of collecting a random sample of the same size from the same population that yields a test statistic at least as extreme as the one calculated from the sample; if the p value is below the alpha, you can conclude that the null hypothesis of your test is probably not true; if the p value is greater than the alpha, you do not have sufficient evidence to reject the null hypothesis
   a. Level of significance (alpha)—probability value arbitrarily chosen by the researcher as the desired level of probability at which one may feel secure in rejecting the null hypothesis; most researchers use 0.05 (5%) or 0.01 (1%) values for alpha in order to minimize the chances of incorrectly rejecting the null hypothesis; 0.05 is a 1 in 20 chance that the given observation could occur by chance variation alone
4. Rejection region—of a test of hypothesis, specifies which values of the test statistic are sufficiently large to warrant rejection of the null hypothesis
5. Confidence interval (CI)—a CI is the estimated range of values that is likely to include an unknown population parameter, the estimated range being calculated from a given set of sample data. The CI is usually calculated to be 95% but can be 90%, 99% or 99.99%

E. Data Presentation
1. Methods
   a. Tables—set of data that is arranged in rows and columns
      (1) Show frequency with which event occurs
      (2) Present information in different categories/subdivisions of a variable or factor
   b. Graphs—method of showing quantitative data using a system of coordinates
      (1) Consist of two sets of lines that intersect at right angles to each other
      (2) Each axis (line) has a scale of measurement and a label
      (3) Horizontal (X) axis (or abscissa) often reflects the time intervals
      (4) Vertical (Y) axis (or ordinate) usually reflects the frequency of occurrence of the event
      (5) When more than one factor (or variable) is shown on a graph, each should be clearly labeled by legend or key
      (6) Types of line graphs—arithmetic scale line graph (equal distances along the Y-axis represent equal quantities anywhere on that axis), semi-logarithmic scale line graph (Y-axis is measured in logarithms of units), histogram (graph of a frequency distribution; uses bars), frequency polygon (uses lines and points instead of bars; can show two sets of data on one graph)

Figure 2–5. Elements of a well-constructed table

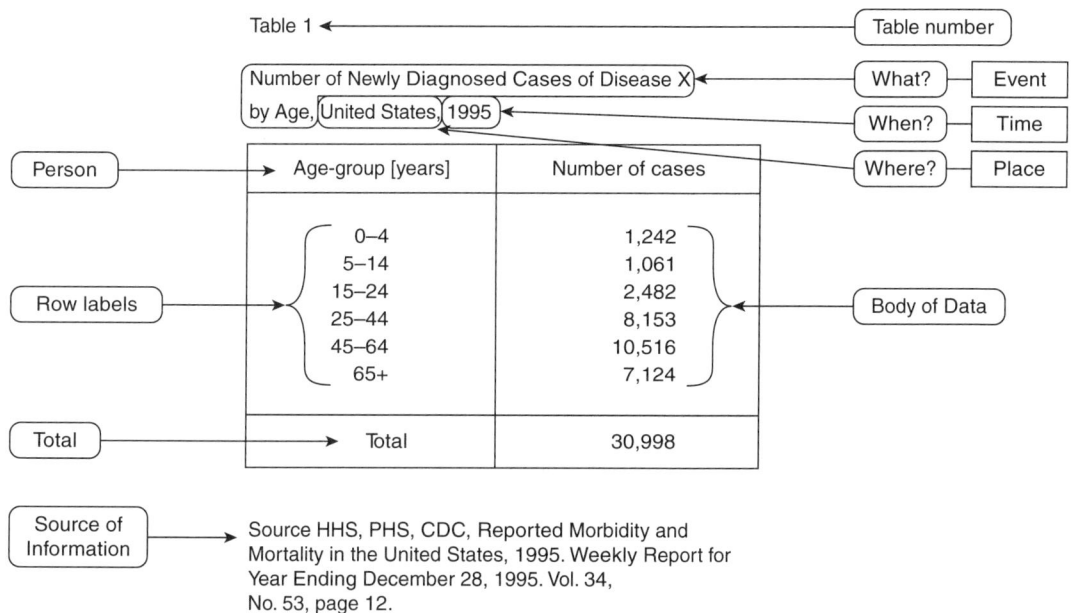

Figure 2–6. Elements of a well-constructed graph

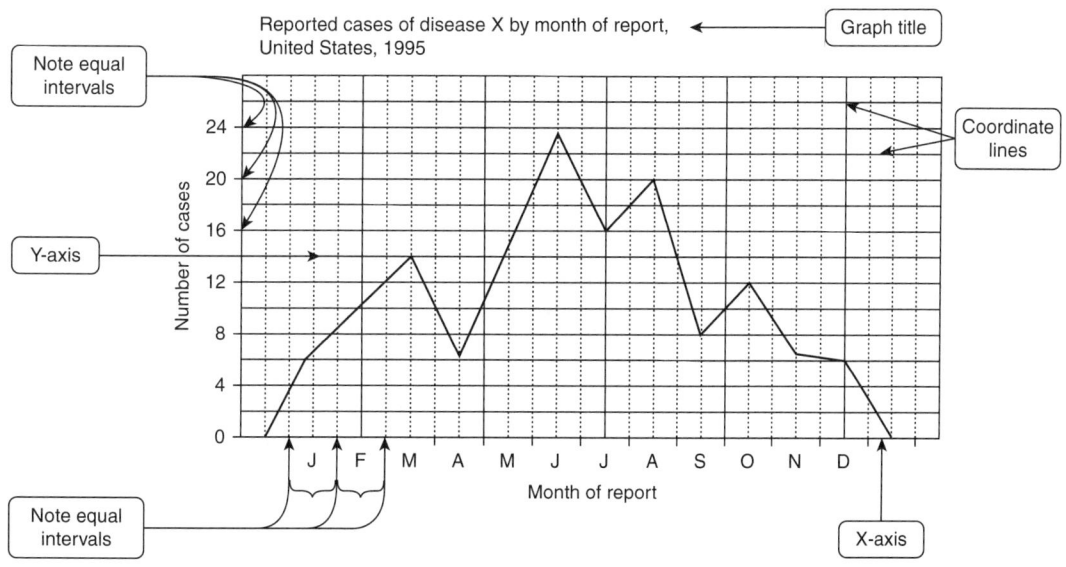

Figure 2-7. Elements of a properly constructed histogram

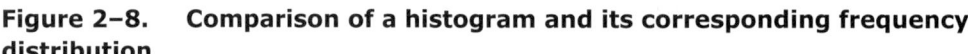

Figure 2-8. Comparison of a histogram and its corresponding frequency distribution

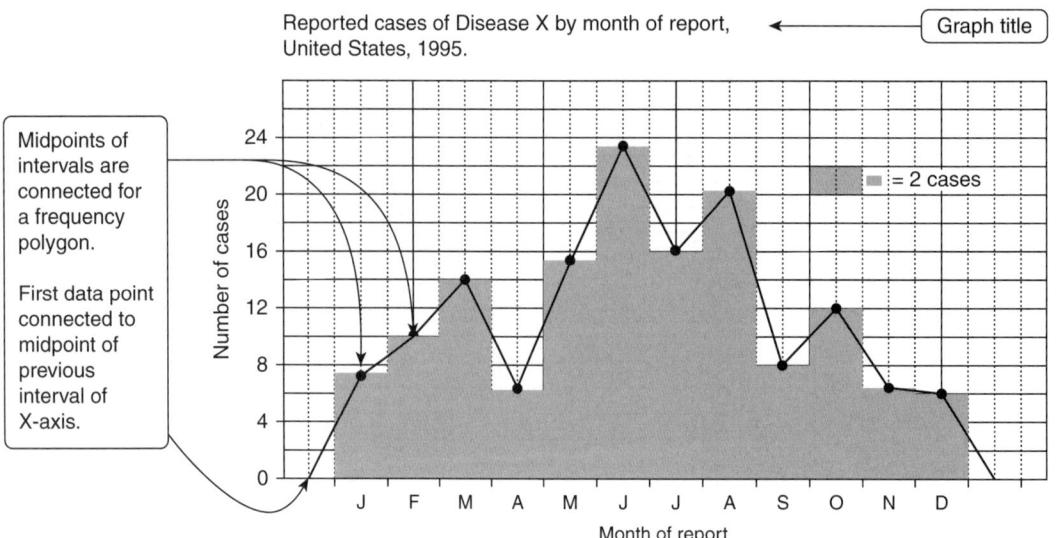

Figure 2-9. Components of a well-constructed bar chart. A comparison of the percent distribution of the age of the population in a sample survey and the census population of Jonesville, June 1995.

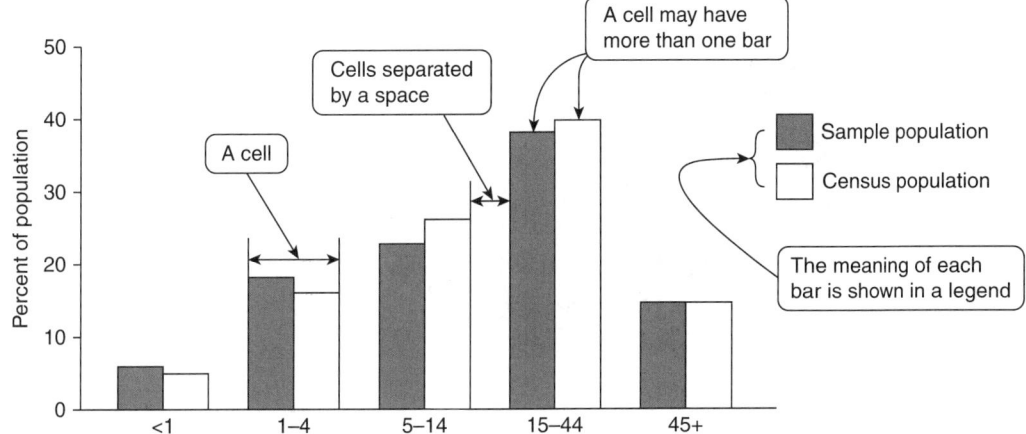

(Source for Figures 2-5 through 2-9: *APIC Text of Infection Control and Epidemiology 2002 and 2005* eds, 2-12 through 2-14.)

    c. Charts—method of illustrating information using only one coordinate
       (1) Bar chart—uses bars to depict event being studied
       (2) Geographic coordinate chart—represents occurrence of events using maps
          (a) Spot map—uses dots or symbols at location where event took place
          (b) Area map—uses shaded or coded areas to show distributions of some condition
       (3) Pictogram—variation of bar chart that uses a series of small identifying symbols to represent the data
       (4) Pie chart—based on proportion that uses wedge-shaped portions of a circle for comparison; each wedge is a percentage of the whole

Figure 2–10. Example of a pie chart

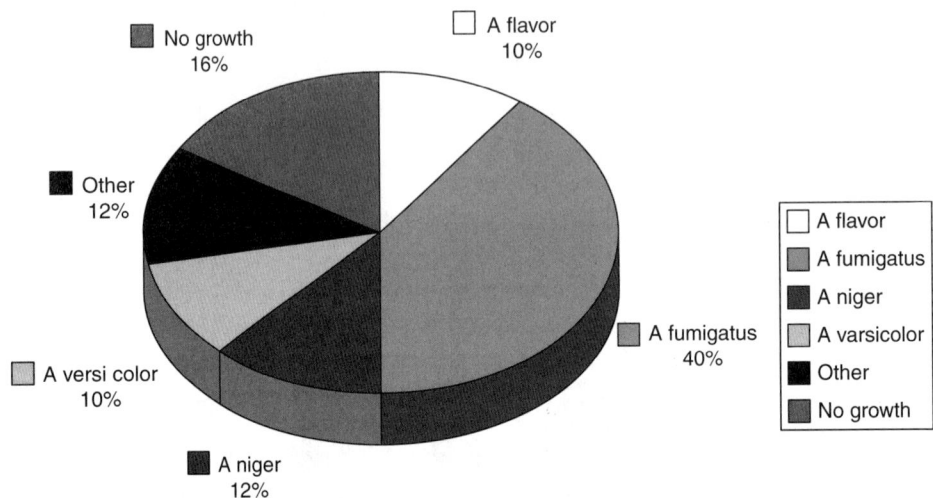

(Source: *APIC Text of Infection Control and Epidemiology*, 2009; 5–10.)

F. Statistical Process Control (SPC)

1. Definition—purpose is to ensure that each process is performed consistently and correctly within predetermined parameters; focuses on process and is based on the principle of random variation
2. SPC used in infection control programs to monitor outcomes (rates of healthcare-associated infection [HAI]) or to monitor the process of care, facilitating the determination of common cause (expected) variation versus special cause (something that creates instability, therefore unpredictability) variation
3. Tools of SPC—control charts; types of data and frequency of events determine type of control chart
    a. Two types of data—continuous and discrete
    b. Events that occur frequently usually follow a normal distribution; those that occur infrequently may not (e.g., Poisson distribution)
    c. Type of data, frequency of the event being monitored and stability of the denominator (sample) are used to determine which type of control chart is applicable to the situation being studied
4. Types of statistical process control charts
    a. The "X-R" chart (mean, range) is used to monitor continuous data
    b. The "p" chart is used to monitor discrete data such as defects

c. The "np" chart is used to monitor the number of defects within a constant sample size
d. The "c" and "u" charts are used when the sample and events being monitored fit the Poisson distribution; used if the event of interest occurs infrequently but the sample size (denominator) is large; the "c" chart is used when the sample is relatively constant and the "u" is used when the sample size is variable over time

5. Steps in constructing a control chart
   a. Collect the data; key aspects must be defined for measurement; data may be collected retrospectively or prospectively
   b. After a sufficient sample is available, calculate the mean
   c. Calculate the standard deviation
   d. Set up the control chart, indicating the mean and control limits; customarily, 3 standard deviations above and below the mean are applied as the upper control limit (UCL) and the lower control limit (LCL)
   e. Determine the scale for the Y-axis to most effectively display the data; label the Y-axis; the X-axis usually represents units of time or subgroups of the sample; the X-axis scale should also be determined and labeled
   f. Draw a horizontal line at the mean value, the UCL, and the LCL
   g. Interpret the data as they are entered onto the control chart to determine whether the process is "in control" or "out of control"

Figure 2–11. Emergency department needle sticks baseline data: 1994, p chart.

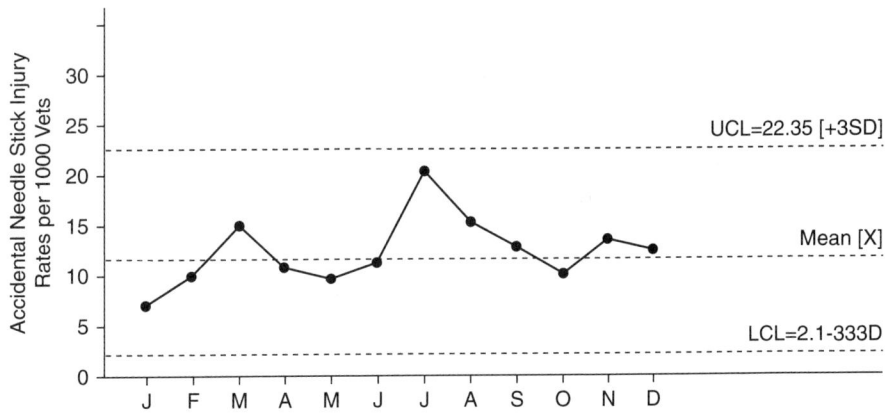

(Source: *APIC Text of Infection Control and Epidemiology*, 2002; 21–2.)

6. Interpretation of control chart data
   a. Data points are examined to see if they are within the UCL and LCL; trends in data are also considered
   b. Process is "out of control"
      (1) One data point above the UCL or below the LCL–
      (2) Two of 3 consecutive points are –2 SDs but –3 SDs on one side of the mean
      (3) Four of 5 consecutive points are –SD but –2 SDs on one side of the mean
      (4) Nine consecutive points on one side of the mean
      (5) Six consecutive points increasing or decreasing
      (6) 14 consecutive points alternating up or down
      (7) 15 consecutive points within 1 SD above or below the mean
   c. Threshold of 3 SDs may not be sensitive in clinical situations; may select 2 SDs, but experts in SPC consider this as "tampering" and over-control of the system

III. Design of Surveillance Systems

A. Surveillance

1. An essential component of an effective infection prevention and control program. It can be defined as a systematic methods of collecting, consolidating and analyzing data concerning the distribution and determinants of a given disease or event, followed by the dissemination of that information to those who can improve the outcomes.[2,3]
2. Use of surveillance
   a. Determine baseline and endemic rates of occurrence of a disease or event
   b. Detect and investigate clusters or outbreaks
   c. Assess the effectiveness of prevention and control measures
   d. Monitor the occurrence of adverse outcomes to identify potential risk factors
   e. Provide information that can be used to target performance improvement activities
   f. Observe practices such as hand hygiene to promote compliance with recommendations and standards
   g. Detect and report notifiable diseases
   h. Identify organisms and disease of epidemiological importance to prevent their spread
   i. Establish mechanisms for identifying those with communicable diseases requiring follow-up and/or isolation
   j. Identify critical/significant laboratory results and implement a notification system
   k. Ensure compliance with federal regulators (such as the Occupational Safety and Health Administration), state regulations (such as infectious waste laws) and mandatory reporting requirements

CHAPTER TWO: SURVEILLANCE AND EPIDEMIOLOGICAL INVESTIGATION | 101

   l. Meet requirements of accrediting agencies such as the Joint Commission
   m. Provide information for the education of healthcare personnel
   n. Detect a bioterrorist event or an emerging infectious disease
   o. Provide data to conduct a facility risk assessment for diseases such as tuberculosis
3. Surveillance programs in healthcare facilities should be integrated to include infection prevention, performance improvement, patient safety, and public health activities.

B. Surveillance Program Design[4-10]

1. Should be designed in accordance with current recommended practices and consist of defined elements
2. Should be based on the population served, services provided, and regulatory or other requirements
3. Approaches to surveillance
   a. Total (or whole) house surveillance—all HAIs are monitored in the entire population of the facility; rates should be calculated for specific HAIs in defined populations such as central line–associated bloodstream infections in an intensive care unit (ICU); overall infection rates should not be calculated
   b. Targeted surveillance—focuses on particular care units, infections related to medical devices, invasive procedures and organisms of epidemiological significance; programs usually focus on high-risk, high-volume procedures and on potentially preventable HAIs and adverse outcomes
   c. Combination surveillance strategy—many infection prevention programs use a combination of targeted and modified total house surveillance; many programs monitor targeted events that occur in a defined population while concurrently monitoring selected HAIs and laboratory reports from house-wide locations
4. Elements of an effective surveillance plan
   a. Select the surveillance methodology—program may measure all infections (e.g., total surveillance) or may be focused (targeted) on events selected by an organization
   b. Assess and define the study population—identify which populations have the greatest risk for infection or other adverse outcome
   c. Choose the indicators (events) to monitor: programs should measure outcomes of healthcare, processes of healthcare, and selected events of importance to the organization; it is common to choose indicators that monitor high-volume, high-risk events in a specific population, especially if the information obtained can be used to guide performance improvement activities; surveillance program should monitor a variety of outcomes (e.g., HAIs such as bloodstream, urinary tract, pneumonia, surgical site; infection or colonization with a specific organism; decubitus ulcers; patient falls; sharps injuries and blood/body fluid exposures in

healthcare providers), processes (e.g., medication errors, influenza vaccination rates; personnel compliance with infection prevention protocols such as hand hygiene, environmental cleaning), and events (e.g., occurrence of reportable disease and conditions, communicable diseases in personnel, biological monitoring of sterilizers); some indicators should focus on personnel; an effort should be made to select some indicators that have validated, nationally available benchmark data that can be used for meaningful comparison, such as the National Healthcare Safety Network (NHSN).

d. Determine time period for observation—surveillance data for each indicator should be collected consistently and for defined periods, such as a month, quarter or year

e. Identify surveillance criteria—surveillance criteria (e.g., case definitions) must be used consistently to determine the presence of an HAI, occurrence of an event or compliance with a process

f. Identify data elements to be collected; limit data collection to those elements that are needed to identify a case and determine whether the case criteria are met for the condition or event being studied

g. Determine methods for data analysis—before data collection is initiated, the statistical measures that will be used to analyze the data must be determined so the appropriate data can be collected; if rates or ratios will be calculated, the values corresponding to each numerator and denominator must be defined and the appropriate data needed to calculate each rate or ratio must be collected; whenever possible, data should be expressed as rates or ratios that are calculated using the same methodology as a nationally validated surveillance system (such as NHSN).

h. Determine methods for data collection and management—data may be collected concurrently (while a person is still under the care of the organization) or retrospectively (closed-record review after discharge); data sources include:
(1) Medical records
(2) Daily reports generated by the laboratory
(3) Admission lists
(4) Monthly reports of census data and patient-days
(5) Nursing care plan
(6) Isolation lists
(7) Interviews with caregivers
(8) List of prescribed medications from the pharmacy
(9) Radiology reports
(10) Incident reports
(11) Employee health reports
(12) Procedure and activity logs

(13) Reports from others who review medical records (such as performance improvement personnel)
5. Design an interpretive surveillance report—a written report provides a mechanism to interpret and disseminate surveillance data to stimulate performance improvement activities
   (1) Tables, graphs and charts are effective tools for organizing, summarizing and displaying data and should be used as applicable
   (2) A surveillance report should:
       (a) Define the event, population, setting and time period studied
       (b) State the criteria used for defining a case
       (c) Specify the number of cases or events identified and the number in the population studied
       (d) Explain the methodology used to identify cases
       (e) Identify the statistical methods and calculations used, when appropriate
       (f) State the purpose for conducting surveillance
       (g) Interpret the findings in a manner that is understandable to those who read the report
       (h) Describe any actions taken and recommendations made for prevention and control measures
       (i) Identify the author and date of the report
       (j) Identify the recipients of the report
6. Identify recipients of the surveillance report
   (a) The report should be disseminated to those managers and healthcare providers who can use the findings to influence performance improvement activities.
7. Develop a written surveillance plan
   (a) Surveillance plan should include: type of facility, services provided and populations served; the purpose of the surveillance program, goals and objectives; the indicators and criteria used; the reason for selecting each indicator (outcome, process and other event); the methodology used for case identification, data collection and analysis; the types of reports generated and to who they are provided; and the process used to evaluate the surveillance program
8. Establish mechanisms for identifying those with communicable diseases requiring follow-up or isolation
9. Evaluate surveillance program
   (a) Evaluate program periodically to assess its usefulness and ability to meet the organization's objectives
   (b) Revisions should be made as needed
   (c) The program structure and activities should be compared with current practices and published recommendations for surveillance programs in similar settings
   (d) Regulatory and accrediting agency requirements should be incorporated

(e) The resources needed to manage the program (such as personnel, technology, provision of ongoing training, office supplies, reference materials and related services) should be assessed and allocations made as needed
10. Integrate surveillance activities within healthcare settings
   (a) The majority of the current literature has focused on the acute care hospital; however, information has been published for surveillance in out-of-hospital settings
   (b) Infection prevention and control programs are now required by accrediting and regulatory agencies in a variety of healthcare settings including hospitals, long-term care, rehabilitation, ambulatory surgery, dialysis, home care, mental health and corrections facilities

IV. Collection and Compilation of Surveillance Data

A. Use Standard Definitions for the Identification of Outcomes and Processes

1. Criteria used should reflect generally accepted definitions of the disease or event being monitored; criteria have been published for defining HAIs in hospitals, long-term care and home care settings[11-13]
2. Use a systematic approach to record surveillance data
   a. Data collection forms should be standardized to eliminate duplicate efforts and prevent misinterpretation by the data collector(s). The form should be designed so that the data elements (e.g., yes/no, procedures, treatments, and risk factors) can be circled, checked, or otherwise selected. Limit narrative entries.
   b. Data should be entered into a computer spreadsheet or database so that they can be sorted and analyzed; ideally, data should be entered directly into a laptop computer or personal digital assistant (PDA) when collected
3. Determine numerators, denominators and constants for calculations of rates of outcomes and processes
4. Organize and manage data in preparation for analysis
   (a) IPs collect and manage large amounts of data; effective use of the data is the fundamental element of a successful program
   (b) Once collected, data must be put in an accessible and stable database to be useful
   (c) Information technology provides a means by which data can be collected, stored, analyzed and reported.
5. Determine the incidence or prevalence of infections
   (a) Calculate specific infection rates (e.g., provider-specific, unit-specific, device-specific, procedure specific)
   (b) Calculate risk-stratified rates to adjust for differences in patients' risks, to account for small numbers of operations performed or to control for differences in the distributions of operations in the comparison and standard population

6. Facilities should implement postdischarge surveillance of HAIs, especially SSIs; these data should be incorporated into calculation of rates

V. Interpretation of Surveillance Data

A. Generate, Analyze and Validate Surveillance Data

1. Data should be collected, managed, analyzed and reported using computers and computerized technology
    a. Specialized infection prevention software is available commercially, although basic software packages that contain word processing, spreadsheet, graphics and database program may be used as well
2. Use basic statistical techniques to describe data (e.g., mean, standard deviation, rates, ratios, proportions)
3. Recognize statistical significance of surveillance data
    a. If the p value is small, the null hypothesis of the test is probably not true and there is sufficient evidence to support that sampling variation or chance is an unlikely explanation for the result; this does not prove that the null hypothesis is true; if the p value is large, there is not sufficient evidence to reject the null hypothesis
4. Monitor and interpret antibiotic resistance patterns
    a. Surveillance of antimicrobial resistance is an essential first step in identifying priority areas for managing antimicrobial use
5. Recognize the need for an epidemiological study to investigate a problem (e.g., case-control, cohort studies)
    a. The choice of study design depends on the available samples (e.g., frequencies of the exposures and outcomes), the populations available for study and the hypothesis or study question being addressed
    b. Each study design has strengths and weaknesses and should be carefully matched to the type of data collected and the desired information
6. Compare surveillance results to published data or other benchmarks
    a. Benchmarking is the process of comparing oneself to others performing similar activities, so as to continuously improve[14]
    b. The following conditions should first be met:
        (1) Criteria for defining a case are standardized and up-to-date
        (2) Criteria are used consistently by all participants and all data collectors
        (3) The population and time period for study are well defined
        (4) The surveillance methodology is standardized and consistently used by all participants over time
        (5) Rates and ratios are calculated using the same numerators (number of cases) and denominators (e.g., population at risk, device-days, patient-days)

(a) The size of the population studied (denominator) is large enough to provide an accurate estimate of the true rate
(b) A standardized risk adjustment method is used by all participants
(c) All data collectors receive training on how to collect data and use a standardized form
(d) The facility and population being compared are similar to the types and facilities and populations in an aggregate database used for external comparison (e.g., data from a neonatal ICU is compared with data from other neonatal ICUs)
(e) The aggregating organization has a mechanism for ensuring the accuracy, sensitivity and specificity of the data submitted
(f) The analysis and interpretation of the data provided by the benchmarking system are accurate and in a form that is understandable to users
(g) Feedback will be disseminated to those who can effect change
(h) The data provided by an organization to an external aggregating system are coded for confidentiality, and the reports provided to the organization or to others do not contain facility identifiers unless the data are being used for a public reporting program
7. Prepare and report findings of surveillance or epidemiological investigation to customers using analyzed data tables, graphs or charts, as appropriate. Feedback is an important intervention; report the data to appropriate committees, physicians and staff as needed to educate for changes needed and to fulfill standards and regulations

B. Other Applications for the Surveillance Process

1. Non–healthcare-associated infections
   a. Communicable diseases that are designated reportable to the public health department
   b. Community outbreaks of infectious disease
   c. Monitoring of important organisms, such as drug-resistant organisms
   d. Surveillance of employee infections with potential for transmission to patients or other staff
2. Noninfectious events
   a. Occupational health—needle/sharps injuries, TB skin test conversions (without TB disease), immunization rates
   b. Surgical case review—intraoperative injuries, unplanned returns to surgery, cesarean-section rates, indications for procedures
   c. Medication use evaluation—prescribing indications, drug selection, administration and medication errors, adverse drug reactions
   d. Miscellaneous noninfectious patient events—falls, decubiti

VI. Outbreak Investigation

A. Outbreak

Defined as an increase over the expected occurrence of an event; exception—one case of an unusual disease (e.g., botulism) may constitute an epidemic. The term "pseudo-outbreak" is generally applied to situations in which there is a rise in test results (e.g., positive microbiology cultures) without actual clinical disease.

B. Components of an Outbreak Investigation

1. Components of initial outbreak investigations
   a. Confirm presence of an outbreak—confirm that what is being reported indeed represents an increase in the outcome by reviewing records; if no records are available, confirmation may be based on general perception
   b. Alert key partners about the investigation—facility administration, risk management, public affairs, microbiology laboratory, health department officials; collaborate with appropriate persons to establish the case definition, period of investigation and case-finding methods
   c. Perform a literature review—help identify possible sources, provide insight into investigative methodology
   d. Establish an initial case definition—develop specific criteria for a definition of a case; should be narrow enough to focus investigation but broad enough to capture the majority of cases; careful consideration should be given to including microbiological results; problem should be defined using time, place, person and risk factors
   e. Develop a methodology for case finding—use laboratory records, IP records or discussions with healthcare personnel; consider the need to identify colonized cases as well
   f. Prepare an initial line list and epidemic curve—line list may include signs and symptoms, medication, procedures, consults, patient location, contact with healthcare personnel and host factors; line lists can be resource-intensive to create, so components should be considered carefully; epidemic curves are histograms of the infection dates that help identify the mode of transmission
   g. Observe and review potentially implicated patient care activities—use line list to identify where observations should take place; initial observations should be free-form (without detailed observation forms) to note any deviations from good IP practice; collaborate with healthcare personnel and look for practices that differ among personnel
   h. Consider whether environmental sampling should be performed—environmental cultures are potentially misleading and often negative; discuss with the

microbiology laboratory before obtaining samples, only culture those items that are possible vectors and make sense as a likely reservoir
  i. Implement initial control measures—during an outbreak it is important to implement a variety of IP measures to halt the adverse event; these measures may be chosen from the line list or observations
 2. Components of the follow-up investigation
    a. Refine the case definition—the definition may be narrowed or expanded to detect all cases that are associated with the outbreak
    b. Continue case finding and surveillance—should continue for some period of time after the outbreak is terminated to ensure it is truly over
    c. Regularly review control measures—regularly review compliance with control measures; those that are time-consuming or resource intensive should be assessed to determine if and when they can be loosened
    d. Considering whether an analytical study should be performed—most often case-control studies; often done to provide statistical support to the causes identified by the line list and observations
    e. Prepare and disseminate reports

C. The Epidemic Curve
 1. An epidemic curve is a graph in which the cases of a disease that occurred during an epidemic (outbreak) are plotted according to the time of onset of illness in the cases. The shape of the curve is determined by the epidemic pattern. The epidemic curve is used to:
    a. Determine whether the source of the infection was common, propagated (continuing) or both
    b. Identify the probable time of exposure of the cases to the source(s) of infection
    c. Identify the probable incubation period
    d. Determine if the problem is ongoing

Figure 2-12. Epidemic curves—common versus propagated source outbreak.
A. Propagated source: single exposure, no secondary cases (e.g., measles) B. Propagated source—secondary and tertiary cases (e.g., hepatitis A). C. Common source—point exposure (e.g., salmonellosis following a company picnic) D. Common source—intermittent exposure (e.g., bacteremia associated with contaminated blood product). (Source: APIC Text of Infection Control and Epidemiology, 2009; Figure 4-1.)

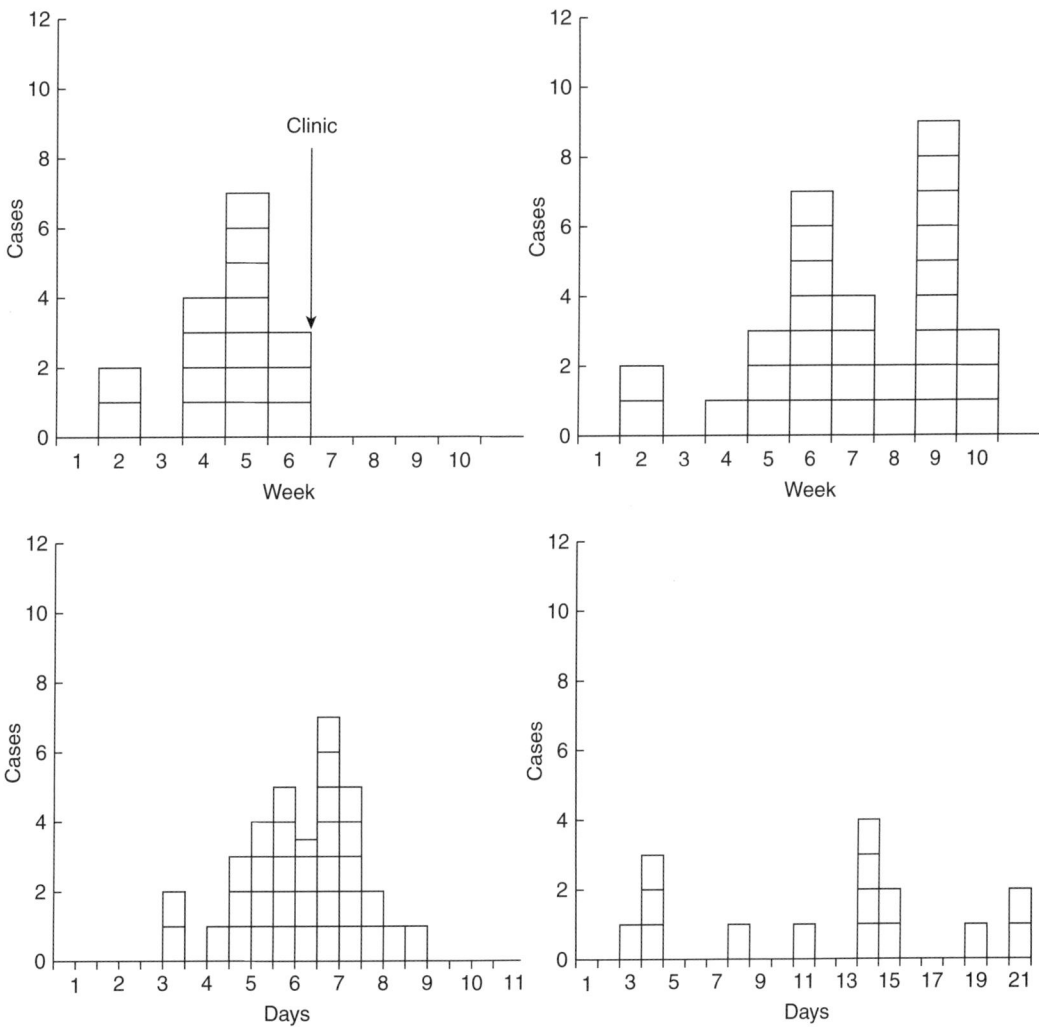

An epidemic curve is a histogram. Cases are plotted by date of onset of illness. Time intervals (x axis) must be based on the incubation or latency period of the disease and the length of the period over which cases are distributed

2. Common source (same origin)—curve approximates a normal distribution curve if there are a sufficient number of cases and if cases are limited to a short exposure with maximum incubation of a few days or less (point source)
   a. Exposure may be continuous or intermittent. Intermittent exposure to a common source produces a curve with irregularly spaced peaks
3. Propagated (continuing) source—cases occur over a longer period of time; explosive epidemics resulting from person-to-person transmission may occur
   a. If secondary cases occur, intervals between peaks usually approximate average incubation periods

VII. CDC Definitions of Healthcare-Associated Infections

A. Healthcare-Associated Infection

1. Definition—an infection meeting the following criteria:
   a. Not present or incubating on admission
   b. Develops during the course of receiving treatment for other conditions
   c. Incubating at the time of admission that is related to previous hospitalization at the same facility or identified in an admission following performance of a procedure during a previous admission
   d. Healthcare workers acquire while performing their duties within a healthcare setting
   e. HAIs include those that occur in the course of care in acute care hospitals, long-term care, behavioral health, correction facilities, dental care, home health, outpatient medical and surgical clinics, dialysis centers, radiology centers, etc.
2. Community-associated versus iatrogenic infection
   a. Community-associated infections—present or incubating on admission to the healthcare facility and not associated with previous treatment/procedures at that healthcare facility
   b. Iatrogenic infection—infection arising from the actions or treatments of a physician or healthcare provider or a secondary condition arising from treatment of a primary condition
      (1) May be healthcare-associated or community-associated (e.g., corticosteroid injections)
3. CDC definition of HAIs[15]

UTI—URINARY TRACT INFECTION

B. SUTI—Symptomatic Urinary Tract Infection

1. Patient with an indwelling urinary catheter at the time of specimen collection—must have a positive urine culture $\geq 10^5$ colony-forming units (CFUs)/mL, with no more than two species of microorganisms *and* at least one of the following with no other recognized cause: fever ($>38°C$), suprapubic tenderness, costovertebral angle pain or tenderness (SUTI Criterion 1a CAUTI)

    or

    A positive urinalysis demonstrated by one of the following:
    a. Positive dipstick for leukocyte esterase and/or nitrate
    b. Pyuria (urine specimen with ≥ 10 white blood cells (WBC)/mm^3 or ≥ 3 WBC/high-power field of unspun urine)
    c. Organisms seen on Gram stain of unspun urine (SUTI Criterion 2a CAUTI)

2. Patient had an indwelling urinary catheter discontinued within 48 hours before specimen was obtained—must have a positive urine culture $\geq 10^5$ CFU/mL, with no more than two species of microorganisms *and* at least one of the following with no other recognized cause: fever ($>38°C$) in a patient ≤ 65 years of age (fever is not part of the criterion for those >65 years of age), urgency, frequency, dysuria, suprapubic tenderness, costovertebral angle pain or tenderness (SUTI Criterion 1a CAUTI)

    or

    A positive urinalysis demonstrated by one of the following:
    a. Positive dipstick for leukocyte esterase and/or nitrate
    b. Pyuria (urine specimen with ≥ 10 WBC/mm^3 or ≥ 3 WBCs/high-power field of unspun urine)
    c. Organisms seen on Gram stain of unspun urine (SUTI-Criterion 2a-CAUTI)

3. Patient did not have an indwelling urinary catheter at the time of specimen collection nor within 48 hours before specimen collection: must have a positive urine culture $\geq 10^5$ CFU/ml with no more than two species of microorganisms *and* at least one of the following with no other recognized cause: fever ($>38°$) in a patient ≤ 65 years of age (fever is not part of the criterion for those >65 years of age), urgency, frequency, dysuria, suprapubic tenderness, costovertebral angle pain or tenderness (SUTI Criterion 1a)

    or

    A positive urinalysis demonstrated by one of the following:
    a. Positive dipstick for leukocyte esterase and/or nitrate
    b. Pyuria (urine specimen with ≥ 10 WBCs/mm^3 or ≥ 3 WBCs/high-power field of unspun urine)
    c. Organisms seen on Gram stain of unspun urine (SUTI Criterion 2a)

4. Patient ≤1 year of age (with or without an indwelling urinary catheter) must have a positive urine culture of $\geq 10^5$ CFUs/mL, with no more than two species of microorganisms *and* at least one of the following with no other recognized cause: fever (>38° core), hypothermia (<36°C core), apnea, bradycardia, dysuria, lethargy, vomiting (SUTI Criterion 3)

   or

   A positive urinalysis demonstrated by one of the following:
   a. Positive dipstick for leukocyte esterase and/or nitrate
   b. Pyuria (urine specimen with ≥10 WBCs/mm³ or ≥3 WBCs/high-power field of unspun urine)
   c. Organisms seen on Gram stain of unspun urine (SUTI Criterion 4)
5. Additional comments
   a. A positive culture of a urinary catheter tip is not an acceptable laboratory test to diagnose a urinary tract infection
   b. Urine cultures must be obtained using appropriate technique, such as clean catch collection or catheterization
   c. In infants, a urine culture should be obtained by bladder catheterization or suprapubic aspiration; a positive urine culture from a bag specimen is unreliable and should be confirmed by a specimen aseptically obtained by catheterization or suprapubic aspiration

C. ABUTI—Asymptomatic Bacteremic UTI

1. Patient with or without an indwelling urinary catheter must have a positive urine culture $\geq 10^5$ CFUs/mL, with no more than two species of microorganisms *and* at least one of the following with no other recognized cause: fever (>38°C) in a patient ≤65 years of age (fever is not part of the criterion for those >65 years of age), urgency, frequency, dysuria, suprapubic tenderness, costovertebral angle pain or tenderness

   and

   A positive blood culture with at least one matching uropathogen microorganism to the urine culture
2. Additional comments
   a. A positive culture of a urinary catheter tip is not an acceptable laboratory test to diagnose bacteriuria
   b. Urine cultures must be obtained using appropriate technique, such as clean catch collection or catheterization

D. OUTI—Other Infections of the Urinary Tract (Kidney, Ureter, Bladder, Urethra or Tissues Surrounding the Retroperineal or Perinephric Spaces)

Must meet at least one of the following criteria:
1. Patient has organisms isolated from culture of fluid (other than urine) or tissue from affected site
2. Patient has an abscess or other evidence of infection seen on direct examination, during a surgical operation or during a histopathological examination
3. Patient has at least two of the following signs or symptoms with no other recognized cause: fever (>38°C), localized pain or localized tenderness at the involved site *and* at least one of the following:
   a. Purulent drainage from affected site
   b. Organisms cultured from blood that are compatible with suspected site of infection
   c. Radiographic evidence of infection, for example, abnormal ultrasound, computed tomography (CT) scan, magnetic resonance imaging (MRI), or radiolabel scan (gallium, technetium)
4. Patient ≤1 year of age has at least one of the following signs or symptoms with no other recognized cause: fever (>38°C rectal), hypothermia (<37°C rectal), apnea, bradycardia, lethargy or vomiting *and* at least one of the following:
   a. Purulent drainage from affected site
   b. Organisms cultured from blood that are compatible with suspected site of infection
   c. Radiographic evidence of infection, for example, abnormal ultrasound, CT scan, MRI, or radiolabel scan (gallium, technetium)
   d. Physician diagnosis of infection of the kidney, ureter, bladder, urethra or tissues surrounding the retroperitoneal or perinephric space
   e. Physician institutes appropriate therapy for an infection of the kidney, ureter, bladder, urethra or tissues surrounding the retroperitoneal or perinephric space

SURGICAL SITE INFECTION

E. SIP/SIS—Superficial Incisional Surgical Site Infection

1. Superficial incisional infection (SIP and SIS)—must meet the following criteria: Infection occurs within 30 days after the operative procedure *and* involves only skin and subcutaneous tissue of the incision *and* patient has at least one of the following:
   a. Purulent drainage from the superficial incision
   b. Organisms isolated from an aseptically obtained culture of fluid or tissue from the superficial incision

c. At least one of the following signs or symptoms of infection: pain or tenderness, localized swelling, redness or heat *and* superficial incision is deliberately opened by surgeon and is culture positive or not cultured; a culture-negative finding does not meet these criteria
d. Diagnosis of superficial incisional SSI by the surgeon or attending physician
e. Reporting instructions
   (1) There are two specific types of superficial incisional SSI, superficial incisional primary (SIP) and superficial incisional secondary (SIS)
   (2) Do not report a stitch abscess (minimal inflammation and discharge confined to the points of suture penetration) as an infection
   (3) Do not report a localized stab wound infection as an SSI; instead report as skin (SKIN) or soft tissue (ST) infection, depending on its depth
   (4) Report infection of the circumcision site in newborns as CIRC, not an SSI
   (5) Report infection of the episiotomy site as a skin and soft tissue infection, not an SSI
   (6) If the incisional site infection involves or extends into the fascia and muscle layers, report as a deep incisional SSI
   (7) Classify infection that involves both superficial and deep incisional sites as deep incisional SSI

2. Deep incisional infection—must meet the following criteria: infection occurs within 30 days after the operative procedure if no implant (a non–human derived implanted foreign body that is permanently placed in a patient during surgery) is left in place or within 1 year if implant is in place and the infection appears to be related to the operative procedure, *and* involves deep soft tissues (e.g., fascial and muscle layers) of the incision *and* patient has at least one of the following:
   a. Purulent drainage from the deep incision but not from the organ/space component of the surgical site
   b. A deep incision spontaneously dehisces or is deliberately opened by a surgeon and is culture-positive or not cultured when the patient has at least one of the following signs or symptoms: fever (>38°C), or localized pain or tenderness. A culture-negative finding does not meet this criterion
   c. An abscess or other evidence of infection involving the deep incision is found on direct examination, during reoperation or by histopathological or radiological examination
   d. Diagnosis of a deep incisional SSI by a surgeon or attending physician
   e. Reporting instructions:
      (1) Classify infection that involves both superficial and deep incision sites as deep incisional SSI

(2) There are two specific types of deep incisional SSI, deep incisional primary (DIP) and deep incisional secondary (DIS)
3. Organ/space—SSI (organ/space) involves any part of the body, excluding the skin incision, fascia, or muscle layers, that is opened or manipulated during the operative procedure. Infection occurs within 30 days after the operative procedure if no implant is left in place or within 1 year if implant is in place and the infection appears to be related to the operative procedure *and* infection involves any part of the body, excluding the skin incision, fascia, or muscle layers, that is opened or manipulated during the operative procedure *and* patient has at least one of the following:
   a. Purulent drainage from a drain that is placed through a stab wound into the organ/space
   b. Organisms isolated from an aseptically obtained culture, fluid or tissue in the organ/space
   c. An abscess or other evidence of infection involving the organ/space that is found on direct examination, during reoperation or by histopathological or radiological examination
   d. Diagnosis of an organ/space SSI by a surgeon or attending physician
   e. The following are specific sites of an organ/space SSI:
      (1) Osteomyelitis
      (2) Breast abscess or mastitis
      (3) Myocarditis or pericarditis
      (4) Disc space
      (5) Ear, mastoid
      (6) Endometritis
      (7) Endocarditis
      (8) Eye, other than conjunctivitis
      (9) Gastrointestinal (GI) tract
      (10) Intra-abdominal, not specified elsewhere
      (11) Intracranial, brain abscess or dura
      (12) Joint or bursa
      (13) Other infections of the lower respiratory tract
      (14) Mediastinitis
      (15) Meningitis or ventriculitis
      (16) Oral cavity (mouth, tongue, or gums)
      (17) Other male or female reproductive
      (18) Other infections of the urinary tract
      (19) Spinal abscess without meningitis
      (20) Sinusitis
      (21) Upper respiratory tract, pharyngitis

(22) Arterial or venous infection
(23) Vaginal cuff

F. PNEU—Pneumonia

Criteria for defining nosocomial pneumonia—general comments applicable to all pneumonia specific site criteria

1. Physician's diagnosis of pneumonia alone is **not** an acceptable criterion for nosocomial pneumonia
2. Although specific criteria are included for infants and children, pediatric patients may meet any of the other pneumonia specific site criteria
3. Ventilator-associated pneumonia (i.e., pneumonia in persons who had a device to assist or control respiration continuously through a tracheostomy or by endotracheal intubation within the 48-hour period before the onset of infection, inclusive of the weaning period) should be so designated when reporting data
4. When assessing a patient for presence of pneumonia, it is important to distinguish between changes in clinical status (caused by other conditions, such as myocardial infarction, pulmonary embolism, respiratory distress syndrome, atelectasis, malignancy, chronic obstructive pulmonary disease, hyaline membrane disease, bronchopulmonary dysplasia, etc.).
    a. Care must be taken when assessing intubated patients to distinguish between tracheal colonization, upper respiratory tract infections (e.g., tracheobronchitis) and early onset pneumonia
    b. It may be difficult to determine nosocomial pneumonia in the elderly, infants and immunocompromised patients because such conditions may mask typical signs or symptoms associated with pneumonia
    c. Alternative specific criteria for the elderly, infants and immunocompromised patients have been included in this definition of nosocomial pneumonia
5. Nosocomial pneumonia can be characterized by its onset—early or late; early-onset pneumonia occurs during the first 4 days of hospitalization and is often caused by *Moraxella catarrhalis, Haemophilus influenzae* and *Streptococcus pneumoniae*
    a. Causative agents of late-onset pneumonia are frequently gram-negative bacilli or *Staphylococcus aureus*, including methicillin-resistant *S. aureus*
    b. Viruses (e.g., influenza A and B or respiratory syncytial virus) can cause early- and late-onset hospital-associated pneumonia
    c. Yeasts, fungi, *Legionella* and *Pneumocystis carinii* are usually pathogens of late-onset pneumonia
6. Pneumonia resulting from gross aspiration (e.g., in the setting of intubation in the emergency room or operating room) is considered hospital-associated if it meets any

specific criteria and was not clearly present or incubating at the time of admission to the hospital
7. Multiple episodes of hospital-associated pneumonia may occur in critically ill patients with lengthy hospital stays
   a. When determining whether to report multiple episodes of nosocomial pneumonia in a single patient, look for evidence of resolution of the initial infection
   b. The addition of or change in pathogen alone is not indicative of a new episode of pneumonia
   c. The combination of new signs and symptoms and radiographic evidence or other diagnostic testing is required
8. Positive Gram stain for bacteria and positive potassium hydroxide (KOH) mount for elastin fibers and/or fungal hyphae from appropriately collected sputum specimens are important clues that point toward the etiology of the infection
   a. Sputum samples are frequently contaminated with airway colonizers and therefore must be interpreted cautiously; in particular, *Candida* is commonly seen on stain, but infrequently causes nosocomial pneumonia

BSI—BLOODSTREAM INFECTION

G. LCBI—Bloodstream Infection, Laboratory-Confirmed (LCBI)

LCBI criteria 1 and 2 may be used for patients of any age, including patients ≤1 year of age

Must meet at least one of the following criteria:
1. Patient has a recognized pathogen cultured from one or more blood cultures, *and* organism cultured from blood is not related to an infection at another site
2. Patient has at least one of the following signs or symptoms: fever (>38°C), chills or hypotension *and* signs and symptoms and positive laboratory results are not related to an infection at another site, *and* at least one of the following:
   a. Common skin contaminant (e.g., diphtheroids, *Bacillus* sp., *Propionibacterium* sp., coagulase-negative staphylococci, or micrococci) is cultured from two or more blood cultures drawn on separate occasions
3. Patient ≤1 year of age has at least one of the following signs or symptoms: fever (>38°C), hypothermia (<37°C), apnea or bradycardia, *and*
   a. Signs and symptoms and positive laboratory results are not related to an infection at another site *and*
   b. Common skin contaminant is cultured from two or more blood cultures drawn on separate occasions

BJ—BONE AND JOINT INFECTION

H. Bone—Osteomyelitis

Must meet at least one of the following criteria:
1. Patient has organisms cultured from bone
2. Patient has evidence of osteomyelitis on direct examination of the bone during a surgical operation or histopathological examination
3. Patient has at least two of the following signs or symptoms with no other recognized cause: fever (>38°C), localized swelling, tenderness, heat or drainage at suspected site of bone infection *and* at least one of the following:
   a. Organisms cultured from blood
   b. Positive blood antigen test
   c. Radiographic evidence of infection

I. JNT—Joint or Bursa

Must meet at least one of the following criteria:
1. Patient has organisms cultured from joint fluid or synovial biopsy
2. Patient has evidence of joint or bursa infection seen during a surgical operation or histopathological examination
3. Patient has at least two of the following signs or symptoms with no other recognized cause: joint pain, swelling, tenderness, heat, evidence of effusion or limitation of motion *and* at least one of the following:
   a. Organisms *and* WBCs seen on Gram stain of joint fluid
   b. Positive antigen test on blood, urine or joint fluid
   c. Cellular profile and chemistries of joint fluid compatible with infection and not explained by an underlying rheumatological disorder
   d. Radiographic evidence of infection

CNS—CENTRAL NERVOUS SYSTEM INFECTION

J. DISC—Disc Space Infection, Vertebral

Must meet at least one of the following criteria:
1. Patient has organisms cultured from vertebral disc space tissue obtained during a surgical operation or needle aspiration
2. Patient has evidence of vertebral disc space infection seen during a surgical operation or histopathological examination
3. Patient has fever (>38°C) with no other recognized cause or pain at the involved vertebral disc space *and* radiographic evidence of infection
4. Patient has fever (>38°C) with no other recognized cause and pain at the involved vertebral disc space *and* positive antigen test on blood or urine

CHAPTER TWO: SURVEILLANCE AND EPIDEMIOLOGICAL INVESTIGATION | 119

K. IC—Intracranial Infection (Brain Abscess, Subdural or Epidural Infection, Encephalitis)

Must meet at least one of the following criteria:
1. Patient has organisms cultured from brain tissue or dura
2. Patient has abscess or evidence of intracranial infection seen during a surgical operation or histopathological examination.
3. Patient has at least two of the following signs or symptoms with no other recognized cause: headache, dizziness, fever (>38°C), localizing neurological signs, changing level of consciousness, or confusion, *and* if diagnosis is made antemortem, physician institutes appropriate antimicrobial therapy, *and* at least one of the following:
    a. Organisms seen on microscopic examination of brain or abscess tissue obtained by needle aspiration or by biopsy during a surgical operation or autopsy
    b. Positive antigen test on blood or urine
    c. Radiographic evidence of infection
    d. Diagnostic single antibody titer (IgM) or 4-fold increase in paired sera (IgG) for pathogen
4. Patient ≤1 year of age has at least two of the following signs or symptoms with no other recognized cause: fever (>38°C), hypothermia (<37°C), apnea, bradycardia, localizing neurological signs or changing level of consciousness, *and* if diagnosis is made antemortem, physician institutes appropriate antimicrobial therapy, *and* at least one of the following:
    a. Organisms seen on microscopic examination of brain or abscess tissue obtained by needle aspiration or by biopsy during a surgical operation or autopsy
    b. Positive antigen test on blood or urine
    c. Radiographic evidence of infection
    d. Diagnostic single antibody titer or 4-fold increase in paired sera (IgM) for pathogen

L. MEN—Meningitis or Ventriculitis

Must meet at least one of the following criteria:
1. Patient has organisms cultured from cerebrospinal fluid (CSF)
2. Patient has at least one of the following signs or symptoms with no other recognized cause: fever (>38°C), headache, stiff neck, meningeal signs, cranial nerve signs or irritability *and* if diagnosis is made antemortem, physician institutes appropriate antimicrobial therapy, *and* at least one of the following:
    a. Increased WBCs, elevated protein and/or decreased glucose in CSF
    b. Organisms seen on Gram stain of CSF
    c. Organisms cultured from blood

d. Positive antigen test of CSF, blood or urine
e. Diagnostic single antibody titer or 4-fold increase in paired sera for pathogen
3. Patient ≤1 year of age has at least one of the following signs or symptoms with no other recognized cause: fever (>38°C), hypothermia (<37°C), apnea, bradycardia, stiff neck, meningeal signs, cranial nerve signs or irritability *and* if diagnosis is made antemortem, physician institutes appropriate antimicrobial therapy, *and* at least one of the following:
   a. Positive CSF examination with increased WBCs, elevated protein and/or decreased glucose
   b. Positive Gram stain of CSF
   c. Organisms cultured from blood
   d. Positive antigen test of CSF, blood or urine
   e. Diagnostic single antibody titer or 4-fold increase in paired sera for pathogen

M. SA—Spinal Abscess without Meningitis

An abscess of the spinal epidural or subdural space, without involvement of the CSF or adjacent bone structures

Must meet at least one of the following criteria:
1. Patient has organisms cultured from an abscess in the spinal epidural or subdural space
2. Patient has an abscess in the spinal epidural or subdural space seen during a surgical operation or autopsy or evidence of an abscess seen during a histopathological examination
3. Patient has at least one of the following signs or symptoms with no other recognized cause: fever (>38°C), back pain, focal tenderness, radiculitis, paraparesis or paraplegia *and* if diagnosis is made antemortem, physician institutes appropriate antimicrobial therapy, *and* at least one of the following:
   a. Organisms cultured from blood
   b. Radiographic evidence of a spinal abscess

CVS—CARDIOVASCUALR SYSTEM INFECTION

N. VASC—Arterial or Venous Infection

Must meet at least one of the following criteria:
1. Patient has organisms cultured from arteries or veins removed during a surgical operation *and* blood culture not done or no organisms cultured from blood

2. Patient has evidence of arterial or venous infection seen during a surgical operation or histopathological examination
3. Patient has at least one of the following signs or symptoms with no other recognized cause: fever (>38°C), pain, erythema or heat at involved vascular site *and* >15 colonies cultured from intravascular cannula tip using semi-quantitative culture method *and* blood culture not done or no organisms cultured from blood
4. Patient has purulent drainage at involved vascular site *and* blood culture not done or no organisms cultured from blood
5. Patient ≤1 year of age has at least one of the following signs or symptoms with no other recognized cause: fever (>38°C), hypothermia (<37°C), apnea, bradycardia, lethargy or pain, erythema or heat at involved vascular site *and* >15 colonies cultured from intravascular cannula tip using semi-quantitative culture method *and* blood culture not done or no organisms cultured from blood

O. ENDO—Endocarditis Involving Either a Natural or Prosthetic Heart Valve

Must meet at least one of the following criteria:
1. Patient has organisms cultured from valve or vegetation
2. Patient has two or more of the following signs or symptoms with no other recognized cause: fever (>38°C), new or changing murmur, embolic phenomena, skin manifestations, congestive heart failure or cardiac conduction abnormality *and* if diagnosis is made antemortem and physician institutes appropriate antimicrobial therapy, *and* at least one of the following:
    a. Organisms cultured from two or more blood cultures
    b. Organisms seen on Gram stain of valve when culture is negative or not done
    c. Valvular vegetation seen during a surgical operation or autopsy
    d. Positive antigen test on blood or urine
    e. Evidence of new vegetation seen on echocardiogram
3. Patient ≤1 year of age has two or more of the following signs or symptoms with no other recognized cause: fever (>38°C rectal), hypothermia (<37°C rectal), apnea, bradycardia, new or changing murmur, embolic phenomena, skin manifestation, congestive heart failure, or cardiac conduction abnormality *and* if diagnosis is made antemortem physician institutes appropriate antimicrobial therapy, *and* at least one of the following:
    a. Organisms cultured from two or more blood cultures
    b. Organisms seen on Gram stain of valve when culture is negative or not done
    c. Valvular vegetation seen during a surgical operation or autopsy
    d. Positive antigen test on blood or urine
    e. Evidence of new vegetation seen on echocardiogram

P. CARD—Myocarditis or Pericarditis

Must meet at least one of the following criteria:
1. Patient has organisms cultured from pericardial tissue or fluid obtained by needle aspiration or during a surgical operation
2. Patient has at least two of the following signs or symptoms with no other recognized cause: fever (>38°C), chest pain, paradoxical pulse or increased heart size *and* at least one of the following:
    a. Abnormal EKG consistent with myocarditis or pericarditis
    b. Positive antigen test on blood
    c. Evidence of myocarditis or pericarditis on histological examination of heart tissue
    d. Four-fold rise in type-specific antibody with or without isolation of virus from pharynx or feces
    e. Pericardial effusion identified by echocardiogram, CT scan, MRI or angiography
3. Patient ≤1 year of age has at least two of the following signs or symptoms with no other recognized cause: fever (>38°C rectal), hypothermia (<37°C rectal), apnea, bradycardia, paradoxical pulse or increased heart size, *and* at least one of the following:
    a. Abnormal EKG consistent with myocarditis or pericarditis
    b. Positive antigen test on blood
    c. Histological examination of heart tissue shows evidence of myocarditis or pericarditis
    d. Four-fold rise in type-specific antibody with or without isolation of virus from pharynx or feces
    e. Pericardial effusion identified by echocardiogram, CT scan, MRI or angiography

Q. MED: Mediastinitis

Must meet at least one of the following criteria:
1. Patient has organisms cultured from mediastinal tissue or fluid obtained during a surgical operation or needle aspiration
2. Patient has evidence of mediastinitis seen during a surgical operation or histopathological examination
3. Patient has at least one of the following signs or symptoms with no other recognized cause: fever (>38°C), chest pain or sternal instability, *and* at least one of the following:
    a. Purulent discharge from mediastinal area
    b. Organisms cultured from blood or discharge from mediastinal area
    c. Mediastinal widening on radiograph

4. Patient ≤1 year of age has at least one of the following signs or symptoms with no other recognized cause: fever (>38°C rectal), hypothermia (<37°C rectal), apnea, bradycardia or sternal instability *and* at least one of the following:
   a. Purulent discharge from mediastinal area
   b. Organisms cultured from blood or discharge from mediastinal area
   c. Mediastinal widening on radiograph

EENT—EYE, EAR, NOSE, THROAT OR MOUTH INFECTION

R. CONJ—Conjunctivitis

Must meet at least one of the following criteria:
1. Patient has pathogens cultured from purulent exudate obtained from the conjunctiva or contiguous tissues, such as eyelid, cornea, meibomian glands or lacrimal glands
2. Patient has pain or redness of conjunctiva or around *eye and* at least one of the following:
   a. WBCs and organisms seen on Gram stain of exudate
   b. Purulent exudate
   c. Positive antigen test on exudate or conjunctival scraping
   d. Multinucleated giant cells seen on microscopic examination of conjunctival exudate or scrapings
   e. Positive viral culture
   f. Diagnostic single antibody titer or 4-fold increase in paired sera for pathogen

S. EYE—Eye, Other Than Conjunctivitis

Must meet at least one of the following criteria:
1. Patient has organisms cultured from anterior or posterior chamber of vitreous fluid
2. Patient has at least two of the following signs or symptoms with no other recognized cause: eye pain, visual disturbance or hypopyon *and* at least one of the following:
   a. Physician's diagnosis of an eye infection
   b. Positive antigen test on blood
   c. Organisms cultured from blood

T. EAR—Ear and Mastoid Infections

Must meet the following applicable criteria: Otitis externa
1. Patient has pathogens cultured from purulent drainage from ear canal
2. Patient has at least one of the following signs or symptoms with no other recognized cause: fever (>38°C), pain, redness or drainage from ear canal *and* organisms seen on Gram stain of purulent material from ear canal

Otitis media
1. Patient has organisms cultured from fluid from middle ear obtained by tympanocentesis or at surgical operation
2. Patient has at least two of the following signs or symptoms with no other recognized cause: fever (>38°C), pain in the eardrum, inflammation, retraction or decreased mobility of eardrum or fluid behind eardrum

Otitis interna
1. Patient has organisms cultured from fluid from inner ear obtained at surgical operation
2. Patient has a physician's diagnosis of inner ear infection

Mastoiditis
1. Patient has organisms cultured from purulent drainage from mastoid
2. Patient has at least two of the following signs or symptoms with no other recognized cause: fever (>38°C), pain, tenderness, erythema, headache or facial paralysis *and* at least one of the following:
    (a) Organisms seen on Gram stain of purulent material from mastoid
    (b) Positive antigen test on blood

U. ORAL—Oral Cavity (Mouth, Tongue, Gums)

Must meet at least one of the following criteria:
1. Patient has organisms cultured from purulent material from tissues or oral cavity
2. Patient has an abscess or other evidence of oral cavity infection seen on direct examination, during a surgical operation or during a histopathological examination
3. Patient has at least one of the following signs or symptoms with no other recognized cause: abscess, ulceration or raised white patches on inflamed mucosa or plaques on oral mucosa *and* at least one of the following:
    a. Organisms seen on Gram stain
    b. Positive KOH stain
    c. Multinucleated giant cells seen on microscopic examination of mucosal scrapings
    d. Positive antigen test on oral secretions
    e. Diagnostic single antibody titer or 4-fold increase in paired sera for pathogen
    f. Physician diagnosis of infection and treatment with topical or oral antifungal therapy

V. SINU—Sinusitis

Must meet at least one of the following criteria:
1. Patient has organisms cultured from purulent material obtained from sinus cavity
2. Patient has at least one of the following signs or symptoms with no other recognized cause: fever (>38°C), pain or tenderness over the involved sinus, headache, purulent exudate or nasal obstruction *and* at least one of the following:

a. Positive transillumination
b. Positive radiographic examination

W. UR—Upper Respiratory Tract, Pharyngitis, Laryngitis, Epiglottitis

Must meet at least one of the following criteria:
1. Patient has at least two of the following signs or symptoms with no other recognized cause: fever (>38°C), erythema of pharynx, sore throat, cough, hoarseness, purulent exudate in throat *and* at least one of the following:
   a. Organisms cultured from the specific site
   b. Organisms cultured from blood
   c. Positive antigen test on blood or respiratory secretions
   d. Diagnostic single antibody titer or 4-fold increase in paired sera for pathogen
   e. Physician's diagnosis of an upper respiratory infection
2. Patient has an abscess seen on direct examination, during a surgical operation or during a histopathological examination
3. Patient ≤1 year of age has at least two of the following signs or symptoms with no other recognized cause: fever (>38°C rectal), hypothermia (<37°C rectal), apnea, bradycardia, nasal discharge or purulent exudate in throat *and* at least one of the following symptoms:
   a. Organisms cultured from the specific site
   b. Organisms cultured from blood
   c. Positive antigen test on blood or respiratory secretions
   d. Diagnostic single antibody titer or 4-fold increase in paired sera for pathogen
   e. Physician's diagnosis of an upper respiratory infection

GI—GASTROINTESTINAL SYSTEM INFECTION

X. GE—Gastroenteritis

Must meet at least one of the following criteria:
1. Patient has an acute onset of diarrhea (liquid stools for >12 hours) with or without vomiting or fever (>38°C) and no likely noninfectious cause
2. Patient has at least two of the following signs or symptoms with no other recognized cause: nausea, vomiting, abdominal pain, fever (>38°C) or headache *and* at least one of the following:
   a. An enteric pathogen is cultured from stool or rectal swab
   b. An enteric pathogen is detected by routine or electron microscopy
   c. An enteric pathogen is detected by antigen or antibody assay on blood or feces
   d. Evidence of an enteric pathogen is detected by cytopathic changes in tissue culture (toxin assay)
   e. Diagnostic single antibody titer or 4-fold increase in paired sera for pathogen

Y. GIT—GI Tract Infections (Esophagus, Stomach, Small and Large Bowel, and Rectum, Excluding Gastroenteritis and Appendicitis)

Must meet at least one of the following criteria:
1. Patient has an abscess or other evidence of infection seen during a surgical operation or histopathological examination
2. Patient has at least two of the following signs or symptoms with no other recognized cause and compatible with infection of the organ or tissue involved: fever (>38°C), nausea, vomiting, abdominal pain or tenderness *and* at least one of the following:
   a. Organisms cultured from drainage or tissue obtained during a surgical operation or endoscopy or from a surgically placed drain
   b. Organisms seen on Gram or KOH stain or multinucleated giant cells seen on microscopic examination of drainage or tissue obtained during a surgical operation or endoscopy or from a surgically placed drain
   c. Organisms cultured from blood
   d. Evidence of pathological findings on radiological examination
   e. Evidence of pathological findings on endoscopic examination

Z. HEP—Hepatitis

Must meet the following criteria:
1. Patient has at least two of the following signs or symptoms with no other recognized cause: fever (>38°C), anorexia, nausea, vomiting, abdominal pain, jaundice or history of transfusion within the previous 3 months *and* at least one of the following:
   a. Positive antigen or antibody test for hepatitis A, hepatitis B, hepatitis C or delta hepatitis
   b. Abnormal liver function tests (alanine aminotransferase [ALT]/aspartate aminotransferase [AST], bilirubin)
   c. Cytomegalovirus (CMV) detected in urine or oropharyngeal secretions
2. Do not report noninfectious hepatitis, biliary obstruction or toxin-induced hepatitis

AA. IAB—Intra-abdominal (Including Gallbladder, Bile Ducts, Liver, Spleen, Pancreas, Peritoneum, Subphrenic or Subdiaphragmatic Space, or Other Intra-abdominal Tissue or Area Not Specified Elsewhere [Excluding Viral Hepatitis])

Must meet at least one of the following criteria:
1. Patient has organisms cultured from purulent material from intra-abdominal space obtained during a surgical operation or needle aspiration
2. Patient has abscess or other evidence of intra-abdominal infection seen during a surgical operation or histopathological examination

3. Patient has at least two of the following signs or symptoms with no other recognized cause: fever (>38°C), nausea, vomiting, abdominal pain or jaundice *and* at least one of the following:
   a. Organisms cultured from drainage from surgically placed drain
   b. Organisms seen on Gram stain of drainage or tissue obtained during surgical operation or needle aspiration
   c. Organisms cultured from blood or radiographic evidence of infection

BB. NEC—Necrotizing Enterocolitis in Infants

Must meet the following criteria:
1. Infant has at least two of the following signs or symptoms with no other recognized cause: vomiting, abdominal distention or prefeeding residuals *and* persistent microscopic or gross blood in stools *and* at least one of the following abdominal radiographic abnormalities:
   a. Pneumoperitoneum
   b. Pneumatosis intestinalis
   c. Unchanging rigid loops of small bowel

LRI—LOWER RESPIRATORY TRACT INFECTION, OTHER THAN PNEUMONIA

CC. BRON—Bronchitis, Tracheobronchitis, Bronchiolitis, Tracheitis, without Evidence of Pneumonia

Must meet at least one of the following criteria:
1. Patient has no clinical or radiographic evidence of pneumonia *and* patient has at least two of the following signs or symptoms with no other recognized cause: fever (>38°C), cough, new or increased sputum production, rhonchi, wheezing *and* at least one of the following:
   a. Positive culture obtained by deep tracheal aspirate or bronchoscopy
   b. Positive antigen test on respiratory secretions
2. Patient ≤1 year of age has no clinical or radiographic evidence of pneumonia *and* patient has at least two of the following signs or symptoms with no other recognized cause: fever (>38°C rectal), cough, new or increased sputum production, rhonchi, wheezing, respiratory distress, apnea or bradycardia *and* at least one of the following:
   a. Organisms cultured from material obtained by deep tracheal aspirate or bronchoscopy
   b. Positive antigen test on respiratory secretions
   c. Diagnostic single antibody titer or fourfold increase in paired sera for pathogen

DD. LUNG—Other Infections of the Lower Respiratory Tract

Must meet at least one of the following criteria:
1. Patient has organisms seen on smear or cultured from lung tissue or fluid, including pleural fluid
2. Patient has a lung abscess or empyema seen during a surgical operation or histopathological examination
3. Patient has an abscess cavity seen on radiographic examination of lung

REPR—REPRODUCTIVE TRACT INFECTION

EE. EMET—Endometritis

Must meet at least one of the following criteria:
1. Patient has organisms cultured from fluid or tissue from endometrium obtained during surgical operation, by needle aspiration or by brush biopsy
2. Patient has at least two of the following signs or symptoms with no other recognized cause: fever (>38°C), abdominal pain, uterine tenderness or purulent drainage from uterus
3. Report postpartum endometritis as a nosocomial infection unless the amniotic fluid is infected at the time of admission or the patient was admitted 48 hours after rupture of the membrane

FF. EPIS—Episiotomy Infections

Must meet at least one of the following criteria:
1. Postvaginal delivery patient has purulent drainage from the episiotomy
2. Postvaginal delivery patient has an episiotomy abscess

GG. VCUF—Vaginal Cuff Infections

Must meet at least one of the following criteria:
1. Posthysterectomy patient has purulent drainage from the vaginal cuff
2. Posthysterectomy patient has an abscess at the vaginal cuff
3. Posthysterectomy patient has pathogens cultured from fluid or tissue obtained from the vaginal cuff

HH. OREP—Other Infections of the Male or Female Reproductive Tract (Epididymis, Testes, Prostate, Vagina, Ovaries, Uterus, or Other Deep Pelvic Tissues, Excluding Endometritis or Vaginal Cuff Infections)

Must meet at least one of the following criteria:
1. Patient has organisms cultured from tissue or fluid from affected site
2. Patient has an abscess or other evidence of infection of affected site seen during a surgical operation or histopathological examination

3. Patient has two of the following signs or symptoms with no other recognized cause: fever (>38°C), nausea, vomiting, pain, tenderness or dysuria *and* at least one of the following:
   a. Organisms cultured from blood
   b. Diagnosis by physician

SST—SKIN AND SOFT TISSUE INFECTION

II. SKIN—Skin Infections

Must meet at least one of the following criteria:
1. Patient has purulent drainage, pustules, vesicles or boils
2. Patient has at least two of the following signs or symptoms with no other recognized cause: pain or tenderness, localized swelling, redness or heat *and* at least one of the following:
   a. Organisms cultured from aspirate or drainage from affected site; if organisms are normal skin flora, they must be a pure culture
   b. Organisms cultured from blood
   c. Positive antigen test performed on infected tissue or blood
   d. Multinucleated giant cells seen on microscopic examination of affected tissue
   e. Diagnostic single antibody titer or fourfold increase in paired sera

Must meet at least one of the following criteria:
1. Patient has organisms cultured from tissue or drainage from affected site
2. Patient has purulent drainage at affected site
3. Patient has an abscess or other evidence of infection seen during a surgical operation or histopathological examination
4. Patient has at least two of the following signs or symptoms at the affected site with no other recognized cause: localized pain or tenderness, redness, swelling or heat *and* at least one of the following:
   a. Organisms cultured from blood
   b. Positive antigen test performed on blood or urine
   c. Diagnostic single antibody titer or 4-fold increase in paired sera for pathogen

JJ. DECU—Decubitus Ulcer, Including Both Superficial and Deep Infection

Must meet the following criteria:
1. Patient has at least two of the following signs or symptoms with no other recognized cause: redness, tenderness or swelling of decubitus wound edges *and* at least one of the following:
   a. Organisms cultured from properly collected fluid or tissue (needle aspiration of fluid or biopsy of tissue from the ulcer margin)
   b. Organisms cultured from blood

KK. Burn Infections

Must meet one of the following criteria:
1. Patient has a change in burn wound appearance or character, such as rapid eschar separation or dark brown, black or violaceous discoloration of the eschar or edema at wound margin *and* histological examination of burn biopsy shows invasion of organisms into adjacent viable tissue
2. Patient has a change in burn wound appearance or character, such as rapid eschar separation, or dark brown, black or violaceous discoloration of the eschar or edema at wound margin *and* at least one of the following:
   a. Organisms cultured from blood in the absence of other identifiable infection
   b. Isolation of herpes simplex virus, histological identification of inclusions by light or electron microscopy or visualization of viral particles by electron microscopy in biopsies or lesion scrapings
3. Patient with a burn has at least two of the following signs or symptoms with no other recognized cause: fever (>38°C), hypothermia (<37°C), hypotension and oliguria, hyperglycemia at previously tolerated level of dietary carbohydrate or mental confusion *and* at least one of the following:
   a. Histological examination of burn biopsy shows invasion of organisms into adjacent viable tissue
   b. Organisms cultured from blood
   c. Isolation of herpes simplex virus, histological identification of inclusions by light or electron microscopy or visualization of viral particles by electron microscopy in biopsies or lesion scrapings

LL. BRST—Breast Abscess or Mastitis

Must meet at least one of the following criteria:
1. Patient has a positive culture of affected breast tissue or fluid obtained by incision and drainage or needle aspiration
2. Patient has a breast abscess or other evidence of infection seen during a surgical operation or histopathological examination
3. Patient has fever (>38°C), local inflammation of the breast *and* physician's diagnosis of breast abscess

MM. UMB—Omphalitis in a Newborn (≤30 Days Old)

Must meet at least one of the following criteria:
1. Patient has erythema and/or serous drainage from umbilicus *and* at least one of the following:
   a. Organisms cultured from drainage or needle aspirate
   b. Organisms cultured from blood

2. Patient has both erythema and purulence at the umbilicus
3. Report as nosocomial if infection occurs in a newborn within 7 days of hospital discharge

NN. PUST—Infant Pustulosis (≤1 Year Old)

Must meet at least one of the following criteria:
1. Infant has one or more pustules *and* physician diagnosis of skin infection
2. Infant has one or more pustules *and* physician institutes appropriate antimicrobial therapy

OO. CIRC—Newborn Circumcision Infection (≤30 Days Old)

Must meet at least one of the following criteria:
1. Newborn has purulent drainage from circumcision site
2. Newborn has at least one of the following signs or symptoms with no other recognized cause at circumcision site: erythema, swelling, or tenderness *and* pathogen cultured from circumcision site
3. Newborn has at least one of the following signs or symptoms with no other recognized cause at circumcision site: erythema, swelling or tenderness, *and* skin contaminant is cultured from circumcision site *and* physician diagnosis of infection or physician institutes appropriate therapy
4. Do not report as an SSI

SYS—SYSTEMIC INFECTION

PP. DI—Disseminated Infection

Defined as infection involving multiple organs or systems, without an apparent single site of infection; usually of viral origin, and with signs or symptoms with no other recognized cause and compatible with infectious involvement of multiple organs or systems

Practice Questions for Chapter Two

Chapter Two:

Surveillance and Epidemiologic Investigation

1. A 73-year-old woman resides in an extended care facility (ECF). Yesterday, she enjoyed a lengthy visit with her grandson. Her grandson calls you—the IP at his grandmother's ECF—today because he was just informed that he was recently exposed to N. meningitidis. The grandson is asymptomatic. However, after a careful evaluation by his physician today, he was strongly urged to start a prophylactic course of rifampin immediately. What should you do?
   a. Nothing at this point
   b. Start a line listing of all the people with whom the boy came in contact during his visit with his grandmother
   c. Confirm the diagnosis and explore the boy's "infectiousness"
   d. Start the grandmother on rifampin

2. The use of influenza vaccines in school-aged children to decrease the number of cases in the community uses the principle of:
   a. Epizootic
   b. Endemic
   c. Herd immunity
   d. Epidemic

3. You are the local public health director for a small town in Connecticut. You get a call today from a resident. The resident complains that his mother and most of his neighbors have Lyme disease. He wants you to support reducing the deer population via hunting and birth control. What action should you take first?
   a. Go visit the resident and bring educational material
   b. Call the state and local newspapers to avoid media attention
   c. Review state and local incidence data to determine if there is a problem
   d. Plan and implement a Lyme disease educational update

4. On September 1, there were 30 surgical patients in the hospital. Two of these were postoperative patients with an SSI. A total of 75 surgeries were performed in September. Six additional SSIs occurred in patients who had surgery in September. What was the numerator for an incidence rate in September?
   a. 30
   b. 6
   c. 8
   d. 75

5. You are the IP at a small rural hospital and have been monitoring all surgical cases for infection. You want to know if your SSI rates are acceptable. What would be your best action?
   a. Network with other local hospitals of the same size and compare your rates using a t test
   b. Calculate a total SSI rate and compare to previous rates for your facility
   c. Look for specific high-volume surgeries and compare to the published literature for each type
   d. Review the CDC SSI rates that have been published (NNIS or NHSN) and compare individual surgery types using a z test

6. You are the consulting IP for a corporation of LTC facilities. You have been asked to investigate whether residents who have an indwelling urinary catheter are at increased risk for a urinary tract infection (UTI). The baseline data that you have is a line listing of all of the residents with an annotation if they have an indwelling urinary catheter or have had a UTI. What is the best first choice of action?
   a. Design and implement a comprehensive and systematic surveillance program
   b. In-service program for nurses and nursing technicians on urinary catheter care
   c. Set up a contingency table and compute a chi-square to see if there is a problem
   d. Do a cross-sectional point prevalence study immediately to assess the validity of a problem

7. The NICU medical director has requested the NICU nosocomial infection rate for bloodstream infections (BSI). He wants baseline data and asks you to design and implement a handwashing campaign, using the BSI rate as one of the outcome indicators. He wants these data presented to the Performance Improvement Program. In the NICU, what information do you need to best risk stratify data?
   a. Birth weight
   b. Length of stay
   c. Age
   d. Gender

8. An ICU reports three cases of VAP during the first quarter of the year. There were 600 ventilator days in the time period. The VAP rate per 1000 vent days is:
   a. 0.005
   b. 200
   c. 3
   d. 5

9. A major difference between a prospective and a retrospective study is that the prospective study:
   a. Requires a relatively small number of subjects
   b. Is usually used for testing initial hypotheses
   c. May require a long follow-up period
   d. Is usually less costly

10. An advantage of a case-control study over a cohort study is that a case-control study:
    a. Is considered less biased than a cohort study
    b. Provides stronger evidence for a causal association
    c. Is less time consuming and less expensive
    d. Is more valid

11. Fifteen persons were infected with *Salmonella* at a picnic at which 75 ate egg salad sandwiches. What was the attack rate of *Salmonella* among those who ate the egg salad sandwiches?
    a. 15%
    b. 0.20
    c. 18%
    d. 20%

12. A measles exposure from a patient in a clinic was identified and an exposure workup was initiated. A staff exposure was defined as "a non-immune HCW with more than 5 minutes of same-room contact or face-to-face contact with the index patient." Forty-eight HCWs were identified as possible exposures. Of these, 44 had documented immunity to measles. Of the remaining HCWs, 3 did not have the same room or face-to-face contact. How many HCWs were at risk for developing measles because of this exposure?
    a. 4
    b. 45
    c. 1
    d. 48

13. In order to formulate a hypothesis on the possible cause of an outbreak, the cases should be characterized by:
    (1) Patient age
    (2) Diagnosis
    (3) Common time periods
    (4) Medical procedures
    (5) Caregivers
       a. 1, 3, 5
       b. 1, 2, 4
       c. 2, 3, 4
       d. 3, 4, 5

14. In 2009, 565 persons died from influenza-related illness in a large metropolitan area with a population 1.8 million. What was the cause-specific mortality rate?
    a. 31 per 100,000
    b. 5.3 %
    c. 31%
    d. 0.0003%

15. All of the 72 patients in a chronic hemodialysis center were tested for hepatitis C. Eight of the patients were identified as HCV positive. What is the prevalence of HCV among the patients at the hemodialysis center?
    a. 0.9%
    b. 9%
    c. 1%
    d. 11%

16. Continuation of Question 15: During the following year, two of the dialysis center's patients who previously tested negative for HCV converted to HCV positive. What was the incidence for that year?
    a. 2.8%
    b. 3.1%
    c. 13.8%
    d. 7.2%

17. The chi-square test can be used:
    (1) To evaluate the effect of a variable on outcomes
    (2) To analyze continuous data
    (3) To calculate an odds ratio or relative risk
    (4) If each cell of the table is greater than 5
    a. 1, 2, 3
    b. 1, 2, 4
    c. 2, 3, 4
    d. 1, 3, 4

18. In 2009, a total of 3254 persons died of all causes in a large metropolitan area with a population of 1.8 million. What was the crude mortality rate?
    a. 18 per 100,000
    b. 0.0018%
    c. 180 per 1000
    d. 180 per 100,000

19. One hundred preschool children were monitored for colds during the winter. Eighteen of them have asthma. Of the children with asthma, 65% had two or more colds. Of the children who did not have asthma, 30% had two or more colds. What type of study was this?
    a. Case-control
    b. Cohort
    c. Cross-sectional
    d. Period prevalence

20. When analyzing control chart data, a process is considered "out of control" if any of the following are present EXCEPT:
    a. Two of three consecutive data points are above the upper control limit or below the lower control limit
    b. Four of five consecutive data points are between 1 and 2 standard deviations above or below the mean
    c. Six consecutive data points are increasing or decreasing
    d. Nine consecutive data points are on one side of the mean

21. You are the IP coordinator for a 400-bed acute care facility that has had an outbreak of orthopedic infections. You begin gathering information about all of the cases. You should characterize the cases according to:
    a. Person, place and time
    b. Agent, host and environment
    c. Agent, host and date of onset
    d. Time, person and date of onset

22. The Employee Health Service has notified the IP that seven employees have *Pseudomonas aeruginosa* folliculitis. Initial investigation reveals that six of the seven cases belong to the same health club. Working on the hypothesis that the whirlpool at the health club is associated with the infections, the IP has decided to conduct a case-control study using two controls for each case. Which of the following groups is the MOST appropriate control?
    a. Non-ill family members of the ill employees
    b. Non-ill hospital employees matched for age and sex
    c. Hospitalized patients with skin disease matched for age and sex
    d. Non-ill members of the health club matched for age and sex

23. What is the range for the following numbers?

    2, 4, 5, 8, 9, 10, 11, 15, 18
    a. 16
    b. 18
    c. 9
    d. 2

24. Pneumonia in the elderly in the long-term care facility is usually identified by:
    a. Sputum cultures
    b. Chest radiograph
    c. Rapid-onset chills, fever and increased respiratory rate
    d. Heavy, productive cough

25. The IP designs a survey to assess the effectiveness of an Infection Prevention and Control in-service course. The choices after each question are: Unsatisfied, Satisfied or Very Satisfied. This is an example of what scale?
    a. Nominal
    b. Equal interval
    c. Continuous
    d. Ordinal

26. What is the probability of committing a Type I error if the P value is 0.10?
    a. 1 in 10
    b. 1 in 100
    c. 1 in 5
    d. 1 in 20

27. The IP is investigating a cluster of surgical site infections on a unit. Which of the following rates describes an epidemic, is expressed as a percent, used for particular populations and observed for a limited period of time?
    a. Attack
    b. Mortality
    c. Incidence
    d. Prevalence

28. Epidemiology is:
    (1) The study of the distribution and determinants of disease
    (2) The study of the frequency, types and factors that influence types of illness and/or injury in groups
    (3) Both a body of knowledge and a method of study
    (4) The study of epidemics of disease that occur in humans
       a. 2, 3, 4
       b. 1, 3, 4
       c. 1, 2, 3
       d. 1, 2, 4

29. Surveillance as used by IP professionals is a process that includes all of the following EXCEPT:
    a. Analysis
    b. Data collection
    c. Causation
    d. Correlation

30. During an outbreak of ventilator-associated pneumonia (VAP) in a medical ICU, the IP gathers risk factor information on the patients involved. All of the following would probably be found as host-related risk factors EXCEPT:
    a. Age
    b. History of chronic disease
    c. Occupations of the patients
    d. Gender

31. During the month of February, the IP finds that there were three sternal wound infections among patients undergoing coronary artery bypass grafts (CABG). Dr. A performed 28 surgeries, Dr. B performed 26 surgeries and Dr. C performed six surgeries. What was the surgical site infection attack rate for CABGs in February?
   a. 3%
   b. 4%
   c. 5%
   d. 20%

32. What additional information would the IP need in order to calculate a surgeon-specific infection rate for each surgeon?
   (1) Additional procedures each surgeon performed for predetermined time period (i.e., 6 months, 1 year)
   (2) Total number of infections for each surgeon during the set time period
   (3) Total number of procedures performed by all surgeons
   (4) Total number of surgical site infections for all surgeons
      a. 2, 4
      b. 2, 3
      c. 1, 2
      d. 4, 5

33. The measure of central tendency MOST affected by outliers is:
   a. Mean
   b. Median
   c. Mode
   d. Range

34. If chance is a likely explanation for the difference between a sample statistic and the corresponding null hypothesis population value, then:
   a. The difference is not statistically significant
   b. The sample result is not compatible with the null hypothesis
   c. The difference is statistically significant
   d. The null hypothesis can be rejected

35. When presenting device-associated infection data to the hospital administration, what data do you benchmark?
    1. Infection rates for area hospitals of similar size
    2. NNIS/NHSN rates for specific device-associated infections
    3. Facility's previous infection rate for specific infection and device
    4. Published rates from literature for largest and most widely respected hospitals in the nation
        a. 2, 4
        b. 1, 4
        c. 2, 3
        d. 1, 3

36. Reviewing culture and sensitivity data best serves which purpose of epidemic investigation?
    a. Indicates appropriateness of antibiotic therapy
    b. Indicates cause of infections
    c. Not usually used in epidemic investigations
    d. Identifies patterns

37. The p value in statistical test results indicate:
    a. Causation
    b. The probability of having committed a Type I error
    c. The probability of having committed a Type II error
    d. The probability of data being accurate and valid

38. On a normally distributed data set, what percentage of values lies within 3 standard deviations from the mean?
    a. 68.2
    b. 95.5
    c. 92.4
    d. 99.7

39. A typical method of collecting data used in qualitative research includes all the following EXCEPT:
    a. Mail out questionnaires
    b. Tape recorded interviews
    c. Focus group meetings
    d. Observations

40. Which statistical test is used when the data are small in numbers?
    a. Fisher's exact
    b. t test
    c. Chi-square
    d. z test

41. Statistical process control (SPC) charts are used for all of the following purposes EXCEPT:
    a. Monitor the process of care
    b. Facilitate the determination of variation
    c. Eliminate natural variation
    d. Monitor outcomes

42. When planning the surveillance program for the next year, which of the following issues should be considered?
    (1) Employee infections or prevention measures
    (2) High-risk surgical procedures performed at the facility
    (3) High-cost infections
    (4) Patient demographics
    (5) Employee staffing patterns
       a. 3, 4, 5
       b. 2, 3, 4
       c. 1, 3, 4, 5
       d. 1, 2, 3, 4

43. You decide to design an experimental epidemiological study of patients who have undergone coronary catheterization. You want to study which skin prep solution results in the least amount of post–heart catheterization site infections. In an experimental study:
    a. The study is usually retrospective
    b. The study and control groups are comparable with respect to every factor
    c. The investigator randomly assigns who shall be exposed to factors and who shall not be exposed
    d. The study population must be large to be valid

44. The frequency measures MOST commonly used in healthcare epidemiology are:
    a. Mean, median and mode
    b. Risk ratio and odds ratio
    c. Incidence rate, prevalence rate and incidence density
    d. Variance, standard deviation and range

Questions 45–47 Seventy-five patients were admitted to the medical-surgical intensive care unit (MS-ICU) in January. Forty were on the surgical service and 35 were on the medical service. Fifteen patients developed a nosocomial infection with methicillin-resistant *Staphylococcus aureus* (MRSA). Nine of the patients with MRSA infection were on the surgical service. The ICU patient days for January were 230 for the surgical patients and 325 for medical patients.

45. The overall attack rate for MRSA in the unit is:
    a. 20%
    b. 2%
    c. 53%
    d. 5%

46. The MRSA attack rate for patients on the medical service is:
    a. 8%
    b. 2%
    c. 17%
    d. 15%

47. The incidence density of MRSA infection for patients on the surgical service is:
    a. 29 infections per 1000 patient days
    b. 26 infections per 1000 patient days
    c. 19 infections per 100 patient days
    d. 39 infections per 1000 patient days

48. You have developed the surveillance program for your department for the next year. It contains surveillance for the employee health program, a device-associated infection study, four targeted surveillance projects, and continuous monitoring of all surgery patients. The impact of this surveillance program would be enhanced LEAST by:
    a. Feedback provided to medical personnel caring for patients in focus projects
    b. Device-related rates calculated and reported to intensive care staff
    c. Surgeon-specific infection rates reported to each surgeon
    d. Monthly calculation of a house-wide infection rate

49. You receive a microbiology report from a urine culture that is growing *Klebsiella oxytoca* ≥10 CFU/ml from a patient in the ICU with an indwelling urinary catheter. The patient also has a matching positive blood culture with the same organism. You discover that the patient has no signs or symptoms of infection. You would classify this as:
    a. Symptomatic urinary tract infection (SUTI)
    b. Other urinary tract infection (OUTI)
    c. Asymptomatic bacteremic urinary tract infection (ABUTI)
    d. This would not be classified as an HAI

50. Which of the following studies is experimental rather than observational?
    a. Cohort
    b. Clinical trial
    c. Case-control
    d. Cross-sectional

51. When a normal distribution is graphed, which of the following are true?
    1. There is a continuous, symmetrical distribution in which both tails extend to infinity
    2. The arithmetic mean, median and mode are identical
    3. The shape of the curve is determined by the mean and standard deviation
    4. 95.5% of the area lies between the mean and ±2 standard deviations
        a. 1 and 2
        b. 2 and 4
        c. 1, 3, and 4
        d. 1, 2, 3, and 4

52. Because of the potential for rapid spread, one confirmed case of this disease is considered an urgent public health situation, and the IP should immediately report suspected and confirmed cases to the health department.
    a. Chickenpox
    b. Influenza
    c. Measles
    d. Legionnaires' disease

Questions 53–57

During the month of October, 20 patients were admitted to the ICU and placed on ventilators for varying periods. Patient A (age 79) was a surgical patient who had a CVA during surgery. She remained on the ventilator for 21 days. Patient B (age 68) had undergone CABG and was intubated for surgery and extubated 36 hours later. Patient C was a trauma patient (age 52) who was on and off the ventilator a total of 9 days during his 2 weeks of treatment in the unit. Patient D (age 84) was admitted with CHF and was on the ventilator for 3 days. Patient E was a pediatric patient (age 4) who had pneumonia and was on the ventilator for 2 days. The total number of vent days for all the patients in the unit was 110. The total number of patient days for the unit was 331. Patients A, B, C and E had sputum cultures during their hospital stay that were positive for *Acinetobacter calcoaceticus*. Patient D had a normal sputum sample on admission, but did not have one collected afterward. Patient D did have a blood culture positive for *A. calcoaceticus* after leaving the unit.

53. In the early stages of the outbreak investigation, the first action the IP should take is:
    a. Notify his/her immediate supervisor of the probable outbreak
    b. Notify the attending physicians of each patient of a probable outbreak
    c. Report the outbreak to the infection prevention and control chair so she/he can support you in closing the unit
    d. Develop a timeline with each patient admission date and culture date graphed

54. While evaluating the culture and sensitivity for each patient, the IP and microbiology director note that all organisms are resistant to the same four antibiotics and Patient A's organism is resistant to two additional antibiotics. Without knowing more information, what might be suspected about Patient A's infection?
    a. Patient A probably has a different organism and source and, therefore, is not part of an outbreak
    b. Four of the patients probably have the same organism in their infection
    c. Transmission of the organism has probably occurred from one patient to each of the other four
    d. Patient A may have developed additional resistance to antibiotics and may be part of the outbreak

55. Which of the following would NOT be done to ascertain which patients might be linked to this potential infection outbreak?
    a. Request sputum be collected for patient D
    b. Request that all isolates be sent for genotyping
    c. Request that all *A. calcoaceticus* isolates be saved
    d. Request that all employees who cared for these patients have nares cultures

56. When searching for possible causes of infection transmission to these patients, one area of initial suspicion should be:
    a. Employees and aseptic technique
    b. Ventilator equipment and therapy devices
    c. Common patient devices: thermometers, blood pressure cuffs, electrode wires, etc.
    d. Ill employees

57. When evaluating the risk factors for pneumonia in these patients, the following characteristics are noted: immunosuppression, trauma and overuse of antibiotics; intubation followed by time spent on the ventilator; elderly; chronic disease; and lack of proper nutrition for an extended period of time. With the information given, which patient probably had the least number of risk factors?
    a. Patient B
    b. Patient D
    c. Patient E
    d. Patient C

58. In February, the employee health nurse complains to you that she has seen five employees lately with scabies. They do not all work on the same unit but have been pulled to various departments during the recent staffing shortages. She wants you to assist in finding the problem before more employees need to be treated. Sources to investigate should include which of the following?
    a. The environment and patients
    b. Other nurses and visitors
    c. Patients and visitors
    d. Other nurses and patients

59. A causal association is
    1. A false association that can be due to chance or bias in study methods
    2. Mixing of effects among exposures, disease and a third factor that is associated with the exposure and independently affects the outcome
    3. When evidence indicates that one factor is clearly shown to increase the probability of occurrence of a disease
    4. Determined through a set of criteria including strength of identification, consistency and biological plausibility
        a. 1 and 2
        b. 2 and 4
        c. 1 and 3
        d. 3 and 4

60. The device utilization rate for a facility that has 600 ventilator days and 3000 patient days is:
    a. 20
    b. 200
    c. 0.2
    d. 5

61. An epidemic curve is an example of a:
    a. Pie chart
    b. Histogram
    c. Frequency polygon
    d. Semi-logarithmic scale line graph

Questions 62–63 Use the following table to answer questions 62–63

	Gold standard positive	Gold standard negative
New test positive	100	3
New test negative	40	500

62. What is the negative predictive value of the above data?
    a. 82.9%
    b. 83.3%
    c. 92.5%
    d. 71.4%

63. What is the positive predictive value of the above data?
    a. 97.0%
    b. 92.5%
    c. 96.2%
    d. 99.4%

64. You are evaluating your control chart and notice that several points in a row are above the mean line. This probably indicates:
    a. The mean is incorrectly calculated
    b. You should investigate potential sources of special cause variation
    c. There is common cause variation in your process, and you should just ignore it for now
    d. You are using the incorrect type of control chart

65. Plague is endemic in parts of the Southwest. The word "endemic" means:
    a. Natives are immune to plague
    b. An expected number of cases occur each year in a given geographical area
    c. Plague has become resistant to all forms of treatment for this population
    d. The disease is seen in a seasonal pattern each year for this area

66. A pandemic differs from an epidemic in that:
    a. Only one disease is involved
    b. It is usually vector borne
    c. There is a higher mortality rate
    d. Several countries or continents are involved

67. Sensitivity may be defined as:
    a. The ability of a test to detect true positives (persons with the disease) when applied to a population with the disease
    b. The ability of a test to detect the true negatives (persons without the disease) when applied to a population without the disease
    c. The ability of a test to detect true positives (persons with disease) when applied to a population without the disease
    d. The percent of persons with true positive results when the test is applied to persons without the disease

68. The IP is called to the hospital day care center for a possible outbreak of hepatitis A. The public health nurse is assisting her in investigating the outbreak. Prophylactic administration of immunoglobulin to the day care workers and noninfected children would be an example of:
    a. Passive immunity
    b. Active immunity
    c. Herd immunity
    d. Nonspecific immunity

69. In a city of 250,000, 2000 persons died during the year, of which 12 died from HIV/AIDS. The crude mortality rate for this city would be:
    a. 8 deaths per 1000 population
    b. 4.8 deaths per 100,000 population
    c. 4.8 deaths per 1000 population
    d. 8 deaths per 100,000 population

70. The IP lives in a community of 100,000 persons. There have been over 1000 cases of hepatitis C with 200 resultant deaths in 1 year. The case fatality rate for this is:
    a. 800 per 1000
    b. 800 per 10,000
    c. 200 per 1000
    d. 200 per 100,000

71. When a test has a higher specificity than sensitivity, it means the test:
    a. Will be more accurate when predicting who is ill
    b. A negative result will be more accurate than a positive
    c. A positive result will be more accurate than a negative
    d. It should only be done as a secondary testing procedure to rule out disease

72. Point-source epidemics usually occur on the basis of transmission by:
    a. A vector
    b. A vehicle
    c. Person-to-person
    d. Droplet infection

CHAPTER TWO: SURVEILLANCE AND EPIDEMIOLOGIC INVESTIGATION | 149

Questions 73–74   In developing a screening test to detect the presence of diabetes, the screening level for a positive blood sugar is set at 160 mg/100 mL in test A and at 120 mg/100 mL in test B.

73. The sensitivity is:
    a. Greater in test A
    b. Greater in test B
    c. Equal in tests A and B
    d. Insufficient information is given

74. The number of false negatives found would be:
    a. Greater in test A
    b. Greater in test B
    c. Equal in tests A and B
    d. Insufficient information is given

75. Incidence rate is defined as:
    a. The number of new cases of a disease divided by the number at risk during a given time and multiplied by a constant
    b. The number of existing cases of a disease in a given time period
    c. The number of new cases of disease in a time period divided by the population at the end of the period
    d. The number of new cases divided by the number of old cases

76. The IP monitors all patients who have CABG for infections and pneumonia. The probability or likelihood of an event occurring is the:
    a. Risk
    b. Attack rate
    c. Host factor
    d. Incidence

77. On a given day, the number of healthcare-associated *Pseudomonas* pneumonias in a 520-bed teaching hospital was seven. The census for that day was 487. The measurement that can be obtained from these data is the:
    a. Attack rate
    b. Prevalence rate
    c. Incidence rate
    d. Relative risk

Questions 78–79 You are the IP in an acute care facility that has five recent heart catheterization site infections. Two patients' catheter sites have cultured *Staphylococcus epidermidis*, one cultured S. aureus, and two cultured S. hominis.

78. You are advised to develop a case-control study to assist in analysis of the problem. A case-control study:
    a. Moves forward from risk factor to disease
    b. First identifies persons with and without disease and then measures degrees of exposure to the risk factor
    c. Follows populations from exposure to risk factor and development of disease
    d. Uses prospective study methods to follow cases of infection that have occurred involving the common risk factor

79. Given the organism information, you might focus on:
    a. A healthcare worker
    b. The technique of the physicians and personnel
    c. The skin prepping procedure and technique
    d. The sensitivity of the organisms to see if they are similar

80. When a study is completed, a report should be written to give the results and evaluation of the study. A good way to display data is by charts or tables. A table is used to illustrate data:
    a. Using only one coordinate
    b. Arranged in rows and columns
    c. Using a system of coordinates
    d. Showing multiple complex factors at one time

81. A characteristic of a good table is that it:
    a. Uses a series of small identifying symbols to represent the data
    b. Compares the magnitude of various events
    c. Is self-explanatory
    d. Presents only raw data

82. The IP plans to show the needle-stick injuries for each department for the year, compared to the previous year. The best type of graph to display this information would be a:
    a. Histogram
    b. Bar chart
    c. Pie chart
    d. Pareto

83. The local health department nurse has asked you to help her develop a graph to display the number of cases of tuberculosis in your state. The trend has been increasing and she wants this to be dramatically shown in the graph. The best graph for this would be a:
    a. Frequency polygon
    b. Bar chart
    c. Histogram
    d. Normal distribution

84. Specificity of a test for infection or disease is defined as:
    a. The number of true negatives divided by the number of positives found, times 100
    b. The number of true negatives divided by the total number of persons with disease, times 100
    c. The number of true positives divided by the total number of persons with disease, times 100
    d. The number of true negatives divided by the total number of persons without disease, times 100

85. Ten per every 100 patients admitted to the oncology unit develop *Candida* infections. The number of *Candida* infections in the total hospital population is 2 for every 100 admissions. The comparison of these events, noted as 5:1, is known as the:
    a. Attack rate
    b. Ratio
    c. Prevalence
    d. Frequency

86. A measure of dispersion that reflects the variability in values around the mean is called the:
    a. Variance
    b. Standard deviation
    c. Range
    d. Bell curve

87. A p value expressed as p <.01 indicates:
    a. The possibility of these results occurring by chance alone is so small; therefore, the result is not significant
    b. The possibility of these results occurring by chance alone is less than 1 in 100 and, therefore, significant enough to prove causality
    c. The null hypothesis should be rejected and the alternative hypothesis should be accepted
    d. The null hypothesis should be accepted

88. Which of the following statements about testing for statistical significance is true?
    a. A p value of .05 means that the probability that the observation occurred by chance alone is 1 in 20
    b. A p value of .05 increases the likelihood of making a type 2 error
    c. The size of the p value indicates the power of the results
    d. The research hypothesis is the basis of significance

89. The median for the following set of values (7, 12, 6, 9, 15, 11) is:
    a. 11
    b. 10
    c. 9
    d. 13

90. The "epidemiological triangle" model for disease causation does NOT include:
    a. Agent
    b. Host
    c. Time
    d. Environment

91. The critical care classes have 48 new students. There are eight male students. The ratio of female to male students is:
    a. 1:5
    b. 5:1
    c. 6:1
    d. 1:6

CHAPTER TWO: SURVEILLANCE AND EPIDEMIOLOGIC INVESTIGATION | 153

Questions 92–93 During the month of January, there were three cases of pneumonia in the neurological intensive care unit. All three were there during the first week and part of the second week of the month. A total of 25 patients were discharged from the unit that month. During February, there were four cases of pneumonia and 20 discharges.

92. What was the prevalence rate for the first week in January per 100 patients?
   a. 120/100 patients
   b. 12/100 patients
   c. 83/100 patients
   d. There are insufficient data to calculate a prevalence rate

93. What was the attack rate for the months of January and February?
   a. 15.5%
   b. 16%
   c. 18%
   d. There are insufficient data to calculate an attack rate

94. If a factor and a disease appear to be related only because of a common underlying condition, but the association disappears when the condition is controlled, the association is:
   a. Indirect
   b. Causal
   c. Spurious
   d. Direct

95. You have identified a cluster of *Candida* bloodstream infections in two adjoining ICUs. You want to look at risk factors that these patients may have had in common. Which study design would you use?
   a. Cross-section study
   b. Cohort study
   c. Case-control study
   d. Clinical trial

96. In using statistical data, it is important to remember that:
   a. Statistical data can be used to disprove the null hypothesis and prove your hypothesis
   b. Statistical data cannot be used to prove an association, only suggest that it exists
   c. Conclusions can be accepted as clinically significant
   d. Conclusions can be accepted as scientific validation of your research methods

97. To determine the attack rate for a defined population, divide the number of new cases of disease for a specified time period by the population at risk for the same time period and multiply by:
    a. 1000
    b. 100
    c. 100,000
    d. Either 100 or 1000 can be used

98. A frequency polygon:
    (1) Is useful for showing two sets of data on a single graph
    (2) Uses bars
    (3) Uses lines and points
    (4) Uses a histogram
    (5) Can show two, three or four sets of data on a single graph
        a. 1, 3, 4
        b. 2, 3, 5
        c. 3, 4, 5
        d. 1, 2, 3

Questions 99–103 You are conducting a prevalence survey on an intensive care unit that has a census of 10 at midnight. You examine all 10 charts between 6 am and 9 am. At 9:30 pm, there is one admission. At 10 am, two additional patients are admitted to the unit. At 11 am, three patients are transferred to a medical-surgical unit. At 3 pm, there is a death resulting from pneumonia. During your survey, you find two urinary tract infections, one pneumonia and one wound infection. All infections are considered healthcare-associated, except the pneumonia.

99. What denominator should be used when computing prevalence?
    a. 10
    b. 11
    c. 13
    d. 9

100. What is the attack rate for urinary tract infections?
    a. 20%
    b. 10%
    c. 10
    d. There are insufficient data to calculate an attack rate

101. What is the prevalence for urinary tract infections in this survey per 1000 patients?
    a. 20
    b. 200
    c. 100
    d. 10

102. What is the overall prevalence of hospital-associated infections per 1000 patients in your survey?
    a. 300
    b. 30
    c. 3%
    d. 33.3%

103. What was the mortality rate from hospital-associated infections per 1000 patients in this survey?
    a. 10%
    b. 100
    c. 0
    d. 10

104. What type of surveillance is the monitoring of bloodstream infection rates?
    a. Outcome surveillance
    b. Mandatory reporting
    c. Process surveillance
    d. Combined surveillance

105. In July, there were six surgical site infections among 120 patients undergoing vascular bypass surgery to the femoral, popliteal or iliac arteries. What was the vascular surgical site infection attack rate for July?
    a. 3%
    b. 4%
    c. 5%
    d. 20%

106. Analysis of quantitative research may be used to:
    a. Suggest an association
    b. Prove causality
    c. Establish a numerical basis of proof
    d. Prove similarities among groups

107. You are interested in the different types of persons who come to the emergency room for treatment of STDs. You have noticed that there are a number of young people who are treated in late December and early June. You theorize they are college students who are at home during semester breaks. What type of study would you perform to develop a description of this population?
    a. Experimental
    b. Case-control
    c. Community trial
    d. Ethnographic

108. An outbreak of RSV occurs in the pediatric unit. You start a descriptive study of the patient and employee population. An example of a descriptive study is a study that:
    a. Proves causality
    b. Includes cohort studies and case-control studies
    c. Characterizes populations by time, person and place
    d. Includes only prevalence

109. When conducting surgical site infection surveillance, all of the following should be performed EXCEPT:
    a. Maintain strict security with surgeon-specific infection rates
    b. Each chart should be reviewed closely for demographics and signs of infection
    c. A printout of patients with discharge coding for surgical site infections can begin the chart investigation process
    d. All positive wound cultures should be investigated and counted as probable surgical site infections

110. The IP classifies surgical site infections by the CDC definitions used for the NHSN system. The criteria for an organ/space infection includes:
    1. Purulent drainage from subcutaneous tissue surrounding the incision
    2. Purulent drainage from a drain that is placed in a stab wound
    3. An abscess found on radiological examination
    4. The incision is packed open with fluff gauze until the wound can heal from the inside out
    5. Purulent drainage is noted coming from the incision after the second surgery in a week
        a. 1, 2, 3
        b. 2, 3
        c. 4, 5
        d. 2, 3, 4

111. You receive an incident report that states a pediatric nurse received an exposure. The report is incomplete. It states the nurse was scratched by a "needle" in a patient's room, while she was spiking an IV bag. You cannot tell at what point the exposure occurred or type of "needle" involved. Your first action should be:
    a. Determine if the source patient is infectious or high risk for blood-borne infectious diseases
    b. Determine if a blood or body fluid exposure actually occurred
    c. Determine who the source patient was and what his/her medical diagnosis was
    d. Determine if correct personal protective equipment was used or improper technique used

112. The qualitative research process can be used to:
    a. Study events that occur infrequently
    b. Study people's perceptions and experiences
    c. Establish incidence and prevalence rates
    d. Identify cases during an outbreak investigation

113. The IP is training a new surveillance nurse. He explains why the facility uses priority-directed surveillance. The main advantage of this type of surveillance is:
    a. The IP has an overall knowledge of the infections that are occurring on each unit
    b. The IP focuses on specific problems or procedures in order to perform a more in-depth study
    c. It allows identification of a cluster of infections before a true outbreak condition exists
    d. It gives the IP more time to perform other duties of the job (e.g., staff education, policy and procedure development or product management)

114. The purpose of a post-discharge surgical surveillance program is to:
    a. Obtain a more accurate picture of the number of surgical site infections
    b. Promote customer relations with the surgical patients
    c. Conduct a performance improvement project that fulfills the requirements of the facility
    d. Perform a valuable research project

115. An experimental study design includes all of the following characteristics EXCEPT:
    a. It is a prospective study
    b. Experimental design helps to prove causation
    c. The researcher manipulates one or more variables
    d. The experimental design often uses the technique of double blinding

116. Surgeon-specific wound infection rates should include:
    a. Stratification by risk factors
    b. Small denominators
    c. Interhospital comparison
    d. Intrahospital comparison

117. You are an infection prevention practitioner at an outpatient surgery center. You are developing the surveillance plan for the center. Which of the following should you take into consideration?
    1. The state laws regarding required surgical site infection rate reporting
    2. The risks associated with the specialized population your center serves
    3. The concerns brought to you regarding the prepping technique of one of the operative nurses
    4. The risks associated with the new surgical technique one of your surgeons is using
        a. 1 and 2
        b. 1 and 4
        c. 1, 2 and 3
        d. 1, 2 and 4

118. Which of the following indicates a strong positive correlation?
    a. $r = 0$
    b. $r = -0.793$
    c. $r = 0.913$
    d. $r = 0.45$

119. The range of the correlation coefficient is?
    a. -1 to 0
    b. 0 to 1
    c. -1 to 1
    d. None of the above

120. Which of the following is not a criterion for mediastinitis?
    a. Patient has organisms cultured from mediastinal tissue or fluid obtained during a surgical operation
    b. Physician diagnoses mediastinitis on the patient's discharge summary
    c. Patient has evidence of mediastinitis seen on surgical operation
    d. Patient has chest pain and purulent discharge from the mediastinal area

Answers for Practice Questions Chapter Two

#		#		#		#	
1.	c	31.	c	61.	b	91.	b
2.	c	32.	c	62.	c	92.	d
3.	c	33.	a	63.	a	93.	a
4.	b	34.	a	64.	b	94.	a
5.	d	35.	c	65.	b	95.	c
6	c	36.	d	66.	d	96.	b
7.	a	37.	b	67.	a	97.	b
8.	d	38.	d	68.	a	98.	a
9.	c	39.	a	69.	a	99.	a
10.	c	40.	a	70.	c	100.	d
11.	d	41.	c	71.	b	101.	b
12.	c	42.	d	72.	b	102.	a
13.	d	43.	c	73.	a	103.	c
14.	a	44.	c	74.	a	104.	a
15.	d	45.	a	75.	a	105.	c
16.	b	46.	c	76.	a	106.	a
17.	d	47.	d	77.	b	107.	d
18.	d	48.	d	78.	b	108.	c
19.	b	49.	c	79.	c	109.	d
20.	a	50.	b	80.	b	110.	b
21.	a	51.	c	81.	c	111.	b
22.	d	52.	c	82.	b	112.	b
23.	a	53.	d	83.	c	113.	b
24.	c	54.	d	84.	d	114.	a
25.	a	55.	d	85.	b	115.	b
26.	a	56.	b	86.	b	116.	a
27.	a	57.	c	87.	c	117.	d
28.	c	58.	d	88.	a	118	c
29.	c	59.	d	89.	b	119.	c
30.	d.	60.	c	90.	c	120.	b

References

1. A Dictionary of Nursing. 2008. Retrieved January 14, 2011, from Encyclopedia.com: http://www.encyclopedia.com/doc/1O62-quantitativeresearch.html.

2. Scheckler, WE, Brimhall D, Buck AS, et al. Requirements for infrastructure and essential activities of infection control and epidemiology in hospitals: a consensus panel report. *Am J Infect Control* 1998;26:47–60.

3. Freidman C, Narnette M, Buck, AS et al. Requirements of infrastructure and essential activities of infection control and epidemiology in out-of-hospital settings: a consensus panel report. *Am J Infect Control* 1999;27:418–430.

4. Centers for Disease Control and Prevention. National Healthcare Safety Network (NHSN) Report, data summary for 2006 through 2008, issued December 2009. *Am J Infect Control* 2009;37:783–805.

5. Gaynes RP, Culver DH, Emori TG, et al. The National Nosocomial Infections Surveillance System: plans for the 1990s and beyond. *Am J Med* 1991;91 (Suppl 3B):116–120.

6. Emori TG, Culver DH, Horan TC, et al. National Nosocomial Infections Surveillance System (NNIS): description of surveillance methods. *Am J Infect Control* 1991;19:19–35.

7. Tokars JL, Miller ER, Stein G. New national surveillance system for hemodialysis-associated infections: initial results. *Am J Infect Control* 2002;30:288–295.

8. Klevens RM, Edwards JR, Andrus ML, et al. NHSN participants in outpatient dialysis surveillance. Dialysis surveillance report: National Healthcare Safety Network (NHSN)- data summary for 2006. *Semin Dial* 2008;21(1):24–28.

9. Friedman C, Barnette M, Buck AS, et al. Requirements for infrastructure and essential activities of infection control and epidemiology in out-of-hospital settings: a consensus panel report. *Am J Infect Control* 1999;27:418–430.

10. Lee TB, Baker OG, Lee JT, et al. APIC Surveillance Initiative Working. Recommended practices for surveillance: Association for Professionals in Infection Control and Epidemiology (APIC), Inc. *Am J Infect Control* 2007;35:427–440.

11. Horan TC, Gaynes RP, Martone WJ, et al. CDC definitions of nosocomial surgical site infections, 1992: a modification of CDC definitions of surgical site infections. *Infect Control Hosp Epidemiol* 1992;13:606–608.

12. Garener JS, Jarvis WR, Emori TG, et al. CDC definitions for nosocomial infections. *Am J Infect Control* 1988;16:128–140.

13. McGeer A, Campbell B, Emori TG, et al. Definitions of infection for surveillance in long-term facilities. *Am J Infect Control* 1991;19:1–7.

14. Lenz S, Myers S, Nordlund S, et al. Benchmarking: finding ways to improve. *Jt Comm J Qual Improv* 1994;20:250–259.

15. Horan TC, Andrus M, Dudeck MA. CDC/NHSN surveillance definition of health care-associated infection and criteria for specific types of infections in the acute care setting. *Am J Infect Control* 2008;36:309–332.

CHAPTER THREE

PREVENTING/CONTROLLING THE TRANSMISSION OF INFECTIOUS AGENTS

CONTENTS

Article	Page
CBIC Content Outline for Preventing/Controlling the Transmission of Infectious Agents	164
Chapter Three: Preventing/Controlling the Transmission of Infectious Agents	165
I. Policy Review	165
II. Disasters and Biological Events	165
III. Hand Hygiene	170
IV. Cleaning, Disinfection and Sterilization	172
V. Specific Care Settings	185
VI. Therapeutic and Diagnostic Procedures and Devices	189
VII. Recalls	195
VIII. Isolation Precautions	196
IX. Environmental Hazards	198
X. Immunization of Patients	200
XI. Construction and Renovation	200
XII. Prevention of Transmission of Tuberculosis	204
XIII. Prevention of Blood-Borne Pathogens (BBP) in Dialysis Units	205
XIV. Elimination of *Clostridium difficile*	207
XV. Prevention and Control of MDROs in Healthcare Settings	208
Practice Questions for Chapter Three	210
References	236

CBIC CONTENT OUTLINE

Preventing/Controlling the Transmission of Infectious Agents (39 Questions)

A. Develop and review infection prevention and control policies and procedures

B. Collaborate with public health agencies in planning community responses to biological agents (e.g., anthrax, influenza)

C. Identify and implement infection prevention and control strategies related to:

1. Hand hygiene
2. Cleaning, disinfection and sterilization
3. Specific direct and indirect care settings (e.g., patient care units, respiratory therapy, operating room, ambulatory care center)
4. Infection risks associated with therapeutic and diagnostic procedures and devices (e.g., intravascular devices, urinary drainage catheter, bronchoscopy, angiography, dialysis, angiography)
5. Recall of potentially contaminated equipment and supplies
6. Initiation and discontinuation of isolation/barrier precautions when indicated
7. Patient placement, transfer and discharge
8. Environmental hazards
9. Use of patient care products and medical equipment
10. Immunization programs for patients
11. Construction and renovation in patient care settings
12. The influx of patients with communicable diseases (e.g., bioterrorism, emerging infectious disease)

Chapter Three: Preventing/Controlling the Transmission of Infectious Agents

I. **Policy Review**

   A. Infection Preventionists (IPs) are responsible for the development and review of infection prevention and control guidelines and policies
   B. Formulation of policies and procedures to control infections should be based on data generated by surveillance and other sources
   C. Professional and practice standards have been defined by APIC[1-3] and should be incorporated into policies. The standards encompass various practice settings and include key indicators to be used in evaluating practice. Three principle goals are described:
      1. Protect the patient
      2. Protect the healthcare worker, visitors and others in the healthcare environment
      3. Accomplish the previous two goals in a cost-effective manner whenever possible
   D. The Healthcare Infection Control Practices Advisory Committee (HICPAC) provides periodic updates of guidelines and other policy statements regarding prevention of healthcare-associated infections (HAIs)
   E. The Centers for Medicare and Medicaid Services (CMS) requires that facilities follow nationally recognized practices and guidelines to prevent HAIs[4]
   F. The Joint Commission (TJC) also publishes infection prevention and control standards, which may be used to establish a framework for an infection prevention program; standards state that the goal is to identify and reduce the risk of infections in patients and healthcare workers. New infection prevention standards in TJC's Standards Improvement Initiative of 2009 includes hand hygiene, sentinel events, prevention of HAIs by multidrug-resistant organisms, central line–associated bloodstream infections and surgical site infections[5]
   G. Written infection prevention policies usually relate to staff and patient-care practices, construction/renovation, disaster planning, employee health and sterilization/disinfection. General polices are applicable to staff in the whole facility and may form the basis of an infection prevention manual. Specific policies may also be developed for each unit/area
   H. Policies must be supported scientifically and address infection prevention needs for the institution

II. **Disasters and Biological Events**

   A. **Definitions**
      1. Bioterrorism: Intentional use of a biological agent or derivative of an agent to inflict harm or death

a. Characteristics of these organisms include:
     (1) Ability to be dispersed in aerosols, which can penetrate the distal bronchioles
     (2) Ability to deliver the aerosols with simple technology
     (3) Feasibility of the agents to infect large numbers of people
     (4) Ability to spread infection, disease, panic or fear[6]
  2. Emerging infections: Infections that are new to a population/geographical region or have increased rapidly
  3. Pandemics: Global outbreaks of disease in humans that exceed expected rates or morbidity/mortality
     a. Six phases:
        (1) Low risk for human cases
        (2) Higher risk for human cases
        (3) No or very limited human-to-human transmission
        (4) Evidence of increased human-to-human transmission
        (5) Evidence of significant human-to-human transmission
        (6) Efficient and sustained human-to-human transmission[7]

B. Preparedness for Biological Events

  1. Collaborate with public health agencies in planning community response to biological agents:
     a. Assessment for hazards and vulnerabilities
     b. Development of an emergency management plan (should address all types of hazards)
     c. Identification of an infectious disease (ID) disaster
     d. Rapid response will often decrease morbidity and mortality
     e. Syndromic surveillance (collection and analysis of syndrome-related data) may be more helpful than traditional active surveillance
     f. Even one case of an unusual disease should be investigated
     g. Vulnerable populations are at higher risk for morbidity and mortality, should be a focus of the preparedness plan
        (1) Pediatrics
        (2) Elderly
        (3) Immunocompromised
        (4) Pregnancy
     h. Educate responding individuals/agencies on the plan
     i. Practice the plan
     j. Evaluate the facility's level of preparedness

C. Mitigation/Infection Prevention Procedures

1. Epidemiological investigation
   a. Follows similar principles to outbreak investigation
   b. Bioterrorism agent identification, as well as the date and location of the release, are key
2. Reporting
   a. Immediately report single cases of unusual disease or syndrome clusters to local health department
   b. If after hours, use emergency numbers
   c. Phone trees should be in place for notification and education with the healthcare facility
3. Triage—quickly identify individuals who need treatment, separate contagious individuals
4. Administer anti-infective therapy, prophylaxis or vaccination
5. Quarantine—separation of individuals who are not yet symptomatic but have been exposed to a contagious person; can be home-based or work-based
6. Surge capacity—plan for a 40% absenteeism rate by:
   a. Having backup contracts for extra staff
   b. Providing incentives to get and keep staff
   c. Prioritizing healthcare workers and their family for treatment, prophylaxis
   d. Cohorting patients to decrease workload
   e. Cohorting staff to patients based on shared illnesses
   f. Cross-training staff
7. Decontamination—most infectious disease disasters will not require patient decontamination
8. Postmortem care—autopsies should be performed using standard precautions

D. Potential Bioterrorism Agents

1. Category A: High-priority agents include organisms that pose a risk to national security because they:
   a. Can be easily disseminated or transmitted from person to person
   b. Result in high mortality rates and have the potential for major public health impact
   c. Might cause public panic and social disruption
   d. Require special action for public health preparedness.
      (1)
         (a) Anthrax
         (b) Botulism
         (c) Plague

(d) Smallpox
(e) Tularemia
(f) Viral hemorrhagic fevers
2. Category B: Second highest priority agents include those that:
    a. Are moderately easy to disseminate
    b. Result in moderate morbidity rates and low mortality rates
    c. Require specific enhancements of CDC's diagnostic capacity and enhanced disease surveillance
        (1)
            (a) Brucellosis
            (b) *Clostridium perfringens* infection
            (c) Food safety threats
            (d) Glanders
            (e) Melioidosis
            (f) Psittacosis
            (g) Q fever
            (h) Ricin toxin
            (i) Staphylococcal enterotoxin B
            (j) Typhus fever
            (k) Viral encephalitis
            (l) Water safety threats
3. Category C: Third highest priority agents include emerging pathogens that could be engineered for mass dissemination in the future because of:
    a. Availability
    b. Ease of production and dissemination
    c. Potential for high morbidity and mortality rates and major health impact
        (1) Emerging infectious diseases such as Nipah virus and hantavirus

E. Agent-Specific Information

1. Most agents of bioterrorism are not transmitted person-to-person (with exception of smallpox and pneumonic plague)
2. Use Standard Precautions with all plus specific additional precautions
    a. Anthrax
        (1) No person-to-person transmission
        (2) Standard Precautions
        (3) After invasive procedures or autopsy, instruments and area should be thoroughly disinfected
        (4) Exposure to powder or dust confirmed to be anthrax spores requires treatment with antibiotics for 6 weeks or more

(5) Nonconfirmed exposures to powder should not be treated or tested until source of exposure is confirmed to be anthrax
b. Plague
   (1) Transmission by droplet (person-to-person)
   (2) Use Standard Precautions plus Droplet Precautions until 72 hours of appropriate antibiotics are started and improvement in patient's condition is seen
   (3) Mask worn within 3 feet of patient, limit transportation
   (4) Private room or cohort patients
   (5) Transmission can occur from skin lesions; use scrupulous hand hygiene
c. Tularemia
   (1) No person-to-person transmission
   (2) Standard Precautions
   (3) Laboratory personnel—wear masks with eye protection, surgical gloves, protective gowns, and show covers when working with pure bacterial cultures
   (4) Blood cultures should be in closed system—biosafety level
d. Q fever
   (1) Transmission person-to-person is very rare
   (2) Standard Precautions
e. Brucella
   (1) Person-to-person transmission by contact with draining lesions, tissue transplantation and sexual contact
   (2) Standard Precautions
   (3) Appropriate personal protective equipment when caring for patients with draining lesions
f. Smallpox
   (1) Transmissible person-to-person by respiratory secretions, aerosols, contact with pox lesions and fomites
   (2) Use Airborne and Contact Precautions
   (3) Use negative pressure room with N95 respirators
   (4) Limit transportation of patient outside of room
   (5) Wear gloves anytime entering the room; remove before leaving, then wash hands immediately with antimicrobial or waterless antiseptic
   (6) Wear gown when entering room and remove before leaving
   (7) Dedicate equipment or thoroughly disinfect before removing
   (8) Use Airborne and Contact Precautions during autopsy and all postmortem examinations (notify mortician)
   (9) Patient is infectious until all scabs have separated

g. Viral encephalitis—Venezuelan equine encephalitis, eastern equine encephalitis, western equine encephalitis
  (1) No person-to-person transmission documented
  (2) Standard Precautions
  (3) Transmission by inhalation or via mosquitoes
h. Botulism
  (1) No person-to-person transmission
  (2) Standard Precautions
i. Staphylococcal enterotoxin B
  (1) No person-to-person transmission
  (2) Standard Precautions
j. Ricin
  (1) No person-to-person
  (2) Standard Precautions
k. Viral hemorrhagic fever
  (1) Person-to-person transmission by inhalation of aerosols or percutaneous injury
  (2) Standard Precautions with Contact Precautions plus mask with eye protection when risk for aerosols or splash is present
  (3) Use Standard Precautions plus mask with eye protection, gown, surgical gloves, etc., during postmortem examinations and autopsy (notify mortician)
l. Cholera
  (1) Transmission by ingestion (contamination from stools)
  (2) Standard Precautions
m. Glanders
  (1) Transmission by inhalation and contact
  (2) Standard Precautions

III. Hand Hygiene

A. Definitions

1. Alcohol-based hand rub—solution containing 60% to 95% alcohol designed to be applied to hands to reduce number of viable microorganisms
2. Antimicrobial soap—contains an antiseptic agent to reduce number of microbial flora
3. Hand antisepsis is either:
   a. Antiseptic hand wash—washing hands with water and antiseptic soap
   b. Antiseptic hand rub—applying antiseptic hand rub to all surfaces of hands without rinsing
4. Hand hygiene includes hand antisepsis and plain lotion soap and water hand-washing

B. **Routine Handwashing and Hand Antisepsis**
1. Product selection
   a. Provision of alcohol-based rubs, as well as sinks with antimicrobial soap, is required in areas with high workloads and high intensity of patient care
   b. Antimicrobial-impregnated wipes are not a substitute for hand antisepsis[8]
   c. Hand lotions or creams should be provided to combat hand skin dryness
2. Dispenser location
   a. Alcohol-based rubs should be at the entrances to patient, examination and treatment rooms; may also be found near bedside or carried in healthcare workers' pockets
   b. Dispensers should not be installed over electrical receptacles or near other potential sources of ignition[9]
   c. Bulk alcohol-based rub supplies should be stored in areas approved for fire safety
3. Indications for hand hygiene
   a. Soap and water handwashing
      (1) If hands are visibly soiled
      (2) Before eating
      (3) After using the restroom
      (4) If exposure to spore-forming organisms
   b. Alcohol-based hand rub
      (1) Before and after direct patient care
      (2) Before donning sterile gloves
      (3) Before inserting invasive devices
      (4) After contact with patient's intact skin
      (5) After removing gloves
      (6) After contact with objects/equipment in patient's vicinity
      (7) When moving from a contaminated body site to a clean site during patient care
4. Technique
   a. Alcohol-based hand rub
      (1) Use manufacturer recommended amount
      (2) Rub all areas of hand surfaces together until dry (15 to 20 seconds)
   b. Soap and water
      (1) Wet hands
      (2) Apply product per manufacturer recommendations
      (3) Rub hands together vigorously, covering all surfaces for at least 15 seconds
      (4) Rinse hands thoroughly
      (5) Dry hands with disposable towel
      (6) Turn off water faucet

C. Surgical Hand Antisepsis

1. Product selection
   a. Antimicrobial soap or alcohol-based hand rub with persistent activity
   b. Order of effectiveness with immediately lowering bacterial counts—alcohol, chlorhexidine gluconate (CHG), iodophors, triclosan, plain soap
   c. Order of effectiveness with persistent antimicrobial activity—CHG, triclosan, iodophors
   d. Combination formulations of alcohol and CHG exceed persistence of alcohol alone
2. Technique
   a. Hand and arm jewelry should be removed
   b. Debris should be removed from under fingernails under running water
   c. Antimicrobial soap and water—hands and forearms should be scrubbed for manufacturer recommended length of time (longer times are not necessary and may lead to dermatitis)
   d. Alcohol-based surgical hand rub—hands and forearms should be prewashed with plain lotion soap and dried; follow manufacture recommendations for product use; allow hands and forearms to dry completely before donning sterile gloves

D. Staff Education and Effective Interventions

1. Provide evidence-based information
2. Multimodal, multidisciplinary strategies may be necessary to improve hand hygiene[10,11]
3. Monitoring for adherence
   a. Centers for Disease Control and Prevention (CDC) and TJC require that healthcare workers' adherence to hand hygiene policies be monitored and feedback provided through:
      (1) Direct observations
      (2) Volume of hand hygiene products used
      (3) Adherence to artificial fingernail policies

IV. Cleaning, Disinfection and Sterilization

A. Definitions

1. Cleaning—removal of all visible dust, soil, and any other foreign material
2. Sanitizing—reduction in microbial population on an inanimate object to a safe or relatively safe level
3. Decontamination—process of removing disease-producing microorganisms and rendering the object safe for handling

4. Disinfection—elimination of many or all pathogenic organisms with the exception of bacterial spores
5. Sterilization—complete elimination, destruction of all microbial life

B. Spaulding Classification System[12]

1. Critical items—involve a high risk for infection if contaminated with microorganism (e.g., surgical instruments, cardiac and urinary catheters, implants, etc.)
    a. Enter sterile tissue or the vascular system
    b. Item should be purchased sterile or be sterilized by steam sterilization if possible
        (1) If heat sensitive, may be treated with ethylene oxide (ETO), with hydrogen peroxide gas plasma or with liquid chemical sterilants if other methods unsuitable (however, liquid sterilization requires that items be cleaned first, may not be wrapped during processing (hard to maintain sterility post-sterilization) and frequently need to be rinsed afterward
2. Semicritical items
    a. Those that will contact mucous membranes or nonintact skin (e.g., respiratory or anesthesia equipment, some endoscopes, etc.)
    b. Should be free of all vegetative microorganisms, but small numbers of spores may be present
    c. Items require high level disinfection using chemical disinfectants
    d. If items contact mucous membranes of respiratory tract or gastrointestinal tract they should be rinsed with water followed by an alcohol rinse; items should be dried and stored in a manner that protects them from contamination or damage[12-14]
3. Noncritical items
    a. Contact intact skin but not mucous membranes
    b. Require intermediate-level and low-level disinfection

C. Methods of Disinfection and Sterilizations

1. Sterilization
    a. Destroys all microorganisms, including spores
    b. Types
        (1) High—steam
        (2) Low—ethylene oxide
        (3) Liquid immersion—chemical sterilants
    c. Advantages and disadvantages of several methods to sterilize patient care items are listed in Tables 3–1 and 3–2.

Table 3-1 Summary of Advantages and Disadvatages of Chemical Agents Used as Chemical Sterilants or as High-level Disinfectants

Sterilization Method	Advantages	Disadvantages
Peracetic acid/Hydrogen Peroxide	• No activation necessary • Odor or irritation not significant	• Material compatibility concerns (lead, brass, copper, zinc) • Limited clinical experience • Potential for eye/skin damage
Glutaraldehyde	• Numerous use studies published • Relatively inexpensive • Excellent material compatibility	• Respiratory irritation from vapor • Pungent/irritating odor • Slow mycobactericidal activity • Coagulates blood/ fixes tissues to surfaces • Allergic contact dermatitis • Vapor monitoring recommended
Hydrogen Peroxide	• No activation necessary • Enhanced removal of organic material/organisms • No disposal issues • No odor/irritation • Does not coagulate blood/fix tissues to surfaces • Inactivates *Cryptosporidium* • Use studies published	• Material compatibility concerns (brass, zinc, copper, nickel/silver plating) • Serious eye damage with contact
Orthophthalaldehyde (OPA)	• Fast-acting high level disinfectant • No activation necessary • Odor not significant • Excellent materials compatibility claimed • Does not coagulate blood/fix tissues to surfaces	• Stains skin, mucous membranes, clothing and environmental surfaces • Repeated exposure may cause hypersensitivity in some patients with bladder cancer • More expensive than glutaraldehyde • Eye irritation with contact • Slow sporicidal activity
Peracetic Acid	• Rapid sterilization cycle time (30-45 min) • Low temperature (50°-55°C) liquid immersion sterilization • Environmentally friendly by-products • Fully automated • Single-use system • Standardized cycle • Enhances removal of organic material & endotoxin	• Potential material incompatibility • Used for immersible instruments only • Biological indicators may not be suitable for routine monitoring • One scope or small number of instruments can be processed in one cycle • More expensive than high-level disinfection • Serious eye and skin damage with contact • Point of-use system, not sterile storage

Table 3-1 Summary of Advantages and Disadvatages of Chemical Agents Used as Chemical Sterilants or as High-level Disinfectants *(continued)*

Sterilization Method	Advantages	Disadvantages
	• No adverse health effects • Compatible with many materials/instruments • Does not coagulate blood/fix tissues to surfaces • Rapidly sporicidal • Provides procedure standardization	

Source: APIC Text of Infection Control and Epidemiology 2009, adapted from Rutala WA, Weber DJ. Disinfection of endoscopes: review of new chemical sterilants used for high-level disinfection. *Infect Control Hosp Epidemiol* 1999;20:69–76.

Table 3-2 Summary of Advantages and Disadvantages of Commonly Used Sterilization Technologies

Sterilization Method	Advantages	Disadvantages
Steam	• Nontoxic • Cycle easy to control, monitor • Rapidly microbicidal • Least affected by organic/inorganic soils • Rapid cycle time • Penetrates medical packaging, device lumens	• Deleterious for heat-sensitive instruments • Microsurgical instruments damaged by repeat exposures • May leave instruments wet, resulting in rust • Potential for burns
Hydrogen Peroxide Gas Plasma	• Safe for environment • No toxic residues • Cycle time 28-73 min, no aeration needed • Used for heat and moisture sensitive items • Simple to operate, install, monitor • Compatible with most medical devices • Only requires electrical outlet	• Cellulose (paper), linens, liquids cannot be processed • Large sterilization chamber size • Some endoscopes/devices with long/narrow lumens cannot be processed • Requires synthetic wrapping, special container tray • May be toxic

Table 3-2 Summary of Advantages and Disadvantages of Commonly Used Sterilization Technologies *(continued)*

Sterilization Method	Advantages	Disadvantages
100% Ethylene Oxide (ETO)	• Penetrates packaging materials, device lumens • Minimizes potential of gas leak and ETO exposure • Simple to operate, monitor • Compatible with most medical materials	• Requires aeration time • Large sterilization chamber • ETO is toxic, a carcinogen and flammable • ETO emissions regulated by states • ETO cartridges must be stored in flammable liquid storage cabinet • Lengthy cycle/aeration cycle
ETO Mixtures	Penetrates medical packaging and many plastics Compatible with most materials Cycle easy to control, monitor	• Some states require ETO emission reductions • Potential hazards to staff, patients • Lengthy cycle/aeration time • ETO is toxic, a carcinogen and flammable
Paracetic Acid	• Rapid cycle time (30-45min) • Low temperature (50°-55°C) liquid immersion sterilization • Environmentally friendly by-products	• Potential material incompatibility • Used for immersible instruments only • Biological indicators may not be suitable for routine monitoring • One scope or small number of instruments can be processed in one cycle • Serious eye and skin damage with contact • Point of-use system, no sterile storage

Source: APIC Text of Infection Control and Epidemiology 2009, adapted from Rutala WA, Weber DJ. Disinfection of endoscopes: review of new chemical sterilants used for high-level disinfection. *Infect Control Hosp Epidemiol* 1999;20:69–76.

2. High-level disinfection
   a. Destroys all microorganisms, except high number of spores
   b. Types
      (1) Heat-automated—pasteurization
      (2) Includes aldehydes, hydrogen peroxide, peracetic acid
3. Intermediate-level disinfection
   a. Destroys vegetative bacteria, mycobacteria, most viruses, most fungi, not spores
   b. Includes phenolics, alcohols, iodophors
4. Low-level disinfection
   a. Destroys most vegetative bacteria, some fungi and viruses, not mycobacteria or spores
   b. Includes quaternary (quats) ammonia products

D. **Principles of Sterilization of Equipment and Supplies**
   1. Factors that affect sterilization process
      a. Duration of exposure: Time—sterilization parameters must be met and maintained for a specific length of time to kill microorganisms
      b. Number and location of microorganisms—the more organisms, the more time a germicide needs to destroy them all; medical instruments with multiple pieces, joints, crevices and channels are more difficult to disinfect
      c. Innate resistance of microorganisms—microorganisms vary in their resistance to germicides and sterilization processes
         (1) Group A—vegetative bacterial cells, fungi, and lipophilic viruses; easiest to kill
         (2) Group B—tubercle bacilli and hydrophilic viruses; more difficult to kill
         (3) Group C—includes bacterial spores (e.g., *Bacillus* spp., *Clostridium* spp.); destruction of spores requires high concentrations and long contact times for most (sporicidal) disinfectants
      d. Concentration and potency of disinfectants: Generally, the more concentrated the disinfectant, the greater its efficacy and the shorter time needed to achieve microbial kill (exception is iodophors)
      e. Physical and chemical factors—temperature, pH, relative humidity and water hardness influence disinfectant procedures
      f. Organic and inorganic matter—interfere with antimicrobial activity of disinfectants
      g. Biofilms—thick masses of cells and extracellular materials that may protect microorganisms from disinfectants
   2. Methods of sterilization
      a. Thermal (heat)
         (1) Moist heat (steam)
         (2) Dry heat (hot-air oven)
      b. Chemical
         (1) Ethylene oxide
         (2) Liquid chemicals (e.g., glutaraldehyde)
         (3) Vaporized hydrogen peroxide
         (4) Plasma sterilization
         (5) Peracetic acid
         (6) Ozone
         (7) Radiation
   3. Steam sterilization
      a. Parameters of steam sterilization
         (1) Pressure—directed into a closed chamber
         (2) Temperature—must reach a specific level to ensure killing the microorganisms (two common temperatures are 250°F (121°C) and 272°F (133°C)

(3) Time—specific temperatures must be maintained for certain time periods to kill microorganisms
  (4) Moisture (100% relative humidity)—longer exposure time and higher temperatures are required for dry heat
 b. Three types of steam sterilizers
  (1) Small tabletop sterilizers—used in dentist offices and clinics; essentially pressure cookers; normal temperature is 250°F (121°C)
  (2) Recessed downward-displacement sterilizers (gravity)—chamber fills with steam, displacing the air downward and forcing it out the drain valve; normally uses 250°F (121°C); flash sterilization usually is 272°F (133°C); may be located in operating suite or substerile room; flash sterilization should be used only under urgent conditions
  (3) High-speed vacuum sterilizers—vacuum pump removes the air from the chamber before the steam is admitted, reducing the penetration time and total cycle time
 c. Advantages/disadvantages
  (1) Advantages—highly effective; rapid heating and rapid penetration of textiles; nontoxic; inexpensive; can be used for liquids
  (2) Disadvantages—items must be heat and moisture resistant; cannot be used to sterilize powders or oils, potential for burns
4. Dry heat sterilization
 a. Types
  (1) Gravity convection
  (2) Mechanical convection—more efficient, temperature more uniform
 b. Temperatures and times required for dry-heat sterilization
  (1) 340°F (171°C)—60 minutes
  (2) 320°F (160°C)—120 minutes
  (3) 300°F (149°C)—150 minutes
  (4) 285°F (141°C)—180 minutes
  (5) 250°F (121°C)—12 hours
 c. Advantages/disadvantages
  (1) Advantages—can be used for powders, anhydrous oils, glass; reaches surfaces of instruments that cannot be disassembled; no corrosion or rust
  (2) Disadvantages—penetrates materials slowly and unevenly; long exposure times necessary; high temperatures damage rubber goods and some fabrics; limited packaging materials; temperature and exposure times may vary depending on article being sterilized

5. Chemical sterilization
   a. Ethylene oxide (ETO)
      (1) Destroys microorganisms by alkylation (replacement of a hydrogen atom in a molecule of the organism with an alkyl group); prevents the cell from metabolizing and/or reproducing
      (2) Parameters—450 to 1500 mg/L gas mixture according to specific sterilizer requirement; no chemical indicators to monitor concentration of ETO during the sterilization cycle
      (3) Temperature—increasing temperature shortens sterilization process; range 67°F (20°C) to 149°F (65°C)
      (4) Humidity—range 40% to 60%; necessary for penetration into the microbial cell
      (5) Time—affected by gas concentration, temperature and humidity; increase in other parameters will allow a decrease in exposure time; cycle time 3 to 6 hours
      (6) Disadvantages
         (a) Difficult to monitor ETO sterilization process
         (b) Requires ETO permeable packaging materials
         (c) Lengthy cycle time
         (d) Cost
         (e) Toxic to patients and personnel
         (f) Must aerate items well before use
         (g) Must have exhaust duct directly to outside
         (h) Room must have 10 air changes per hour; 50% relative humidity; temperature must be 70°F (21°C)
         (i) Occupational Safety and Health Administration (OSHA) mandates maximum of 1 ppm (part per million) per 8 hours of exposure
      (7) Symptoms associated with ETO exposure
         (a) Irritation of eyes, respiratory passages, nose, throat and a "peculiar taste"
         (b) Delayed—headache, nausea, vomiting, dyspnea, cyanosis, pulmonary edema, weakness, unsteadiness, EKG abnormalities, dark urine
         (c) Direct contact—dermal irritation and burns
         (d) Intermittent exposure over several years—elevation of absolute lymphocyte counts, lowered hemoglobin values, chromosomal aberrations
   b. Glutaraldehyde—see Section C.4.f under chemical disinfectants
      (1) Cidex (2.4%)—high-level disinfection in 45 minutes at 25°C or Cidex Plus (3.4%), 20 minutes at 25°C
      (2) Rapicide (2.5%)—high-level disinfection in 5 minutes at 35°C (95°F)
      (3) Wavicide (2.5%)—Metricide (2.5%, 2.6%, 3.4%), Omnicide (2.4%, 3.4%), MedSci (3%), Procide (2.4%), Cetylcide-G (3.2%)

c. Ortho-phthalaldehyde (OPA) 0.55%
   (1) Excellent stability over wide pH range of 3 to 9
   (2) Nonirritating to eyes and nasal passages
   (3) No activation prior to use
   (4) High-level disinfection in 12 minutes at 20°C
d. Sporicidin—glutaraldehyde 1.12% and phenol/phenate 1.93%—high level disinfection in 20 minutes at 25°C
e. Vaporized hydrogen peroxide—see Section C.4.h. under categories of chemical disinfectants for advantages and disadvantages
   (1) Sporicidal at low concentrations (<10 mg/L)
   (2) Temperature usually 38°C but can be as low as 4°C
   (3) Tested with spore strips of *Bacillus stearothermophilus*
f. Gas plasma—hydrogen peroxide—see Section C.4.h. under categories of chemical disinfectants for advantages and disadvantages
   (1) Generated from vapor in a vacuum chamber by application of radio waves, resulting in reactive free radicals that are sporicidal
   (2) Temperature is below 50°C for 1 hour
   (3) The FDA has approved for use for lumens or channels of at least 3 mm and 153 inches length
   (4) Tested with spore strips of *Bacillus subtilis* var. *niger*
g. Liquid peracetic acid sterilization—see Section C.4.i. under categories of chemical disinfectants for advantages and disadvantages
   (1) Intended to sterilize fully immersible instruments
   (2) Chemical delivered in single-use container that contains 35% peracetic acid, buffer, anticorrosive and detergent, which prevents personnel contact with chemicals
   (3) Instruments cleaned with 0.2% solution
   (4) Connectors direct fluid into the channels of endoscopes
   (5) Process completed in 20 minutes at 50°C to 56°C (122°F to 133°F)
   (6) Tested by spore strips of *B. stearothermophilus*
h. Superoxidized water
   (1) Antimicrobial activity affected by the concentration of the active ingredient (free chlorine)
   (2) Nontoxic to biological tissues
   (3) Rapidly effective (<2 minutes) in reducing microorganisms
   (4) Biocidal activity decreased substantially in the presence of organic material
i. Performic acid—under review by FDA
   (1) Wide spectrum, oxidative liquid sterilant; inactivates viruses, bacteria, bacterial spores, mycobacteria and microscopic fungi.
   (2) Drawback is instability

Table 3–3. Decreasing Order of Resistance of Microorganisms to Disinfection and Sterilization and the Level of Disinfection and Sterilization

Resistant	Level
| Prions (Creutzfeldt-Jakob disease)	Prion reprocessing
| Bacterial spores (*Bacillus atrophaeus*)	Sterilization
| Coccidia (*Cryptosporidium*)	
| Mycobacteria (*M. tuberculosis, M. terrae*)	High
| Nonlipid or small viruses (polio, coxsackie)	Intermediate
| Fungi (*Aspergillus, Candida*)	
| Vegetative bacteria (*Staphylococcus aureus, Pseudomonus aeruginosa*)	Low
↓ Lipid or medium-sized viruses (HIV, herpes, hepatitis B)	

Susceptible

(Source: Rutala WA, Weber DJ. *Guideline for disinfection and sterilization in healthcare facilities.* Atlanta: Healthcare Infection Control Practices Advisory Committee, 2000.)

E. Cleaning

1. Items must be cleaned using water with detergents or enzymatic cleaners before processing[15,16]
   a. Removes foreign material that interferes with the sterilization process
   b. Precleaning of heavily soiled object may need to take place at the area of item use
2. Presoaking: prevents soils and proteins from drying on instruments, should be done immediately after the surgical procedure
3. Manual cleaning follows presoaking, uses a neutral detergent and friction; mechanical equipment uses an alkaline detergent
4. Monitoring of cleaning is possible, but not routinely recommended

F. Types of Mechanical Cleaning

1. Washer-sterilizer
   a. Action—cleaning is accomplished by a vigorously agitated detergent bath in which items to be cleaned are immersed

b. Advantages—renders items free of microbial life and safe to handle; removal of gross soil
c. Disadvantages—complete removal of soil depends on amount and kind of serrations in the equipment (equipment must be opened); length of washing cycle; pH of solution; strength and efficacy of the detergent; moisture level of the soil; many instruments cannot tolerate the temperature; equipment requires preventive maintenance and adherence to procedures
2. Ultrasonic cleaner
   a. Action—sonic waves generate minute bubbles for gas nuclei; bubbles expand until they become unstable and then collapse; the implosion produces very localized vacuum areas that dislodge soil from surfaces (cavitation)
   b. Advantages—process can overcome problems of poor equipment design by removing soil from inaccessible crevices
   c. Disadvantages—equipment requires preventive maintenance and attention to operative procedures; if sonic cleaner does not have rinse cycle, loosened particles can remain on equipment and must be hand rinsed; delicate items may be damaged
3. Dishwasher
4. Utensil washer-sanitizer
5. Washer-disinfector and flushing disinfectors

G. Reprocessing of Endoscopes

1. Most common device association with outbreaks[17-19]
2. All heat-sensitive endoscopes must be properly cleaned and high-level disinfected following each use
3. Steps include clean, disinfect, rinse, dry, store
4. Initial and annual competency testing for individuals involved in reprocessing endoscopes should occur[12]
5. Automatic endoscope reprocessors automate the processing steps, reduce the likelihood of steps being skipped and reduce personnel exposure to high-level disinfectants and chemical sterilants; failures have occurred with these

H. Other Considerations

1. Disinfection strategies for other semicritical items (e.g., applanation tonometers, rectal/vaginal probes, cryosurgical instruments and diaphragm fitting rings) vary widely. Device manufactures must include a validated cleaning and disinfection/sterilization protocol in the labeling for their devices; this disinfection strategy should be used by healthcare facilities
2. The CDC recommends tonometers be disinfected by wiping with 3% hydrogen peroxide, 5000 ppm chlorine, 70% ethyl alcohol or 70% isopropyl alcohol; however,

recent data indicated that 3% hydrogen peroxide and 70% isopropyl alcohol is ineffective and should not be used. After disinfection, rinse in tap water and dry
3. The CDC recommends diaphragm fitting rings be cleaned with soap and water wash followed by a 15 minute immersion in 70% alcohol
4. Endocavitary probes, including vaginal probes, should be covered with a new condom/probe cover for each patient, and the probe should also be high-level disinfected
5. Ultrasound probes should be covered with a sterile sheath and be sterilized between each patient use; if this is not possible, the probe should be high-level disinfected and covered with a sterile probe cover
6. Cryosurgical probes are not fully immersible; tip should be immersed in high-level disinfectant; other portions of the probe can be wrapped in a cloth soaked in a high-level disinfectant to allow the recommend contact time, then rinsed with tap water and dried. Nonimmersible probes should be replaced with immersible probes

I. Prions

1. The agents of Creutzfeldt-Jakob disease (CJD) and other human transmissible spongiform encephalopathies (TSEs) are resistant to conventional chemical and physical decontamination methods
2. Special procedures with CJD contaminated items includes:
    a. Critical or semicritical medical devices that have had contact with high-risk tissues from high-risk patients should be cleaned then sterilized by either autoclaving or using a combination of sodium hydroxide and autoclaving using of the four options
    b. Autoclave at 56.6°C (134°F) for 18 minutes in a prevaccum sterilizer
    c. Autoclave at 0°C (32°F) for 1 hour in a gravity-displacement sterilizer
    d. Immerse in 1 N sodium hydroxide for 1 hour, rinse in water, then autoclave in a gravity-displacement sterilizer at 121°C (249.8°F or prevacuum) for 1 hour
    e. Immerse in 1 N sodium hydroxide for 1 hour, rinse and heat in gravity-displacement sterilizer at 121°C (249.8°F) for 30 minutes, clean and subject to routine sterilization or prevacuum for 1 hour
    f. Devices that are difficult to clean can be discarded. If cleaning is desired, soak device in a liquid to prevent the tissues from adhering before decontamination (autoclave at 134°C (273.2°F) for 18 minutes in a prevacuum or at 121°C (249.8°F) for 1 hour and then normal wrapping and sterilization. There are 4 chemicals that reduce the titer by greater than 4 logs: chlorine, phenol, guanidine thiocyanate and sodium hydroxide. Because some chemicals (e.g., chlorine) are highly corrosive, they may not be used with some instruments
    g. Always prevent instruments from drying with tissues and body fluids before cleaning and decontamination
    h. Do not flash sterilize any instruments potentially contaminated by CJD

i. Items that only allow low-temperature sterilization should be discarded
j. Any item that was not processed using these guidelines should be recalled and reprocessed correctly. Neurosurgical instruments used in suspected cases could be disposable
k. Noncritical environmental surfaces (laboratory surfaces) should be cleaned and then spot decontaminated with a 1:10 dilution of hypochlorite solutions
l. Noncritical equipment contaminated should be cleaned and disinfected with a 1:10 solution of sodium hypochlorite or 1 N sodium hydroxide. The equipment should be tagged after use and staff trained to decontaminate properly. Ensure that powered instruments have disposable protective covers or use nonpowered instruments
m. Surfaces that have been contaminated by low-risk or no-risk tissues (from high-risk patients) should be cleaned with standard tuberculocidal disinfectants as mandated by the Occupational Safety and Health Administration (OSHA) (this includes endoscopes)
n. Autopsies should be performed only by facilities that are totally prepared to protect the physicians, technicians, etc. completely from aerosolized particles and should be done following the World Heath Organization (WHO) recommendations. Laboratory testing can be done to increase probability of correct diagnosis (14–3–3 protein of cerebrospinal fluid [CSF] fluid) has been reported in 95% of cases of sporadic CJD and less with familial CJD). The National Prion Disease Pathology Surveillance Center provides a variety of diagnostic test to aid in diagnosis of CJD

J. Sterilization Monitoring Systems

1. Mechanical indicators—recording charts for time and temperature; pressure gauges
2. Chemical indicators—chemically impregnated paper or strips; pellet in glass tube; Bowie Dick test checks removal of air from the sterilizer and efficiency of vacuum pump
3. Biological indicators—spore strips *Bacillus stearothermophilus* or *Bacillus subtilis*; Association for the Advancement of Medical Instrumentation (AAMI) recommends a biological indicator be used in the first load of each day (preferred) but at least once a week
4. Report positive indicators to appropriate persons: IP, director of surgery, surgeons if any instruments have been used, and others as directed per facility policy; take corrective action to remove all instruments/supplies that may not be sterile or are contaminated; resterilize those instruments; determine if company needs to be consulted for service of equipment; keep equipment out of service until biological indicator is determined to be a false positive or corrections are made

5. Causes of false-positive spore tests—accidental contamination of the sterilized test strip in the laboratory; defective biological indicator; contamination of growth medium with a *Bacillus* spp.

K. Performance Indicators

1. Monitor adherence to high-level disinfection and/or sterilization guidelines for endoscopes; should include training for personnel performing reprocessing and annual competency testing
2. Develop mechanism of reporting all adverse occupational health events potentially resulting from exposure to disinfectants and sterilants; review any exposures and implement engineering, work practice and personal protective equipment (PPE) to prevent future exposures
3. Monitor possible sterilization failures; assess whether additional training of personnel or equipment maintenance is required

V. Specific Care Settings

A. Respiratory Therapy

1. Hand hygiene, Standard Precautions, and Isolation Precautions are particularly important for respiratory therapy personnel
2. Nebulizers
   a. Used to apply solutions in liquid particle form directly to the upper airway and lower respiratory tract
   b. Ready vehicles for bacterial contamination[20-22]
   c. Sterile fluids should always be used
   d. Multiuse vials should not be used, if possible
3. Artificial airways
   a. Risk for infection increases because they bypass normal upper airway defense mechanisms
   b. Ventilator-associated pneumonia (VAP) prevention[21]
      (1) Head of bed should be elevated to 30 to 40 degrees
      (2) Daily antiseptic decontamination of the mouth
      (3) Peptic ulcer disease prophylaxis
      (4) Deep venous thrombosis prophylaxis
      (5) Daily sedation vacations/assessment of readiness to extubate
      (6) Institute techniques to ensure cuff pressure
      (7) Subglottic secretion suction ports may be used
   c. Patients should be turned side-to-side every 2 hours
   d. Patients should be encouraged to perform deep breathing to full inflation

4. Suctioning—help protect the airway in patients unable to cough effectively and facilitate secretion material; open suction systems require sterile catheters, gloves and sterile saline (if desired); closed suction systems may reduce VAP and lower cost of mechanical ventilation
5. Sputum induction—involves collecting a deep chest sputum sample; samples should be collected early in the morning and successive samples may be needed
6. Bronchoscopy—direct visualization of airways; pneumonia risk is high; bronchoscopes are difficult to sterilize, many facilities only high-level disinfect
7. Pulmonary function testing instruments—used to measure lung volumes, capacities, flow rates and diffusion rates; low-resistance, high-efficiency filters are placed between a mouthpiece and device to minimize contamination between the device and the patient
8. Incentive spirometry equipment is single-patient use; visible secretions should be rinsed out between uses
9. Manual resuscitator bags should be completely disassembled and sterilized between use
10. End-tidal CO_2 monitoring systems should be high-level disinfected between patients
11. Mechanical ventilators—infections are associated with contamination of the ventilator circuit tubing and humidification systems
    a. High-efficiency bacterial filters should be used on inspiratory and expiratory limbs of the circuit
    b. Circuit changes involve the ventilator tubing and the filter, exhalation valve and humidifier; should only be changed with visible soil or mechanical malfunction
    c. Sterile water should be used in humidifiers
    d. Condensate that collects in tubing should be drained away from patient
    e. Internal circuits are not routinely disinfected or sterilized
    f. Daily sedation vacations and spontaneous breathing trials should be used to facilitate ventilator discontinuation

B. Surgical Services[23-36]

1. Control of air quality and ventilation
    a. Operating rooms should be maintained at a positive pressure with respect to adjacent areas and corridors with 15 air changes per hour, 3 of which must be fresh air
    b. High-efficiency particulate air (HEPA) filters may be used to clean/purify air, consider use when surgical site infection (SSI) rates are high
    c. Laminar airflow is a type of system that produces little turbulence; use of these has not been routinely shown to lower SSI rates
    d. Laminar airflow body suits protect patient from shedding by operating room personnel and operating room personnel from blood-borne pathogen exposure from patients; some data exist for reduction of SSIs

- e. Ultraviolet light decreases microbial air counts, but no effect on SSI has been seen; UV-C lights require more study
- f. Misting and fogging technology for cleaning and disinfection may show effect on SSIs; however, most require precleaning and long turnaround time
- g. Necessity of environmental controls for laser-generated air contaminant from laser and cautery remain unresolved

2. Traffic control
   a. Unrestricted zone—street clothes permitted
   b. Semirestricted areas—hallways, offices and supply rooms adjacent to operating room; surgical attire is required; patients should be in hospital attire with hair covered
   c. Restricted zone—actual operating room and scrub area; surgical attire and face mask required

3. Supplies
   a. Clean and sterile supplies should be on a covered cart; remove from shipping containers before entering operating room; soiled items should be covered when leaving operating room and should not be stored with clean/sterile items

4. Proper surgical attire
   a. Institution-approved laundering
   b. Fleece should not be worn
   c. Hair covering should be donned first, so hair does not fall on clean clothing; all hair should be covered
   d. Sterile gown and gloves are donned for personnel within the sterile field; gown should protect from strikethrough of blood and body fluids
      (1) The gown is considered sterile from the operative area up to within 2 inches of neckline, around sleeves and up to 2 inches above elbow; the back of the gown is not considered sterile
      (2) Gloving may be done through closed or open gloving methods
      (3) Fluid-resistant mask is worn
      (4) Jewelry is confined within scrub attire or removed
      (5) Artificial fingernails or extenders should not be worn; natural nails should be less than ¼ inch long

5. Surgical skin preparation
   a. Patients should perform preoperative cleansing with an antiseptic agent, preferably CHG
   b. Clipping of hair at the surgical site should be done just before the time of surgery, outside of the operating room
   c. Prepping agents are available based on the procedure; proper application method for reducing microbial populations should be used

6. Sterile fields should be prepared where they will be used immediately before the operation; sterile fields should not be covered and should be under continual direct observations[36]
7. Environmental cleaning
    a. Microfiber technology should be used to clean lights and furniture
    b. Floor is cleaned with hospital disinfectant according to manufacturer recommendations
    c. A complete terminal clean should be done at the end of each day
8. Sterilization and disinfection
    a. Knowledge of the use and function of physical and chemical monitors and chemical and biological indicators verifies the effectiveness of sterilization
    b. Comprehensive documentation should be maintained
    c. Anesthesia equipment should be properly cleaned and disinfected, per manufacturer recommendations
    d. Flash sterilization should be used only when there is an urgent need for the items; cleaning, decontamination, inspection and proper arrangement of instruments should be followed; physical layout should ensure direct delivery to the point of use
9. Principles of aseptic practice
    a. Scrubbed persons should wear sterile gown and gloves
    b. Sterile drapes should be used to establish a sterile field
    c. Items used within a sterile field should be sterile
    d. All items introduced onto a sterile field should be opened, dispensed and transferred by methods that maintain sterility and integrity
    e. A sterile field should be constantly monitored and maintained
    f. All personnel moving within or around a sterile field should do so in a manner that maintains the integrity of the sterile field
    g. Policies and procedures for basic aseptic technique should be written, reviewed annually and readily available within the practice setting

C. Intensive Care

1. HAIs are five to ten times more prevalent among critically ill patients than in the general hospital population
2. Risk factors include impaired host defenses, severity of illness, extremes of age, nutritional status, invasive therapeutic devices
3. Infection sites, incidence and prevalence vary by ICU type
4. Infection prevention program should include surveillance, use of standardized definitions, and actions to decrease patient risk
5. Strategies to reduce the transmission of infections include:
    a. Consistent use of transmission-based precautions
    b. Ensure adequate staffing

c. Reduce length of stay by physician–led multidisciplinary rounds, daily meetings to assess bed utilization, use of bundles, and culture changes focusing on team decision making processes
d. Encourage and monitor adherence to hand hygiene practices
6. Provide information, education and intervention tools to the ICU to reduce risk factors for infection

D. Ambulatory Care

1. The basic principles of acute care infection prevention and control apply to ambulatory care; however, these settings may present special challenges due to patient mix, practice environment or highly specialized care.
2. Overall risk of HAI is lower among outpatients
3. Risk factors for exposure to infectious disease in ambulatory care include waiting rooms, invasive procedures
4. Infection prevention and control program responsibilities include:
   a. Program should be responsibility of one person
   b. Infection prevention decisions must be multidisciplinary
   c. Surveillance
      (i) Outcome surveillance:
         (a) No standardized definitions for ambulatory care, however may adapt HAI definitions from other settings
         (b) Outcomes in addition to HAIs include rates of vaccine-preventable diseases in staff, TB skin test conversions, rates of hand hygiene compliance
      (ii) Surveillance of reportable disease
      (iii) Process surveillance (e.g. unit/area surveys)
   d. Education of staff, patients, and visitors
   e. Communication

VI. Therapeutic and Diagnostic Procedures and Devices

The risk for HAI is related to the mode of transmission of the infectious agent, type of patient care activity or procedure being performed and the individual's underlying host defenses.

A. Increased Risk for Infection

1. Associated with stays in the ICU, prolonged hospitalization and antimicrobial use
2. High-risk procedures
   a. Intravascular access, especially central lines
   b. Mechanical ventilation
   c. Surgical and invasive procedures

  d. Intracranial monitoring
  e. Parenteral nutrition (e.g., hyperalimentation)
  f. Urinary tract instrumentation, especially indwelling catheterization
  g. Extracorporeal membrane oxygenation
  h. Ventricular assist devices (used to maintain a patient with a heart transplant)
 3. The risk for infection associated with devices and certain procedures can be reduced by adherence to appropriate infection prevention measures (e.g., hand hygiene, barrier precautions, device-specific bundles)

Figure 3-1.   **Infection types in acute care settings**[41]

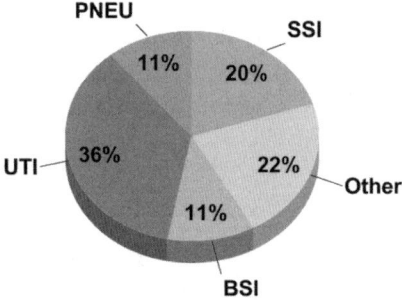

B. Prevention of Surgical Site Infections[23-28]

1. SSIs remain the third most common HAI; most SSIs results from microbial contamination of the wound during surgery.
2. Endogenous bacteria are the primary source of SSI.
3. Exogenous sources include the OR environment, surgical personnel, or seeding of the operative site from a distant focus of infection.
4. Host risk factors include
   a. Age
   b. Obesity
   c. Smoking
   d. Chronic disease and immune status
   e. Nasal carriage of *S. aureus*
   f. Duration of pre-op stay
   g. Nutritional status
   h. Mental status
   i. Presence of infection at another site
   j. Medications

5. Procedure risk factors include:
   a. Operative technique
   b. Hair removal technique
   c. Timing of antibiotic prophylaxis
   d. Duration of procedure
   e. Warmth of patient
   f. Blood glucose levels
   g. Use of flash sterilized instruments
   h. OR room traffic
6. HICPAC guideline
   a. Recommended rankings
      (1) Category IA—strongly recommended for implementation and supported by well designed studies
      (2) Category IB—strongly recommended for implementation and supported by some studies and strong theoretical rationale
      (3) Category II—suggested for implementation and supported by suggestive clinical or epidemiology studies or theoretical rationale
7. Pre-operative control
   a. Measures to improve host factors
      (1) Treat infections before surgery (IA)
      (2) Minimize pre-op stay (IA)
      (3) Control diabetes (IB)
      (4) Stop smoking (IB)
      (5) Lose weight
      (6) Improve nutritional status
8. Pre-op control measures
   a. Surgical site skin prep
      (1) Pre-op shower or bath (IB)
      (2) Do not remove hair (IB)
      (3) Use clippers (IA)
      (4) Alcohol (70%-90%)
      (5) Chlorhexidine (2%, 4%)
      (6) Iodine/iodophors (10% aqueous/1% iodine or formulation with 7.5%)
      (7) Chlorhexidine/alcohol combination
9. Pre-op control measures
   a. Surgical hand scrubs
      (1) Timing of preoperative antibiotic prophylaxis
10. Intra-operative control
    a. Measures

                (1) Surgical technique
                (2) Barriers
                (3) Limit people entering room (II)
                (4) Keep doors closed (IB)
                (5) Equipment in room before surgery
                (6) >15 air exchanges per hour—positive pressure
                (7) Relative humidity 50%–60%
        11. Post-op control measures—incision care
            a. Sterile dressing for 24–48 hrs (IA)
            b. Hand hygiene (IA)
            c. Sterile technique for dressing change (II)
            d. Patient education

    C. **Elimination of Catheter-Related Bloodstream Infections (CRBSI)**[37-40]
        1. Forty percent of all healthcare-associated bacteremia can be attributed to vascular access
        2. CRBSIs carry an attributable mortality of 12% to 25% among critically ill patients
        3. Sources of CRBSIs are device colonization or infusion of contaminated fluid; organism access occurs by:
            a. Invasion of percutaneous tract (during insertion or in subsequent days)
            b. Contamination of catheter hub during guidewire insertion or during manipulation
            c. Seeding from a remote source of localized infection
        4. Risk factors for CRBSI
            a. Prolonged hospitalization
            b. Underlying disease, particularly acquired immunodeficiency syndrome (AIDS), neutropenia
            c. Gastrointestinal disease
            d. Active infection at another site
            e. ICU/critical care unit (CCU) placement
            f. Other intravascular devices
            g. High APACHE III score
            h. Mechanical ventilation
            i. Transplantation
            j. Antibiotic use
            k. Difficulty of insertion
            l. Insertion site (subclavian vs. femoral or internal jugular)
        5. APICs *Guide to the Elimination of Catheter-Related Bloodstream Infections* contains simple, practical implantation tools to eliminate CRBSIs; strategies to prevent CRBSIs should include:

a. General measures
   (1) Healthcare worker and patient education
   (2) Ensure adequate staffing levels in ICUs
       (a) Surveillance—monitor facility infection rate
       (b) At catheter insertion
           (i) Aseptic technique—hand hygiene, clean or sterile gloves, maximum barrier precautions, use all-inclusive catheter kits, insertion checklists, monitor compliance with recommended insertion practices
           (ii) Dedicated interavenous device team
           (iii) Cutaneous antisepsis; chlorhexidine preferred but an iodophor or 70% alcohol acceptable
           (iv) Subclavian site preferred
           (v) Sterile gauze or semipermeable polyurethane dressing to cover site
       (c) Maintenance
           (i) Remove catheter immediately
           (ii) Monitor site daily
           (iii) Change site dressing at least weekly
           (iv) Do not use topical antibiotic ointment
           (v) Replace administration sets no more frequently than every 72 hours
           (vi) Do not routinely replace catheter for prevention of infection

D. Elimination of CAUTIS[41-43]

1. CAUTIS are the most frequent type of infection in acute care settings, comprising 36% of the total HAI estimate
2. A urinary catheter provides a portal of entry into the urinary tract; bacteria may ascend into the tract via either the external or internal surface of the catheter
3. APIC's Guide to the Elimination of Catheter-Associated Urinary Tract Infections (CAUTIS) provides evidence-based practice guidance for the prevention of CAUTI in acute and long-term care settings. Strategies to prevent CAUTIS include:
   a. Use indwelling catheters only when medically necessary
   b. Use aseptic insertion technique with appropriate hand hygiene and gloves
   c. Allow only trained healthcare providers to insert catheters
   d. Properly secure catheters after insertion to prevent movement and urethral traction
   e. Maintain a sterile closed drainage system
   f. Maintain good hygiene at the catheter–urethral interface
   g. Maintain unobstructed urine flow
   h. Maintain drainage bag below level of bladder at all times

i. Remove catheters when no longer needed
  j. Do not change indwelling catheters or urinary drainage bags at arbitrary fixed intervals
  k. Document indication for urinary catheter on each day of use
  l. Use reminder systems to target opportunities to remove catheter
  m. Use external (or condom-style) catheters if appropriate in men
  n. Use portable ultrasound bladder scans to detect residual urine amounts
  o. Consider alternatives to indwelling urethral catheters

E. **Elimination of VAP**[44,45]
  1. Pneumonia accounts for approximately 11% to 15% of all HAIs, and 27% and 24% of all infections acquired in the medical intensive care unit (MICU) and coronary care unit (CCU), respectively
  2. Mechanical ventilation is the primary risk factor for the development of hospital-associated bacterial pneumonia
  3. Risk factors for pneumonia are patient-related; device-related, people-related and procedure-related factors include extremes of age, chronic lung disease, immunosuppression, depressed consciousness
  4. Key prevention strategies
     a. Pay strict attention to hand hygiene and basic infection prevention strategies
     b. Avoid unnecessary antibiotics
     c. Perform routine antiseptic mouth care
     d. Prevent aspiration of contaminated secretions: maintain semirecumbent positioning
     e. Shorten duration of mechanical ventilation—apply weaning protocols and optimal use of sedation
     f. Avoid routine ventilator changes
     g. Remove condensate from ventilatory circuits; keep the ventilatory circuit closed during condensate removal
     h. Disinfect and store respiratory therapy equipment properly
     i. Minimize gastric distention
     j. Educate healthcare personnel who care for patients undergoing ventilation about VAP
     k. Perform direct observation of compliance with VAP-specific process measures
     l. Conduct regular surveillance for outcomes measures

F. **Elimination of Infection Risk Associated with Hemodialysis**
  1. Patients receiving hemodialysis are vulnerable to healthcare-associated infections because of multiple human, environmental and procedural factors related to the dialysis setting, as well as to the multitude of patient comorbidities

2. The infection prevention program should include a bundle of strategies and interventions to reduce the risk for both employees and patients. These include[43]:
   a. Environmental cleaning/disinfection
   b. Equipment cleaning/disinfection
   c. Hand hygiene
   d. Immunizations and screening for patients and employees
   e. Medication/injection safety
   f. Patient/family/employee education
   g. Presurgical/postsurgical infection prevention
   h. Standard/Transmission-Based Precautions
   i. Vascular access—infection prevention during insertion and care
   j. Water treatment/testing
   k. Infection surveillance
   l. Quality improvement program

G. Cardiac Catheterization and Electrophysiology

1. Early onset infections from cardiac catheter-associated procedures due to entry of organisms into bloodstream during vascular access
2. Late onset of infections frequently related to implantable devices
3. Normal skin flora and skin pathogens are often the causative agents of infection
4. To reduce risk of infection:
   a. Follow standard precautions; minimize exposure to blood and body fluids
   b. Patient preparation includes:
      (1) Clipping hair prior to arrival in procedure room
      (2) Facility approved skin antisepsis
      (3) Sterile draping for all vascular access procedures
      (4) Sterile surgical technique
      (5) Antibiotic prophylaxis
   c. Post-procedure closely monitor catheters, remove as soon as indicated
   d. Detect remote infections early and treat appropriately
   e. Implantable device infections require treatment with antibiotics and may require removal of device and hardware

VII. Recalls

A. Contaminated Equipment and Supplies

1. Can lead to outbreaks of infectious disease either at the time of production (intrinsic contamination) or during use (extrinsic contamination)

2. When a contaminated or defective product (including blood and human tissues), device or medication is suspected as the cause of the outbreak, the Food and Drug Administration (FDA) and the CDC should be notified
3. If a product or device is suspected to be contaminated, it should immediately be removed from use
4. If associated with an outbreak, an outbreak investigation must be initiated (see Chapter 2)

VIII. Isolation Precautions

A. Standard Precautions: HICPAC Synthesis of Universal Precautions and Body Substance Isolation

1. Applies to all persons receiving healthcare regardless of medical diagnosis or presumed infection status
2. Basic concept is to treat all patients' blood or body fluids as if they are infectious material; applies to blood, body fluids, secretions and excretions; nonintact skin; and mucous membranes
3. Includes hand hygiene and use of gloves, gowns, masks, eye protection or face shields depending on anticipated exposure
   a. In addition:
      (1) Safer injection practices—use a sterile single-use needle and syringe for each injection; use single-use medication vials when possible, avoid using multiple use vials; avoid reinsertion of used needles in multiple use vials or solutions and use of single-use needles and syringes to administer IV medication to multiple patients
      (2) Use a face mask during spinal procedures (e.g., lumbar puncture, myelogram and spinal anesthesia)
      (3) Respiratory hygiene/cough etiquette—cover mouth and nose during coughing and sneezing with a tissue or offer surgical mask to coughing patients

B. Contact Precautions

1. Used for diseases transmitted by contact with the patient or the patient's environment (e.g., drug-resistant organism isolation, lice, scabies, *C. difficile*); requires direct skin-to-skin contact and physical transfer of microorganisms to a susceptible host from an infected or colonized person; may be patient-to-patient, patient-to-staff, patient-to-contaminated equipment or object
2. Single room is preferred; however, patients with same disease or organism may be cohorted to share a room

3. Gloves and gown required on entry
4. Limit patient transport outside the room to medically necessary purposes
5. Discontinue Contact Precautions when signs and symptoms resolve, unless pathogen-specific recommendations differ

C. Droplet Precautions

1. Prevent transmission of diseases caused by large respiratory droplets generated by coughing, sneezing or talking (e.g., influenza, mumps, bacterial meningitis resulting from *Neisseria meningitideis* infection)
2. Single room is preferred; however, patients with same disease or organism may be cohorted to share a room
3. Wear surgical mask on room entry; use gloves when handling items contaminated with respiratory secretions (e.g., tissues)
4. Limit patient transport outside the room to medically necessary purposes
5. Discontinue droplet precautions after signs and symptoms have resolved or according to pathogen-specific guidelines

D. Airborne Transmission

1. Used to prevent transmission of infectious organisms that remain suspended in air and travel great distances (e.g., chickenpox, tuberculosis, smallpox)
2. Place patient in an airborne infection isolation room with negative air pressure relative to the corridor and at least 6 to 12 air exchanges with direct exhaust of air to the outside; monitor the air pressure daily; keep door shut
3. Wear N95 or higher level respirator when entering room
4. Limit transport of patients to essential medical procedures; if transport necessary, place surgical mask on patient and instruct to observe respiratory hygiene and cough etiquette.
5. Discontinue Airborne Precautions according to pathogen-specific recommendations; state and local health departments may offer further guidance on discontinuing isolation precaution measures for patients with known or suspected pulmonary tuberculosis

E. Protective Environment

1. Recommended for allogenic hematopoietic stem cell transplant recipients
2. Environmental controls—filter incoming air with positive pressure HEPA filtration
3. Limit time spent outside of protected environment
4. Implement Droplet and Contact Precautions as needed

F. **Prevention of Multidrug-Resistant Organisms (MDRO)**
   1. Administrative measures and adherence monitoring
   2. Involvement in decision to complete active surveillance culturing
   3. Activate computer alerts for previously infected/colonized patients
   4. Provide enough handwashing sinks
   5. Maintain staffing levels
   6. Enforce adherence to hand hygiene and Isolation Precautions
   7. Ensure adequate funding for hand hygiene and Isolation Precautions
   8. Education
      a. Facility-wide and unit-specific
      b. Include rates, trends, prevention strategies
      c. Create a culture that supports desired behaviors
   9. Judicious use of antimicrobials through formulary restriction, education, automatic stop orders, antimicrobial cycling and approval programs
   10. Surveillance—including incidence, infection rates, molecular typing for investigations, detection of asymptomatic carriers
   11. Follow recommended isolation precautions—including guidelines for discontinuation
   12. Scrupulous cleaning of environmental reservoirs
   13. Decolonization may be effective, although generally not routinely used or standardized

IX. **Environmental Hazards**

   A. **Linen and Laundry**
   1. General guidelines—all used/soiled linen should be handled as though contaminated
      a. Carry away from the body
      b. Use appropriate barriers to protect skin/clothing
      c. Store in manner to prevent contamination of the environment
      d. Transport in closed hampers that are approved by facility and state regulations
      e. Protect visitors from contact with contaminated linen
   2. Clean linen
      a. Store in closed carts or cabinets
      b. Do not store in open cabinets or in storage room with clean or dirty supplies
      c. Storage must comply with state and local Fire Marshall
      d. Clean linen taken into a patient room but not used should be discarded as soiled linen
   3. Employee garments/uniforms/scrubs
      a. Any garment that is considered to be personal protective equipment (PPE) must be laundered by the facility

b. There are no scientific data that state that home laundering of employee clothing poses any increased risk for infection transmission (provided it is not soiled with blood or other potentially infectious material [OPIM] per OSHA)
c. Employee clothing that is contaminated with blood or OPIM (per OSHA) must be laundered by the facility
d. Train employees to follow correct procedure and removal of scrubs/clothing to prevent contamination of skin

B. Trash and Biohazard Waste
1. Terminology*—for waste to be capable of causing infection, the following specific factors are necessary:
    a. Presence of a pathogen (this does not always result in infection)
    b. Pathogen must be of sufficient virulence
    c. Pathogen must be present in a sufficient dose
    d. Organism must have a portal of entry (into the body)
    e. Must be a susceptible host
2. Categories of infectious waste
    a. Contaminated sharps
    b. Microbiological cultures and stocks of infectious agents
    c. Animal wastes
    d. Blood and blood products
    e. Selected isolation wastes—materials contaminated
    f. Pathology wastes
3. Waste management plan
    a. Definition of infectious waste
    b. Designation—policies/procedures
    c. Segregation
    d. Packaging
    e. Storage
    f. Transport
    g. Treatment
    h. Disposal
    i. Contingency planning
    j. Training

* Medical waste is regulated by federal, state and local agencies using different terms and definitions (e.g., biomedical waste, infectious waste). Fluids should be disposed of with methods that minimize the possibility of leakage in the environment, splashing or exposure to trained trash handlers who are protected by appropriate barriers. Refer to local regulations for specific medical waste disposal information.

C. Needles and Sharps

1. Place used needles and sharps in puncture-resistant containers designated for sharps only and located as near the point of use as possible
2. Avoid unnecessary recapping—when recapping is necessary, the one-handed scoop method or a recapping device should be used as defined by policy
3. Use needle and sharps safety devices; mandated by OSHA Needlestick Safety and Prevention Act of 2000 and OSHA Bloodborne Pathogen Standard (2001)

D. Laboratory Specimens and Tissue Samples

1. Handle all specimens as if they were known to be infectious
2. Wear gloves when handling specimen containers until container can be placed into a biohazard bag
3. Transport specimens in a manner that minimizes the chance of spillage
4. Label all specimen containers, freezers, incubators and refrigerators with "biohazard"

X. Immunization of Patients

A. Standing Orders Programs

1. Authorize nurses and pharmacists to administer vaccinations according to an institution- or physician-approved protocol without a physician's examination
2. These programs have documented improved vaccination rates among adults
3. Can be used in inpatient and outpatient facilities, long-term-care facilities, managed-care organizations, assisted living facilities, correctional facilities and home health-care agencies
4. The Advisory Committee on Immunization Practices (ACIP) recommends standing orders for influenza and pneumococcal vaccinations[46,47]
5. Other vaccines that should be offered to adults as necessary include hepatitis A, hepatitis B, MMR (mumps, measles and rubella), Td/Tap, meningococcal, human papillomavirus (HPV), zoster
6. Children and teens may require the following vaccines: varicella, DTap, hepatitis A, hepatitis B, *Haemophilus influenzae* type b, HPV, MMR, Td/Tap, meningococcal, inactivated polio vaccine (IPV), HPV, rotavirus (infants)

XI. Construction and Renovation

A. Main Areas of Focus

1. Planning and design—IP input is necessary to ensure the design of the finished construction project facilitates desired infection prevention program practices (e.g., must have enough airborne isolation rooms, use of materials that are able to be properly cleaned/disinfected)

2. Construction hazard and risk mitigation—airborne microbial contamination or water-related contamination associated with construction resulting in HAIs have been described; systematic approach to construction activity is essential to improve safety and reduce risk associated with chemicals, dust, allergens and transmission of infectious agents to vulnerable patients[48-51]

B. Infection Prevention Risk Assessment (ICRA)
1. Elements related to building design features
    a. Number, location and type of airborne isolation and protective environment rooms
    b. Location of special ventilation and filtration of heating, ventilation and air-conditioning (HVAC) serving emergency department areas
    c. Air handling and ventilation needs in surgical services and other special needs areas
    d. Water systems to limit *Legionella*
    e. Finishes and surfaces
2. Elements related to building site areas affected by construction
    a. Impact of disrupting essential services to patients and employees
    b. Determination of the specific hazards and protection levels for each
    c. Location of patients based on susceptibility to infection and definition of risks to each
    d. Impact of potential outages or emergencies and protection of patients during planned or unplanned outages, movement of debris, traffic flow, cleanup and testing and certification
    e. Assessment of external and internal construction activities
    f. Location of known hazards
3. Preparation for actual construction
    a. Patient placement and relocation
    b. Standards for barriers and other protective measures required to protect adjacent areas and susceptible patients from airborne contaminants
    c. Temporary provision or phasing for construction or modification of heating, ventilating, air-conditioning and water supply systems
    d. Protection of occupied patient areas from demolition
    e. Measures to be taken to train healthcare facility staff, visitors and construction personnel on maintenance of interim life safety and risk mitigation recommendations

C. Construction and Renovation Policy (CRP)
1. Ensures timely notification to the IP for early program planning efforts
2. Provides for an ICRA evaluation of the project from concept to completion

3. Plan for communication of projects provided by the construction coordinator to the IP; should include:
   a. Authority and responsibility for establishing orientation, training, coordination and accountability for general and subcontractors
   b. Strategic planning for air and water quality for each building, including types of barriers and monitors
   c. Authority for determining unit closure issues
   d. Specific expectations for contractor accountability in the event of breaches in infection prevention program practices and related written agreements
   e. Communication linkages, including documentation responsibilities
   f. Criteria for emergency work stoppages and processes to stop and start
   g. Educational needs for whom and by whom
   h. Occupational health expectations for contractors and subcontractors before start, as appropriate
   i. General traffic patterns for construction personnel, patients, visitors and healthcare workers
   j. Transport and manifest approval, if required, of waste materials and supplies
   k. Noise and vibration issues related to the project
   l. Emergency preparedness plans for major utility failures—location and responsibilities
   m. Phasing and commissioning

D. IP Role
   1. Facilitation and communication among health agencies and facility administration regarding essentials for safe practice and infection control guidelines, in the absence of clear-cut regulations
   2. Consultation related to current and future patient populations and care delivery systems; this includes need and number of airborne isolation and necessity of protective environment, scope of services, etc.
   3. Evaluation of plans considering system policies related to structural design and needs for patient and healthcare workers
   4. Determination of impact on infection prevention program aspects based on scope of project
   5. Review of proposed construction, in light of infection prevention program-related standards and regulations that will need to interface with federal, state and local codes issued by the appropriate authorities having jurisdiction
   6. Review and recommendations for optimal use of space and design, while ensuring positive infection prevention program outcomes, particularly for air and water quality

7. Determination of environmental monitoring needs and budgeting for appropriate consultants
8. Determination of types and methods of educational provisions for internal and external contractors
9. Development of infection prevention program expectations into initial agreements and project checklists and contractor accountability in the event of breaches in infection program practices

E. Input
1. Design phase
   a. Air and water quality
   b. Fixtures
   c. Sharps and waste disposal placement
   d. Surfaces (ceiling to floor)
   e. Utility rooms
   f. Storage areas
   g. Adjacency and flow of people, patient care items, laundry and waste
2. Preconstruction phase
   a. Patient risk assessment
   b. Remove furniture/supplies (protect from dust)
   c. Block off air feed ducts and dampen returns
   d. Reduce dust (misting)
   e. Determine access routes
3. Construction phase
   a. Provide appropriate barriers between construction zone and patient care areas
   b. Monitor all dust and floor contamination; construction area should have mats at exits of renovation areas
   c. Maintain negative pressure in construction area with fans and air scrubbers
   d. Monitor all trash and debris removal for potential environment contamination; carts must be covered when taking them out of construction area
   e. Place severely immunocompromised patients in proper room with positive pressure
   f. Monitor filters for adequate ventilation, change more often during times of renovation and demolition; alarm systems notify engineering of need to change filters
   g. Make rounds to ensure cleanliness of job site and traffic paths
   h. Monitor supplies for water damage (e.g., drywall, insulation)
   i. Monitor all drywall finishing for cracks that would allow dust from interior walls to contaminate facility

j. Monitor handwashing facilities on blueprints for adequate locations and access
k. Monitor disinfection of water lines after construction completed
l. Assess each system of ductwork for contamination after initial cleaning; cover with plastic barriers after initial cleaning to prevent dust from entering before reconnection to main system
m. Inspect exhaust systems to ensure adequate distance from intake air systems as required per state regulations (some states mandate 25 feet)
n. Ensure any interruptions in utilities are planned and prepared for as much as possible (e.g., replacement water available, lines are flushed after water restored, staff are prepared with instructions before interruptions)

4. Postconstruction phase
   a. Windows sealed
   b. Sinks, soap and towel dispensers in place
   c. Ceiling ducts cleaned
   d. Negative/positive pressure rooms working
   e. Plumbing lines and gas lines cleaned/disinfected per state regulations
   f. Terminal cleaning by contractor and then by facility staff

5. Traffic as a contributor to air contamination
   a. Patients and visitors may contribute to air contamination
   b. Waste, linen, supplies and equipment may also create an environmental hazard
   c. Prevention strategies
      (1) Patient movement should cause minimal exposure of patients to others
      (2) Patients who are in isolation should be transported using appropriate precautions
      (3) Visitor traffic routes should minimize contact with patients, and visitors should be assessed for communicable disease
      (4) Routes for transporting clean and sterile supplies from storage should not allow contact or permit temporary storage near contaminated materials
      (5) Laundry/trash chutes are contaminated and bags can rupture during use; chutes should be monitored for potential transmission of infectious agents
      (6) Waste transport must be contained to reduce any risk for contamination

XII. Prevention of Transmission of Tuberculosis

A. Background

1. It is estimated that one third of the world's population is infected with TB
2. A total of 11,545 TB cases (a rate of 3.8 cases per 100,000 persons) were reported in the United States in 2009; the TB rate in 2009 was the lowest recorded since national reporting began in 1953[52]
3. Multidrug resistant (MDR) and extensively drug-resistant (XDR) TB strains have emerged and are more difficult to treat

4. Numerous case reports describe patients and healthcare workers who became infected after exposure to patients with TB[53-56]

B. Prevention Strategies[57]

1. Index of suspicion—isolate when case is suspected in negative pressure isolation room; wear N95 respirator; begin testing to rule out TB; make sure physicians and facility administration are educated about procedure and receive follow-up information related to cases, number of exposures, and statistics for facility
2. Training—education of staff and physicians before suspected case is present (include exposure information, isolation procedure, department notification policy when TB is determined after patient discharged (unknown case), then education of patient and family (should be clear, concise, tailored to individual needs and comprehensive ability and lasting [give written and visual information to back up the verbal to increase the retention of information])
3. Environmental controls—monitor isolation rooms, ventilation checks, documentation of appropriate ventilation before and during TB case visits, traffic of isolated patients
4. Laboratory testing and flow of information—determine what testing can be done locally and ensure that appropriate personnel and physicians are notified rapidly
5. Screening should be done via a PPD skin test conducted in a concentric circle starting with those people who had the closest and most frequent contact with the patient and who have previously tested negative
6. Collaboration and communication with local partners—public health and community—ensure that good communication is maintained with the local health department; allow health department to visit patients in hospital to begin education before they are discharged; make sure nursing personnel know appropriate phone numbers to contact any time patient may be discharged on the weekend
7. Discharge planning—begin planning for the patients' discharge when the patient is suspected of having TB; if patient will be sent home on medicine or isolation, make sure health department has appropriate info about patient when information is available (history and physical, laboratory information, radiography reports, etc.); do not wait until discharge to send; begin teaching patient and family about home early in diagnosis (home visitors, safety in the home, trips to the doctor's office, etc.).

XIII. Prevention of Blood-Borne Pathogens (BBP) in Dialysis Units

A. General Recommendations

1. Staff must follow Standard Precautions
2. PPE must be accessible, in appropriate sizes, available in nonlatex, available also to visitors and used by all; it is recommended that gloves be placed beside each dialysis station

3. Thorough cleaning and disinfection of all surfaces and equipment that may be contaminated by blood or other body fluids (including peritoneal), using an approved tuberculocidal disinfectant
4. Disposable contaminated items are discarded according to state and federal Environmental Protection Agency (EPA) requirements
5. Soiled linen should be treated as infectious and handled following Standard Precautions
6. Personnel exposed to blood or other potentially infectious materials should follow current CDC and Public Health Service recommendations
7. All patients should be tested on admission to a hemodialysis unit for HBsAg, anti-HBc, anti-HBs, anti-HCV and alanine aminotransferase (ALT); patients who are anti-HBc and anti-HBs positive do not require further HBV testing
8. Transmission of HBV and HCV has occurred in hemodialysis units; therefore, infection prevention and control policies/procedures should be reviewed regularly and followed rigorously
9. There should be clear separation of clean and dirty areas. Common carts should not be used within the treatment area

B. Hepatitis B Virus

1. Hepatitis B vaccine is recommended for all susceptible hemodialysis patients and staff
2. Vaccine dose must be larger (patients) because antibody response is poorer in hemodialysis patients; vaccine booster should be given if antibody level falls below 10
3. Unvaccinated hemodialysis patients should be tested monthly for HBsAg and semiannually for anti-HBs; those who are anti-HBs positive should be tested annually for anti-HBs
4. Vaccinated patients should be tested—anti-HBs positive—annually; anti-HBs negative or low levels—monthly for HBsAg and semiannually for anti-HBs
5. Patients who are HBsAg positive should not be included in reuse programs
6. Separation of HBsAg patients by room or area and use of a dedicated machine
7. Nonimmune staff members should be tested semiannually for HBsAg and anti-HBs
8. Transmission of HBV and HCV has occurred in hemodialysis units; therefore infection prevention and control policies/procedures should be reviewed regularly and followed rigorously

C. Hepatitis Delta Virus (HDV)

1. Patients infected with HDV should be dialyzed in separate areas from other dialysis patients

2. Routine screening of patients and staff for HDV is recommended only if there has been a patient known to have HDV or evidence of transmission in the unit
3. HDV-infected patients should not be included in reuse programs

D. Hepatitis C virus (HCV)

1. Standard Precautions should be followed with all patients with HCV
2. All anti-HCV–negative patients should be tested for increased ALT monthly and anti-HCV semiannually
3. HCV-positive patients may be included in reprocessing programs

E. Human Immunodeficiency Virus (HIV)

1. Patients who have been diagnosed as HIV positive or have AIDS do not have to be isolated from other patients or receive treatment on separate machines
2. Standard Precautions should be followed for patients with HIV or AIDS
3. Routine screening of patients and personnel for HIV antibody is not recommended
4. HIV-infected patients may be included in reprocessing programs

XIV. Elimination of *Clostridium difficile*

A. Background

1. Severity of *C. difficile* infection is increasing
2. Associated with increased length of stay by 2.6 to 4.5 days; attributable costs for inpatient care estimated to be $2,500 to $3,500 per episode
3. Attributable mortality rate of 6.9% at 30 days and 16.7% at 1 year[58-63]

B. Prevention Strategies[64]

1. Preventing the development and transmission of CDI is priority for IPs; local data should drive priority setting and choice and timing of interventions
2. CDI bundles should include:
    a. Early recognition of CDI, through appropriate surveillance case-finding methods and microbiological identification
    b. Implementation of Contact Precautions, in addition to Standard Precautions and patient placement
    c. Establishment and monitoring of adherence with environmental controls
        (1) Use EPA-approved germicide for disinfection
        (2) Ensure personnel allow appropriate germicide contact time
        (3) Education of employees on appropriate cleaning and disinfection techniques
        (4) Hand hygiene measures

(5) Patient and family education
(6) Evidence-based methods for patient treatment and management of disease
(7) Antimicrobial stewardship
(8) Education of healthcare workers
(9) Administrative support

XV. Prevention and Control of MDROs in Healthcare Settings[65]

A. Administrative Support

1. Organizational priority
2. Fiscal and human resource support
3. Communication systems—to administrative and public health
4. Multidisciplinary process to monitor adherence to Standard and Contact Precautions
5. System to designate patients colonized or infected with MDRO

B. MDRO Education

1. Provide education on risks/prevention strategies (and facility experience) during periodic updates for healthcare workers

C. Antimicrobial Use

1. Multidisciplinary process to review patterns, agents
2. Implement systems to prompt clinicians to use appropriate agents
3. Provide clinicians with susceptibility reports and analysis of trends
4. Prepare and distribute reports to providers if limited electronic communication systems

D. Surveillance

1. Use standardized laboratory methods and published guidelines for determining antimicrobial susceptibilities
2. System for prompt notification of infection control or medical director
3. Laboratory protocols for storing isolates of selected MDROs
4. System to detect and communicate MDROs
5. Prepare facility specific reports
6. Monitor reports for changing resistance patterns
7. Monitor special-care units for MDROs
8. Monitor trends in target MDROs

E. Infection Control Precautions

1. Standard Precautions
2. Contact Precautions
   a. Acute care—all patients colonized/infected with target MDROs
   b. Long-term care—consider patient's clinical situation and facility resources
   c. Ambulatory and home care—Standard Precautions
   d. Dialysis—follows dialysis-specific guidelines
3. Masks not indicated except for prevention of splash or spray
4. Single-patient rooms (infected or colonized) preferred or cohort patients with same MDRO in same room or (third choice) place with patients at low risk

F. Environmental Measures—Cleaning and Disinfecting

1. Dedicate noncritical medical items to individual patient
2. Prioritize room cleaning of patients on Contact Precautions
3. Focus cleaning and disinfecting on frequently touched surfaces (bed rails, commodes, doorknobs and equipment in immediate vicinity of patient)

G. Decolonization—Not Recommended Routinely

Practice Questions for Chapter Three

Chapter Three:

Infection Prevention and Control

1. Decontamination is the process by which an item is:
   a. Cleaned of all soil and germs
   b. Rendered free from all pathogens and infectious organisms
   c. Sterilized and ready for reuse
   d. Rendered safe for handling without protective attire

Questions 2–3

A 20-year-old college student with a high fever and respiratory problems arrived in the emergency room by ambulance. He required emergency intubation and was transferred to the intensive care unit. A radiograph showed an air-space disease, probably pneumonia. A Gram stain of the bronchoscopy-obtained specimen revealed gram-negative diplococci.

2. What precautions are indicated for this patient?
   a. Standard Precautions only
   b. Standard Precautions plus airborne isolation for the first 24 hours of antibiotic therapy
   c. Standard Precautions plus droplet isolation for the first 24 hours of antibiotic therapy
   d. No precautions indicated

3. The attending physician calls you to assist with both the employees who cared for this patient and the patient's contacts. Those in need of prophylaxis following exposure to this patient are:
   a. The EMTs, the ER staff on duty, the ICU personnel and the radiography technician
   b. The EMT who suctioned the patient, the person who intubated the patient and the patient's girlfriend
   c. The ICU and ER staff, the college students in his dormitory and his family
   d. No special prophylaxis needed

4. What chemical agent should be used in an area where blood might be on the floor?
   a. Ethylene oxide
   b. Peracetic acid
   c. Phenolic
   d. Glutaraldehyde

5. Heat- and moisture-sensitive items are best sterilized by:
   a. Ultrasonic cleaning
   b. Steam
   c. Ethylene oxide
   d. Plasma

6. A laryngoscope blade should be disinfected by the following method:
   a. Cleaning followed by high-level disinfection
   b. Cleaning followed by chlorhexidine for 20 minutes
   c. Cleaning followed by ultrasonic washer
   d. Alcohol disinfection

Questions 7–9

A patient with rust-colored sputum, malaise, weight loss and fatigue is admitted to the medical center from a long-term care (LTC) facility. The doctor orders sputum for AFB smear and culture, fungal and bacterial cultures. A chest radiograph shows right upper lobe infiltrates.

7. What precautions should be instituted?
   a. Standard Precautions only
   b. Standard Precautions plus Airborne Precautions
   c. Standard Precautions plus Droplet Precautions for the first 24 hours of antibiotic therapy
   d. Standard Precautions plus Airborne Precautions with negative pressure ventilation

8. The patient has a negative PPD, and one sputum specimen is smear negative.
   a. The patient can be removed from isolation because he does not have TB
   b. Isolation should continue
   c. Isolation can be discontinued after he has been on antibiotics for 24 hours
   d. Isolation can be discontinued after the second sputum smear is negative

9. The patient is finally diagnosed with TB by culture after three sputum specimens were smear-negative. The IP contacts the LTC facility to inform them of the test results. Screening should be conducted on all those at risk, but how should it be conducted?
    a. Screening should be done via a PPD skin test conducted in a concentric circle starting with those people who had the closest and most frequent contact with the patient and who have previously tested negative
    b. Regardless of contact, all patients in the LTC facility should be screened with a PPD and chest radiograph
    c. PPD testing and chest radiographs should be done on all of those with close, frequent contact with the patient
    d. PPD skin testing should be done on all patients and employees in the LTC facility who have previously tested negative, with chest radiographs and sputum analysis of those who test positive

10. An IP receives notice that the antimicrobial soap his facility is using has been recalled because of potential contamination. What step should be taken first?
    a. Contact each department immediately to tell them to stop using the product
    b. Call the health department to alert them to the potential outbreak and type of organism involved
    c. Tell the nursing department staff to stop using the product because they have patient contact and allow ancillary departments to use up existing stock
    d. Obtain some of the product and send it to the microbiology department for culturing; if negative, continue using product

11. A patient was admitted over the weekend with suspected Creutzfeldt-Jakob disease (CJD). The IP is called to the unit and finds that the patient is in strict isolation with the staff wearing masks, gowns, gloves and hair covers. The IP develops a staff education program that includes:
    (1) The potentially infectious body fluids and tissue include cerebrospinal fluid, brain, spinal cord, eye, and possibly lymph glands, kidneys and lungs
    (2) Noninfectious materials are blood, sweat, tears, saliva, stool and urine.
    (3) The risk for transmission is moderate for the healthcare worker
    (4) Standard Precautions are adequate, except for the operating room and autopsy section

    Which of these statements are true?
    a. 1, 2, 4
    b. 1, 2, 3
    c. 2, 3, 4
    d. 1, 3, 4

12. The IP exits the elevator and finds a major renovation area with nonintact barriers near the operating room and ICUs. Dust and debris are evident in the corridor. A meeting is immediately arranged between the hospital engineering director and the contractor. The IP stresses the following:
    (1) An airtight barrier must be installed from floor to ceiling and taped closed with duct tape
    (2) All debris hauled out of the renovation area must be in tightly closed containers
    (3) All dust tracked outside the area must be removed immediately, either by damp mopping or HEPA-filtered vacuum
    (4) All ventilation ducts must be blocked within the construction area

    Which of these statements are true?
    a. 1, 2, 3
    b. 1, 3, 4
    c. 1, 2, 4
    d. 2, 3, 4

13. The newborn nursery nurses are complaining that there has been an unexplained increase in hyperbilirubinemia in the infants. They also stated that a housekeeper informed them that a new disinfectant was being evaluated. The IP had not been informed but suspects the new agent to be a:
    a. Chlorine compound
    b. Phenolic
    c. Quaternary ammonium compound
    d. Iodophor

14. Your hospital has just purchased a free-standing ophthalmologic care center. The center performs ophthalmologic surgery, which requires difficult-to-clean instruments with multiple crevices. You have been asked to determine the most effective way to clean these instruments before sterilization. You recommend the purchase of:
    a. Washer-sterilizer
    b. Utensil washer sanitizer
    c. Ultrasonic cleaner
    d. Washer-disinfector

15. You are asked to provide advice to an obstetrician's office on the appropriate disinfectant for diaphragm fitting rings. You recommend that the following disinfectant be used, after the diaphragm fitting ring is cleaned:
    a. Isopropyl alcohol (70%)
    b. Sodium hypochlorite (100 ppm)
    c. Glutaraldehyde (2%)
    d. Quaternary ammonium germicide (4%)

16. Antiseptics are regulated by the:
    a. Centers for Disease Control and Prevention
    b. Food and Drug Administration
    c. National Institute of Occupational Health and Safety
    d. Environmental Protection Agency

17. The infection prevention and control chair and the IP are reviewing departmental policies and notice several areas that are performing routine culturing. In which of the following areas is routine culturing recommended?
    a. Dialysis
    b. Rehabilitation
    c. Respiratory therapy
    d. Endoscopy

18. All of the following statements are true concerning 5.25% sodium hypochlorite EXCEPT:
    a. It has a broad spectrum of antimicrobial activity
    b. Used in the proper dilution, sodium hypochlorite is effective against hepatitis B and HIV
    c. Sodium hypochlorite is active in the presence of organic material
    d. Sodium hypochlorite is a fast-acting disinfectant

19. What is the most common device associated with outbreaks?
    a. Endoscopes
    b. Ventilators
    c. Central lines
    d. Pacemakers

20. In reviewing the literature on risk for acquiring postoperative pneumonia, the IP finds that the risk is greatest for patients undergoing what type of surgery?
    a. Total hip replacement
    b. Bowel resection
    c. Coronary artery bypass
    d. Esophagogastrectomy

21. All of the following statements are true concerning steam sterilization EXCEPT:
    a. The temperature inside the autoclave is raised in proportion to the pressure
    b. Steam must be superheated to ensure effective penetration
    c. Steam must be saturated for effective sterilization
    d. Pressure, temperature, time and moisture are the four parameters of steam sterilization

22. Following surgery on a dirty wound, the greatest risk for infection complications is associated with:
    a. Delayed primary closure of the wound
    b. Secondary closure of the wound
    c. Immediate primary closure of the wound
    d. Open wound management

23. A patient was recently diagnosed with *C. difficile* infection of the colon. You are called to institute Contact Precautions and do all of the following EXCEPT:
    a. Gloves and gown required before entry
    b. Move the patient to a single room
    c. The patient is limited in movement outside of the room except when absolutely medically necessary
    d. The patient is moved to a negative pressure room to avoid airborne fomite exposure

24. To facilitate drying and to reduce microbial contamination and proliferation in an endoscope, you should:
    a. Blow dry with compressed air, rinse with tap water and hang vertically to dry
    b. Blow compressed air through the channel and rinse with 70% ethyl or isopropyl alcohol
    c. Rinse with tap water and blow compressed air through the channels
    d. Rinse with alcohol, hang vertically to dry and store in a case to keep clean

25. The hospital is full and the IP is consulted concerning placement of a new admission. Which of the following patients are the BEST candidates for cohorting?
    a. A new patient postoperative from a cholecystectomy and a patient with a decubitus ulcer that was débrided in surgery today
    b. A patient with AIDS and a patient receiving chemotherapy
    c. A new admission with influenza and a patient with pneumonia who was originally admitted with influenza 4 days ago
    d. A premature neonate and a full-term healthy baby, born this morning

26. The nursing director of a local LTC facility is concerned about their urinary tract infection rate and has implemented several measures to reduce infections. You are consulted to direct the surveillance for the facility. You discover that all of the following actions are being performed. The MOST important action that will reduce infections is:
    a. An appropriately trained person performing twice-daily meatal care with a povidone-iodine solution
    b. Maintaining a sterile, closed drainage system
    c. Changing all indwelling catheters every 7 days and obtaining a urine culture on removal
    d. Administering continuous antibiotic bladder irrigation on all patients who must maintain a catheter

27. Your facility has recently combined the labor/delivery, postpartum, nursery, pediatrics, and gynecology areas of the hospital under the title of maternal child services. You have been told that the same housekeeping personnel will clean all areas. The director of the area wants you to recommend one cleaning solution that can be used for all areas. Which of the following disinfectant(s) should be considered?
    (1) Diluted sodium hypochlorite
    (2) Phenolics
    (3) Quaternary ammonium compounds
    (4) Hydrogen peroxide
    a. 1, 2
    b. 2, 3
    c. 1, 3, 4
    d. 1, 3

28. The nursing personnel on the postpartum unit have consulted the IP because they are concerned about their risk for acquiring hepatitis B from postpartum patients who are positive for hepatitis B surface antigen (HBsAg). Which of the following responses is MOST appropriate?
    a. Personnel can reduce risk by using the appropriate PPE during the labor, delivery and postpartum phases of the patients' care
    b. All personnel working on the unit should have the hepatitis B vaccine series
    c. All unit personnel who are exposed should call the employee health department immediately so they can be treated with hepatitis B immune globulin
    d. Pregnant nurses who take care of the postpartum patients should have a hepatitis B titer done before caring for these patients

29. The IP is reviewing the procedure for prepping of the IV site because of some recent IV site infections. Which one of the following agents should NOT be used?
    a. Iodophor
    b. Acetone
    c. Isopropyl alcohol
    d. Chlorhexidine

30. The admitting/registration department has called infection prevention and control to advise on placement of a 14-year-old male who was admitted with copious diarrhea of unknown etiology. Which of the following room assignments is MOST appropriate?
    a. A 16-year-old male with a closed fracture of the femur in traction
    b. A 12-year old male with uncontrolled diabetes mellitus
    c. A 2-year-old male with congenital rubella syndrome
    d. A 14-year-old with Hodgkin's disease

31. During an educational in-service to pediatric nurses, the IP is asked how to manage a patient with cytomegalovirus (CMV). The correct precautions include:
    a. Using Droplet Precautions
    b. Following Standard Precautions
    c. Cohorting all children with CMV
    d. Assigning nonpregnant nurses to care for CMV-infected children

32. When giving an in-service program on hand hygiene following an infection outbreak, which of the following issues is LEAST important to be covered during the lecture?
    a. Amount of contact time for soap
    b. Types of soap to use during specific situations
    c. Types of flora on skin, resident versus transient
    d. Information about protection of skin

33. A home health nurse has called to ask you for advice about a patient with diarrhea from *C. difficile*. The family members are concerned about getting the infection from the patient. Which statement is MOST accurate?
    a. The only persons who are at risk of getting this infection are those on multiple antibiotics
    b. Family members are unlikely to become infected if they wash their hands
    c. The patient's dishes should be washed separately from those of other family members
    d. Because the environment becomes contaminated, it should be cleaned with a germicide or 10% bleach solution and detergent

34. The critical care units meet monthly to review policies. They have asked you to advise them on the policy for central line dressing changes. You read the policy and have several concerns about the present wording. The BEST action for you to take would be to:
    a. Revise the policy the way current literature recommends and take it to the meeting to discuss with the members
    b. Call several area facilities to find out what their current practice is
    c. Summarize the latest guideline for intravenous therapy and take the guideline, summary and your recommendations to the meeting to discuss
    d. Meet with your infection prevention and control committee to ask for a recommendation before going to the critical care meeting

35. A disadvantage to the use of the ultrasonic cleaner is:
    a. The implosion of the tiny bubbles may damage fragile instruments
    b. The heat from the energy caused by the exploding bubbles can damage instruments
    c. The high-frequency sound waves generated by the bubbles will damage the pacemakers of central sterile department employees
    d. The explosions caused by the bubbles can cause small particles of soil to be embedded in grooves and cracks of instruments

36. Which of the following precautions should be used for a patient who is immunocompromised and suspected of having cryptococcal meningitis?
    a. Airborne Precautions for 24 hours after antibiotic is started if the patient is improving
    b. Mask worn when within 3 feet from the bed
    c. Standard Precautions for family and staff
    d. Contact Precautions for staff; family restricted from visiting other patients

37. A disinfectant that can kill organisms in the group C category is a:
    a. High-level disinfectant
    b. Chemical sterilant
    c. Tuberculocidal disinfectant
    d. Bacteriocidal agent

38. The nurses in the ICU have all started using a lotion from a local department store. One of the physicians called you because he does not like the smell and suspects it might not be as good for the staff as a medicated lotion recommended for hospital use. Which of the following would be the MOST appropriate actions?
    (1) Remove the lotion and throw it away
    (2) Culture the lotion to see if is contaminated
    (3) Explain to the physician that it is keeping the nurses' hands in good condition and should be kept
    (4) Talk with the director and then the staff about the use of products not approved by infection prevention and control
    (5) Deliver hospital-approved lotion to the unit
    (6) Educate the staff about the effect of the lotion on antimicrobial residue on hands
    (7) Ask nurses to keep unapproved lotions in their lockers
       a. 1, 2, 4, 5, 6
       b. 2, 3, 4, 7
       c. 4, 5, 6, 7
       d. 2, 4, 5, 6, 7

39. When a patient with severe burns is admitted, which of the following may actually INCREASE the patient's risk for infection?
    a. Using sterile linens for all of the patient's stay in the critical care unit
    b. Frequent nasotracheal suctioning with sterile saline
    c. Immediate tracheostomy upon arrival to the emergency room
    d. Using silver nitrate, antibiotic and antifungal ointments to the burned skin when changing dressings

40. While talking with the director of the surgery department, you learn that most surgery orderlies are still doing a shave prep on all surgical patients with a razor. In an effort to reduce surgical site infections, you schedule a meeting to plan measures to reduce infections. Items most important in the discussion are:
    (1) Current guidelines for surgical site infection prevention from the Centers for Disease Control and Prevention
    (2) Current AORN guidelines for surgical practice
    (3) A list of operative area prep techniques
    (4) Recommendations of the skin disinfectant manufacturer
    (5) Lists of surgeons with types of surgery each one performs
       a. 3, 4, 5
       b. 1, 2, 3
       c. 1, 2, 4
       d. 1, 2, 5

41. For this meeting to be most effective, the following persons should attend:
    (1) Administration personnel
    (2) Surgery department director and education coordinator
    (3) Risk manager
    (4) Chief of surgical services
    (5) Director of surgical ICU
    - a. 2, 3, 4
    - b. 2, 4, 5
    - c. 1, 2, 3
    - d. 1, 2, 4

42. The admissions clerk has called you with concerns about four patients who are being admitted to the respiratory floor and placed in Airborne Precautions with negative pressure ventilation. Which patient is LEAST likely to have TB?
    - a. A 40-year-old male prison inmate who was injured in a fight but has a suspicious left upper lobe nodule on his chest radiograph
    - b. An 84-year-old woman from a nursing home who has pneumonia in the right upper lobe and a history of a positive PPD many years ago
    - c. A 48-year-old homeless man who has a chronic cough but has been coughing up blood for the past 2 weeks and has no medical history records
    - d. A 36-year-old woman being treated for breast cancer who has a positive AFB smear from a bronchial washing and states history of negative PPD skin tests

43. The evening charge nurse of the surgical floor called you at 9 pm to tell you that a man scheduled for surgery is refusing his shave prep. He has a malignant tumor in the right lower lobe. She tells you he is very hairy, and she had an orderly scheduled to shave his chest with electric clippers per hospital policy. Your advice would be:
    - a. Obtain some depilatory cream or gel and use this to remove the hair
    - b. Call the surgeon and ask his advice
    - c. Do not shave the patient; just scrub the skin with the approved antimicrobial cleanser
    - d. Use a regular razor to shave the chest, being very careful not to cause any nicks or cuts in the skin

44. When a patient with AIDS is admitted with possible pneumonia, the physician, who is a general practitioner, orders airborne isolation. What is the correct response?
    a. PCP is not transmitted person-to-person and does not require isolation
    b. A TST skin test should be placed to determine if patient may have TB
    c. A sputum specimen should be collected for AFB daily × 3, if TB is suspected.
    d. If the chest radiograph is clear, isolation can be discontinued

45. The IP is reviewing practices in the ICU after two patients developed an infection with vancomycin-resistant *Enterococcus* (VRE). The IP discovers that the second patient was placed in the first patient's room after the first patient was moved out. Which of the following actions would be the LEAST effective in preventing future infections?
    a. Find out exactly what pieces of equipment the housekeepers/nursing staff are cleaning
    b. Review the cleaning chemicals being used, dilution used and effectiveness of each chemical on different organisms
    c. Determine the cleaning methods used for each piece of equipment (e.g., spray surface of equipment or spray rag and wipe surface)
    d. Do environmental culturing of all surfaces after the patient is moved out of the room

46. You are called late in the afternoon about a patient who is being sent to your facility with an infectious disease about which you know very little. The director of nursing at this nursing home is concerned about her staff and other patients. Your FIRST action would be to:
    a. Call the patient's physician to find out what precautions should be taken for the nursing home residents, staff and your employees
    b. Tell the director of nursing that you will call her back after you have consulted your infectious disease literature and the patient's chart
    c. Tell the director of nursing that you will call her back in the morning after you have had a chance to review the new tests that you will be performing on the patient on arrival
    d. Call the local health department to let them advise the nursing home on precautions

47. When reviewing sputum cultures for your patients during a renovation project, which would concern you the most?
    a. An 80-year-old man with COPD patient for 3 days
    b. An 18-year-old man being treated for leukemia
    c. A 33-year-old woman who has just given birth
    d. A 48-year-old man who just had CABG surgery

48. Which of the following processes should be used for contaminated endotracheal blades?
    a. Cleaning followed by high-level disinfection
    b. Cleaning with chlorhexidine followed by soaking for 20 minutes
    c. Cleaning followed by ultrasonic washer
    d. Alcohol disinfection

49. When giving in-service training on handwashing following an infection outbreak, which of the following issues is LEAST important to be covered during the lecture?
    (1) Amount of contact time for soap with skin to be effective
    (2) Types of soap to use during specific situations, such as body fluid contact, invasive procedures
    (3) Types of flora on skin, resident versus transient
    (4) Information about protection of skin from dermatitis
    (5) Alcohol-based alternatives to soap and water
        a. 3, 4
        b. 4, 5
        c. 2, 3
        d. 1, 2

50. Which of the following healthcare workers is at the LOWEST risk for occupational acquisition of syphilis?
    a. Housekeeping
    b. Laboratory technician
    c. Labor and delivery room nurses
    d. Emergency room nurses

51. Cavitation is a term used to describe the cleaning process used during:
    a. Pasteurization
    b. High-level disinfection by peracetic acid
    c. Cleaning by ultrasonic washer
    d. Cleaning by washer-disinfector

52. When doing in-service training on the nursing units about sterile supplies and instruments, what misconception is MOST likely to be heard from the nurses?
    a. If an indicator has turned black, the package of instruments has been sterilized
    b. Glutaraldehyde should not be used by someone who has not been trained to use it
    c. A sterilizer can kill all the germs on dirty instruments
    d. If an instrument package has not expired but has become moist, it should not be used

53. You are called to a nursing unit because an anesthesiologist has instructed the nurses to place a patient under Airborne Precautions because of MRSA pneumonia. The anesthesiologist has instructed them to wear masks, gowns, gloves, hair covers and shoe covers. Your FIRST action should be:
    a. Call the anesthesiologist to find out where she/he got these recommendations
    b. Review your isolation policy with the infection prevention and control chair and then ask him/her to talk with the anesthesiologist about changing the isolation orders on the patient
    c. Take a copy of the latest guidelines on isolation and resistant organisms with you to the unit to show the charge nurse that your policy has not changed
    d. Leave the patient in isolation until discharged or the attending physician discontinues the isolation

54. A nurse calls you about what articles of personal protection are needed when assisting a physician in draining a large abscess at the bedside. She will have to hold the patient to keep him from jerking during the procedure. You recommend the following articles:
    a. Gloves and face shield
    b. Gloves and gown
    c. Gown, gloves and mask
    d. Gown, gloves and face shield

55. When developing a tube feeding–associated pneumonia study, the ICP decides to stratify the risk factors for pneumonia. Included in the risk factors are:
    (1) Decreased level of consciousness
    (2) Narcotic administration
    (3) Use of antibiotics before surgery
    (4) Physical activity of patient
    (5) History of influenza vaccine
    - a. 2, 3, 4
    - b. 1, 2, 4
    - c. 1, 2, 3
    - d. 3, 4, 5

56. The director of the labor and delivery unit calls you to ask about stopping the use of hospital-laundered scrubs for his personnel. He tells you how much he spends a year in providing scrubs and is planning a cost-analysis study with the supervisor of the laundry. He says that all delivery nurses wear a doctor's gown when assisting in the delivery room suite. When helping him to make the decision, the issues of LEAST importance would be:
    (1) OSHA Blood-Borne Pathogens Standard
    (2) Cost of doctors' gowns for all assisting nurses
    (3) Number of accidental splashes/exposures of amniotic fluid, blood, etc.
    (4) State regulations and recommendations of obstetric/gynecology organizations
    (5) Practices of other facilities in the area or similar-sized institutions
    - a. 2, 5
    - b. 3, 5
    - c. 1, 2
    - d. 1, 3

57. All of the following are sporicidal EXCEPT:
    - a. Glutaraldehyde
    - b. Ethylene oxide
    - c. Alcohol
    - d. Peracetic acid

Questions 58–59 After a recent outbreak of MRSA surgical site infections at your hospital, you perform follow-up reviews on the procedures from the time a patient enters the hospital until they leave. Below are questions relating to your review.

Upon reviewing surgical skin preparation, you discovered that the following were being done. Which would you consider inappropriate?
   a. Patients were given chlorhexidine gluconate scrubs immediately before surgery.
   b. The surgical site was cleaned and clipped/shaved at least 24 hours before arrival to the hospital to allow healing of any cuts/scrapes
   c. Each surgical procedure to be performed had a pre-arranged prepping agent determined by the surgeons, infection control professionals, and the operating room nurses
   d. The operating room had a predetermined method of microbial reduction in place approved by the ICP, surgeons and operating room staff.

58. Your review of the air quality in the operating room areas and preoperative areas revealed several deficits. Which one of the following is the CORRECT means of maintaining air quality?
   a. Operating room air exchanges were set at 12 air changes per hour
   b. Fluorescent lights were replaced with black lights to show where contamination existed
   c. HEPA filters were installed in place of microfiber air filters
   d. Dehumidifiers were placed in each operating room to decrease the risk of *Legionella* infections

59. It is recommended to replace central venous catheters routinely
   a. Every 7 days
   b. Every 3 days
   c. Only when indicated
   d. Never

60. Which of the following statements is FALSE regarding cardiac catheterization and electrophysiology?
   a. Early onset infections are due to the entry of organisms into bloodstream during vascular access
   b. Late onset of infections is frequently related to implantable devices
   c. Flora from the gastrointestinal tract are often the causative agents of infection
   d. Remote infections must be detected early and treated appropriately

Questions 61–64 You receive a call from a frantic nurse on the obstetrics unit. She has a patient who lived with a man who has just been diagnosed with active tuberculosis (TB). She has just been tested by the local health department on her left forearm. There is a raised area in the position where you usually give PPD skin tests. It measures 12 mm across the diameter of the induration.

61. The nurse states that the young woman is in active labor and will probably have the baby within the next 2 hours. She states they do not have any isolation rooms on the labor/delivery unit. Your advice would be:
    a. Do nothing until the infant is born; then get a chest radiograph
    b. Question the mother regarding symptoms of TB and get a chest radiograph after the baby is born
    c. Move the mother to an isolation room with negative pressure, wear N95 respirators and place a trained labor room nurse with her
    d. Place a surgical mask on the mother until after childbirth, when a chest radiograph can be obtained

62. The woman gives birth to a 4-pound, 8-ounce baby girl. The baby develops respiratory distress at birth, is intubated and placed on a ventilator. The mother does well after the birth and a chest radiograph is taken. The chest radiograph is normal and the mother has no signs or symptoms of infection. The obstetrician asks you if you think the mother should be isolated. Your best response would be:
    a. The mother could be isolated, with sputum specimens obtained for AFB, to ease the pediatrician's concerns
    b. The positive skin test represents a probable latent TB infection.
    c. Because the baby has developed respiratory distress, the mother may have pulmonary TB, which did not show up on the radiograph; she should be isolated
    d. Sputum specimens for AFB should be collected each morning for 3 days, but the mother does not need isolation

63. The baby improves and is removed from the ventilator. The mother has been discharged from the hospital. She wants to visit the baby, but the nurses in the neonatal unit refuse to allow her to visit. Your best course of action would be:
    a. Give the mother a mask to wear during visits to the baby
    b. Call the public health department TB coordinator and request that the state epidemiologist or health department physician call the pediatrician to allow visits by the mother
    c. Talk with the mother yourself, explaining the risk to the baby and the need to protect her from all unnecessary germs
    d. Prepare an educational inservice for the unit employees on TB

64. Categorization of a disinfectant as high-, intermediate- or low-level is based on its ability to kill microbes. The easiest microbes to kill are:
    a. Lipid viruses
    b. Hydrophilic viruses
    c. Vegetative bacteria
    d. Mycobacteria

65. You have to review the procedures at an outpatient surgical center. Instruments that will come in contact with mucous membranes or nonintact skin require at least:
    a. Low-level disinfection
    b. Intermediate-level disinfection
    c. High-level disinfection
    d. Sterilization

66. At your infection prevention and control committee meeting, the director of the central sterile processing department reports on plans to change the chemical used for high-level disinfection of endoscopes. The chemical name is unfamiliar to you. Your first action after the meeting would be:
    a. Tell the director that products cannot be changed until researched and approved by the infection prevention and control committee
    b. Go to the Internet to research the product
    c. Go to the director to get the product information they have related to FDA approval, processing time, etc.
    d. Find out the planned implementation time so you will have time to research the product, then present it to the products committee

67. When you review the product information with the director, you both learn that the product does not have FDA clearance for use as a high-level disinfectant. However, you do learn that it is being used as a high-level disinfectant in Europe. The director still intends to use the product because of the time and money savings. Your actions would include:
    (1) Telling the director the chemical cannot be used
    (2) Holding a meeting with the central sterile processing department director, the infection prevention and control chair, the central sterile administrative manager and risk management personnel
    (3) Develop a list of the reasons this product should not be used
    (4) Meet with the central sterile director to review the pros and cons of using an unapproved product
    (5) Contact risk management department to discuss legal issues
    (6) Contact the infection prevention and control chair to solicit his/her opinion
    a. 1, 2, 3
    b. 3, 4, 5, 6
    c. 2, 3, 6
    d. 1, 3, 4, 6

68. You are the IP in a small rural hospital. You have been told to develop a policy for hemodialysis. Your administrator is planning to have a large nearby hospital come to your facility to perform the dialysis. Your first action would be:
    a. Contact the hospital to meet with the dialysis unit director/coordinator to learn about their policies and procedures
    b. Begin researching and reading national guidelines for hemodialysis
    c. Find out what population of patients requires dialysis in your facility and why they cannot be transferred to the other facility
    d. Investigate the patient medical conditions to determine if they could be treated with peritoneal dialysis (in your facility) instead of hemodialysis

69. It is recommended to change the dressing on the central venous catheter insertion site:
    a. Daily
    b. Every 3 days
    c. When indicated and at least weekly
    d. Every 7 days

70. When caring for patients receiving dialysis, the risk for infection is reduced by all of the following EXCEPT:
    a. Knowledgeable, well-trained staff
    b. Strict adherence to aseptic technique during all procedures
    c. Monitoring of patients following procedures for signs of infection
    d. Comprehensive baseline testing of all patients for immune system deficiencies before beginning procedures

Questions 71–72 You have been called to investigate a recent increase in the rates of ventilator-associated pneumonias (VAPs) in your adult ICU. You discover that your staff modified several standard procedures without your notification or approval.

71. Which of the following changes is APPROPRIATE to reduce VAPs?
    a. High-efficiency bacterial filters were placed on the inspiratory and expiratory limbs of the ventilator circuit
    b. Internal circuits were cleaned each shift by respiratory therapists
    c. Tap water was used in tubing to reduce residue buildup
    d. Tubing condensate was drained toward the patient and emptied each shift to reduce humidity

72. Staff received continuing education regarding ventilators, but the instructor missed one key point. Which of the following is INCORRECT?
    a. Emphasis was placed on routine antiseptic mouth care
    b. Weaning protocols were reduced in order to reduce strain on patients
    c. Mechanical ventilation is the primary risk factor for the development of hospital-associated bacterial pneumonia
    d. Nasogastric tube protocols were emphasized to prevent gastric distention

73. Which of the following statements regarding the insertion of urinary catheters is FALSE?
    a. Even though catheter-associated infections are rare, a Foley should be avoided unless absolutely necessary
    b. A condom catheter may be more appropriate if the patient is male
    c. Avoiding indwelling catheters in patients helps prevent catheter-associated infections
    d. If a Foley catheter is placed, it should be removed at the earliest possible moment to avoid infection

74. A leak test on endoscopes is performed between each patient use because:
    a. It can detect damage to the channel
    b. It can detect damage to the exterior
    c. Perforated channels are an infection control risk
    d. All of the above

75. The recommended time of preoperative hair removal in elective surgery is:
    a. Immediately before surgery
    b. ≤12 hours before surgery
    c. Unresolved by lack of evidence
    d. 12 to 24 hours before surgery

76. Elective surgery on patients with remote site infections should be postponed until the infection has resolved.
    a. This is true for all patients
    b. This is true only for debilitated patients
    c. This is true only for patients infected with multiresistant microorganisms
    d. This is false

77. The involvement of an IP during disaster preparation is:
    a. Not as important as safety personnel until after the initial phases of the disaster
    b. Very important in planning stages for bioterrorism disasters only
    c. Important for all types of disaster during planning and preparation but not during actual response phase
    d. Very important when developing the policies and procedures

78. Infection prevention and control priorities in a disaster include all of the following EXCEPT:
    a. Drinking water for employees and victims
    b. Sterilization of instruments and disinfection of equipment
    c. Maintaining ability to prepare food for employees and victims
    d. Obtaining medication from vendors not affected by disaster

79. If a facility is involved in the damage from a disaster, the MOST urgent need for water would include:
    a. Wetting down dust outside the building
    b. Cleaning dust and debris from the emergency room
    c. Testing water pipes, which may be leaking into the walls
    d. Obtaining water to flush toilets or chemical toilets

80. Supplies that the IP would monitor during a disaster include all of the following EXCEPT:
    a. Food
    b. Phones, walkie-talkies
    c. Water
    d. PPE

81. Optimal positioning to prevent ventilator-associated pneumonia (VAP) includes:
    a. Supine positioning
    b. Semirecumbent positioning
    c. The position of the patient does not influence the risk for VAP
    d. Prone positioning

82. During a bioterrorism event, the outside agency that will most benefit the IP are:
    a. Local and state public health departments
    b. Local and national law enforcement agencies
    c. Disaster and emergency services
    d. Centers for Disease Control and Prevention

83. Host risk factors for surgical site infection include all of the following EXCEPT:
    a. Obesity
    b. Age
    c. Hair removal technique
    d. Smoking status

84. You have been notified that a possible smallpox patient has been identified in your community. The patient is being admitted directly to your facility. What type of precautions should your personnel take when caring for this patient?
    a. Droplet Precautions
    b. Resistant Organism Contact Precautions
    c. Airborne Isolation with negative pressure ventilation
    d. Airborne Isolation with positive pressure ventilation

85. Your laboratory notifies you that there are six patients with positive sputum cultures for *Francisella tularensis*. The cultures will be sent to the state laboratory for confirmation, but until confirmed, your best action would be:
    a. Do nothing until cultures are confirmed
    b. Place the patients under Airborne Precautions with negative pressure, and N95 respirators on all caregivers
    c. Make sure patients are in private rooms and Standard Precautions are used
    d. Develop educational modules for patients/staff and notify key hospital and health department personnel

86. Of all the common types of agents used for bioterrorism, one type is primarily transmitted to others by contaminated food/water. Which type is that?
    a. Tularemia
    b. Cholera
    c. Q fever
    d. Anthrax

87. What type of precautions should be used for patients with suspected pneumonic plague?
    a. Surgical mask worn when within 3 feet of the patient, door may be open
    b. Negative pressure isolation room with use of N95 respirator
    c. Normal ventilation, but door must remain closed and N95 respirator mask worn
    d. No mask required, but patient must be in private room and contacts should be treated for exposure

88. If the patient's hair at or around the incision site interferes with the operation, it is recommended to remove it by:
    a. Razor shave
    b. Depilatory agents
    c. Electric clippers
    d. Laser techniques

89. You have just been hired as the IP at a large adolescent behavioral health center. There is no infection prevention and control program in place currently. Which of the following should you perform FIRST:
    a. Write infection definitions and a surveillance plan
    b. Set up an infection prevention and control committee
    c. Perform an infection risk assessment of the facility
    d. Determine your job description and reporting structure

90. The IP has been consulted by a physician because her patient has a positive sputum culture for MRSA. She feels the patient is ready for nursing home placement, but the local nursing home has refused to admit the patient because their isolation room is in use. Which of the following actions is LEAST appropriate?
    a. Recommend that the physician place the patient on vancomycin for 10 days
    b. Review the patient's clinical condition, symptoms and culture reports to determine if the patient has an active infection or is colonized
    c. Talk with the nursing home director about their restrictions related to colonization of MRSA
    d. Identify any additional cultures that may be needed before nursing home placement

CHAPTER THREE: PREVENTING/CONTROLLING THE TRANSMISSION | 235

Answers for Practice Questions Chapter Three

1.	d	31.	b	61.	b
2.	c	32.	c	62.	b
3.	b	33.	d	63.	d
4.	c	34.	c	64.	c
5.	c	35.	a	65.	c
6.	a	36.	c	66.	c
7.	d	37.	b	67.	b
8.	b	38.	c	68.	a
9.	d	39.	c	69.	c
10.	a	40.	b	70.	d
11.	a	41.	d	71.	a
12.	a	42.	d	72.	b
13.	b	43.	a	73.	a
14.	c	44.	c	74.	d
15.	a	45.	d	75.	a
16.	b	46.	b	76.	a
17.	a	47.	b	77.	d
18.	c	48.	a	78.	d
19.	a	49.	a	79.	d
20.	d	50.	a	80.	b
21.	b	51.	c	81.	b
22.	c	52.	c	82.	a
23.	d	53.	c	83.	c
24.	b	54.	d	84.	c
25.	c	55.	b	85.	d
26.	b	56.	a	86.	b
27.	d	57.	c	87.	a
28.	a	58.	c	88.	c
29.	b	59.	c	89.	c
30.	a	60.	c	90.	a

References

1. Scheckler WE, Brimhall D, Buck AS, et al. Requirements for infrastructure and essential activities of infection control and epidemiology in hospitals: a consensus panel report. *Am J Infect Control* 1998;26:47–60.

2. Friedman C, Barnette M, Buck AS, et al. Requirements for infrastructure and essential activities of infection control and epidemiology in out-of-hospital settings: a consensus panel report. *Am J Infect Control* 1999;27:418–430.

3. Friedman C, Curchoe R, Foster M, et al. APIC/CHICA-Canada infection control and epidemiology: professional and practice standards. *Am J Infect Control* 2008;36:385–389.

4. Conditions of Participation for Hospitals. CMS, Code of Federal Regulations 42CFR482, 2007.

5. The Joint Commission. TJC National patient safety goals. Available at: http://www.jcrinc.com/National-Patient-Safety-Goals/. Accessed November 17, 2010.

6. Franz DR, Jahrling PB, Friedlander AM, et al. Clinical recognition and management of patients exposed to biological warfare agents. *JAMA* 1998;278:399–411.

7. U.S. Department of Health and Human Services. Pandemic planning assumptions. 2008. Available at: *www.hhs.gov/pandemicflu/plan/*. Accessed November 17, 2010.

8. Boyce JM, Pittet D. Guideline for hand hygiene in health-care settings. *Morbid Mortal Wkly Rev* 2002;51:1–44.

9. Facilities Guidelines Institute, American Institute of Architecture Academy of Architecture for Health, Services. *2006 guidelines for design and construction of health care facilities*. Washington, DC: American Institute of Architects/Facilities Guideline Institute, U.S. Department of Health and Human Services, 2006.

10. Trick WE, Vernon MO, Welbel SF, et al. Multicenter intervention program to increase adherence to hand hygiene recommendations and glove use and to reduce the incidence of antimicrobial resistance. *Infect Contr Hosp Epidemiol* 2007;28:42–49.

11. Lam BCC, Lee J, Lau YL. Hand hygiene practices in a neonatal intensive care unit: a multimodal intervention and impact on nosocomial infection. *Pediatrics* 2004;114:e565–571.

12. Rutala WA, Weber DJ, Healthcare Infection Control Practices Advisory Committee. Guideline for disinfection and sterilization in healthcare facilities, 2008. Available at: http://www.cdc.gov/hicpac/pdf/guidelines/Disinfection_Nov_2008.pdf. Accessed November 17, 2010.

13. Nelson DB, Jarvis WR, Rutala WA, et al. Multi-society guideline for reprocessing flexible gastrointestinal endoscopes. *Infect Control Hosp Epidemiol* 2003;24:532–537.

14. Gerding DN, Peterson LR, Vennes JA. Cleaning and disinfection of fiberoptic endoscopes: evaluation of glutaraldehyde exposure time and forced-air drying. *Gastroenterology* 1982;83:613–618.

15. Babb JR, Bradley CR. Endoscope decontamination: where do we go from here? *J Hosp Infect* 1995;30:543–551.

16. Merritt K, Hitchins VM, Brown SA. Safety and cleaning of medical materials and devices. *J Biomed Mater Res* 2000;53:131–136.

17. Spach DH, Silverstein FE, Stamm WE. Transmission of infection by gastrointestinal endoscopy and bronchoscopy. *Ann Intern Med* 1993;118:117–128.

18. Weber DJ, Rutala WA. Lessons from outbreaks associated with bronchoscopy. *Infect Control Hosp Epidemiol* 2001;22:403–408.

19. Weber DJ, Rutala WA, DiMarino AJ, Jr. The prevention of infection following gastrointestinal endoscopy: the importance of prophylaxis and reprocessing. In: DiMarino AJ Jr, Benjamin SB, eds. *Gastrointestinal Diseases: An Endoscopic Approach*. Thorofare, NJ: Slack Inc., 2002, pp. 87–106.

20. Haley RW, Culver DH, White JW. The efficacy of infection surveillance and control program in preventing nosocomial infections in U.S. hospitals. *Am J Epidemiol* 1985;121(2):182–205.

21. Implement the ventilator bundle. Available at: http://www.ihi.org/IHI/Topics/CriticalCare/IntensiveCare/Changes/ImplementtheVentilatorBundle.htm. Accessed January 30, 2009.

22. Southwick KL, Hoffmann K, Ferree K, et al. Cluster of tuberculosis cases in North Carolina: possible association with atomizer reuse. *Am J Infect Control* 2001;29(1):1–6.

23. Association of PeriOperative Registered Nurses. *Standards, Recommended Practices, and Guidelines.* Denver: AORN, 2003.
24. Centers for Disease Control and Prevention, U.S. Department of Health and Human Services. Guideline for prevention of surgical site infections: 1999. *Infect Control Hosp Epidemiol* 1999;20:247–278.
25. Atkinson LG, editor. *Berry and Kohn's Operating Room Technique.* 8th ed. St. Louis: Mosby, 1996.
26. Emori TG, Gaynes RP. An overview of nosocomial infections, including the role of the microbiology laboratory. *Clin Microbiol Rev* 1993;6:428–442.
27. Gruendemann BJ, Fernsebner B. *Comprehensive Perioperative Nursing Principles.* Vol. 1. Boston: Jones and Bartlett, 1995.
28. Kluytmans J. Surgical infections including burns. In: Wenzel RP, ed. *Prevention & Control of Nosocomial Infections.* 3rd ed. Baltimore: Williams & Wilkins, 1995:841–867.
29. Sehulster L, Chinn RY, CDC, et al. Guidelines for environmental infection control in healthcare facilities. Recommendations of CDC and Healthcare Infection Control Practices Advisory Committee (HICPAC). *MMWR Recomm Rep* 2003;52:1–42.
30. American Institute of Architects. *Guidelines for Design and Construction of Hospitals and Health Care Facilities.* Washington, DC: American Institute of Architects Press, 2001.
31. Reno D, Association of PeriOperative Registered Nurses, eds. *Standards, Recommended Practices, and Guidelines.* Denver: AORN, 2000 p 341.
32. Ahl T, Dahlen N, Jorbeck H, et al. Air contamination during hip and knee arthroplasties: horizontal laminar flow randomized vs. conventional ventilation. *Acta Orthop Scand* 1995;66:17–20.
33. van Griethuysen AJ, Spies-van Rooijen NH, Hoogenboom-Verdegaal AM. Surveillance of wound infections and a new theatre: unexpected lack of improvement. *J Hosp Infect* 1996;34:99–106.
34. Dharan S, Pittet D. Environmental controls in operating theaters. *J Hosp Infect* 2002;51:79–84.
35. Owers KL, James E, Bannister GC. Source of bacterial shedding in laminar flow theaters. *J Hosp Infect* 2004;58:230–232.

36. Association for periOperative Registered Nurses. Recommended practices for maintaining a sterile field. In: *AORN Perioperative Standards and Recommended Practices*. 2008 ed. Denver, CO: Association for Perioperative Registered Nurses, 2008, p. 56.

37. Crnich CJ, Maki DG. The promise of novel technology for the prevention of intravascular device-related bloodstream infection. I. Pathogenesis and short-term devices. *Clin Infect Dis* 2002;34(9):1232–1242.

38. Association for the prevention of infection control. Guide to the Elimination of Catheter-Related Bloodstream Infections, 2009. Available at: http://www.apic.org/AM/Template.cfm?Section=APIC_Elimination_Guides&Template=/CM/HTMLDisplay.cfm&ContentID=16388. Accessed November 18, 2010.

39. Crnich CJ, Maki DG. The role of intravascular devices in sepsis. *Curr Infect Dis Rep* 2001;3(6):497–506.

40. Raad I, Hanna H, Maki DG. Intravascular catheter-related infections: advances in diagnosis, prevention, and management. *Lancet Infect Dis* 2007;7(10):645–657.

41. Klevens RM, Edwards JR, Richards CL, et al. Estimating healthcare-associated infections and deaths in U.S. hospitals, 2002. *Public Health Rep* 2007; 122:160–167. http://www.cdc.gov/ncidod/dhqp/pdf/hicpac/infections_deaths.pdf

42. Association for the prevention of infection control. Guide to the Elimination of Catheter-Associated Urinary Tract Infections (CAUTIS), 2008. Available at: http://www.apic.org/AM/Template.cfm?Section=APIC_Elimination_Guides&Template=/CM/HTMLDisplay.cfm&ContentID=16388. Accessed November 18, 2010.

43. Association for the prevention of infection control. Guide to the Elimination of Infections in Hemodialysis, 2010. Available at: http://www.apic.org/AM/Template.cfm?Section=APIC_Elimination_Guides&Template=/CM/HTMLDisplay.cfm&ContentID=16388. Accessed November 18, 2010.

44. Association for the prevention of infection control. Guide to the elimination of infections in hemodialysis, 2009. Available at: http://www.apic.org/AM/Template.cfm?Section=APIC_Elimination_Guides&Template=/CM/HTMLDisplay.cfm&ContentID=16388. Accessed November 18, 2010.

45. Kollef M. Prevention of hospital-associated pneumonia and ventilator-associated pneumonia. *Crit Care Med* 2004;32(6):1396–1405.

46. CDC. Prevention of pneumococcal disease: recommendations of the Advisory Committee on Immunization Practices (ACIP). *MMWR* 1997;46(No. RR–8).

47. CDC. Prevention and control of influenza: recommendations of the Advisory Committee on Immunization Practices (ACIP). *MMWR* 1998;47(No. RR–6).

48. Bartley JM. APIC state-of-the-art report: the role of infection control during construction in health care facilities. *Am J Infect Control* 2000;28:156–169.

49. Bartley JM, Olmsted RN, eds. *Construction and Renovation*, 3rd ed. *Toolkit for Professionals in Infection Prevention and Control*. Washington DC: Association for Professionals in Infection Control and Epidemiology, Inc.; 2007.

50. Hota S, Hirji Z, Stockton K. Outbreak of multidrug-resistant *Pseudomonas aeruginosa* colonization and infection secondary to imperfect intensive care unit room design. *Infect Control Hosp Epidemiol* 2009;30:25–33.

51. Drinka PJ, Krause P, Schilling M, et al. Report of an outbreak: nursing home architecture and influenza-A attack rates. *J Am Geriatr Soc* 1996;44:910–913.

52. Centers for Disease Control and Prevention. Trends in Tuberculosis Fact Sheet, 2009. Atlanta: U.S., Department of Health and Human Services, CDC. Available at: http://www.cdc.gov/tb/publications/factsheets/statistics/TBTrends.htm. Accessed November 20, 2010.

53. Jacobsen E, Gurevich I, Cunha BA. Extent of tuberculosis contact investigation [letter]. *J Hosp Infection* 1995;30:75–76.

54. Templeton GL, Illing LA, Young L, et al. The risk for transmission of *Mycobacterium tuberculosis* at the bedside and during autopsy [see comments]. *Ann Intern Med* 1995;122:922–925.

55. Valway SE, Sanchez MPC, Shinnick TF, et al. An outbreak involving transmission of a virulent strain of *Mycobacterium tuberculosis*. *N Engl J Med* 1998;338:633–639.

56. Hutton MD, Stead WW, Cauthen GM, et al. Nosocomial transmission of tuberculosis associated with a draining abscess. *J Infect Dis* 1990;161:286–295.

57. Centers for Disease Control and Prevention. Guidelines for Preventing the Transmission of *Mycobacterium tuberculosis* in Health-Care Settings, 2005. *MMWR* 2005;54(RR-17).

58. Dubberke ER, Reske KA, Olsen MA, McDonald LC, Fraser VJ. Short- and long-term attributable costs of *Clostridium difficile*-associated disease in nonsurgical inpatients. *Clin Infect Dis* 2008;46(4):497–504.

59. Redelings MD, Sorvillo F, Mascola L. Increase in *Clostridium difficile*-related mortality rates, United States, 1999–2004. *Emerg Infect Dis* 2007;13(9):1417–1419.

60. Kenneally C, Rosini JM, Skrupky LP, et al. Analysis of 30-day mortality for *Clostridium difficile*-associated disease in the ICU setting. *Chest* 2007;132(2):418–424.

61. McDonald LC, Owings M, Jernigan DB. *Clostridium difficile* infection in patients discharged from U.S. short-stay hospitals, 1996–2003. *Emerg Infect Dis* 2006;12(3):409–415.

62. O'Brien JA, Lahue BJ, Caro JJ, Davidson DM. The emerging infectious challenge of *Clostridium difficile*-associated disease in Massachusetts hospitals: Clinical and economic consequences. *Infect Control Hosp Epidemiol* 2007;28(11):1219–1227.

63. Kyne L, Hamel MB, Polavaram R, Kelly CP. Healthcare costs and mortality associated with nosocomial diarrhea due to *Clostridium difficile*. *Clin Infect Dis* 2002;34(3):346–353.

64. Association for the prevention of infection control. Guide to the Elimination of *Clostridium difficile* Infections in Healthcare Settings, 2008. Available at: http://www.apic.org/AM/Template.cfm?Section=APIC_Elimination_Guides&Template=/CM/HTMLDisplay.cfm&ContentID=16388. Accessed November 18, 2010.

65. Siegel, JC, Rhinehart E, Jackson M, et al. Healthcare Infection Control Practices Advisory Committee. Management of Multidrug- Resistant Organisms in Healthcare Settings, 2006. Available at: http://www.cdc.gov/hicpac/mdro/mdro_0.html Accessed November 17, 2010.

CHAPTER FOUR

EMPLOYEE/OCCUPATIONAL HEALTH

CONTENTS

Article	Page
CBIC Content Outline for Employee/Occupational Health	244
Chapter Four: Employee/Occupational Health	245
I. Infection Prevention Objectives of an Employee/Occupational Health Program	245
II. Major Components of an Employee/Occupational Health Program	245
Practice Questions for Chapter Four	266
References	276

CBIC CONTENT OUTLINE

Employee/Occupational Health (10 Questions)

A. Review and/or develop screening and immunization programs

B. Provide counseling, follow-up, work restriction recommendations related to communicable disease or following exposures

C. Assist with analysis and trending of occupational exposure incidents and information exchange between occupational health and infection prevention and control departments

D. Assess risk for occupational exposure to infectious diseases (e.g., TB, blood-borne pathogens)

Chapter Four: Employee/Occupational Health

I. Infection Prevention Objectives of an Employee/Occupational Health Program

   a. Educate personnel about the principles of infection prevention and their individual responsibility for infection prevention
   b. Collaborate with the infection prevention department in monitoring and investigating potentially harmful infectious exposures and outbreaks
   c. Provide care to personnel for work-related illnesses or exposures
   d. Identify work-related infection risks and institute appropriate preventive measure
   e. Contain costs by preventing infectious diseases that result in absenteeism and disability[1]

II. Major Components of an Occupational Health Program (OHP)

A. Administration

   1. Organizational issues
   2. Policies, procedures and protocols

B. Operational Issues

   1. Screening
   2. Education and counseling
   3. Occupational illness and injury treatment
   4. Nonoccupational illness treatment
   5. Preventive health services
   6. Environmental assessment and control
   7. Record keeping. The maintenance of OHP records, data management and confidentiality are required by federal, state and local standards; copies of individual records are to be made available to the worker upon request.

C. Communication Between the IP and Personnel in the OHP

   1. Share information related to:
      a. Healthcare worker exposure to communicable diseases
      b. Healthcare worker infections
      c. Community and personnel outbreaks
      d. Development of policies and procedures for occupational health
      e. Educational programs for healthcare workers

D. **Occupational Health Professional**
   1. Coordinates and performs the activities of the OHP

E. **Medical Advisor or Consultant**
   1. Collaborates in the development of protocols
   2. Serves as a resource to the occupational health professional when needed in assessing, screening or treating healthcare workers

F. **Healthcare Personnel**
   1. CDC defines the term *healthcare personnel* as all paid and unpaid persons working in healthcare settings who have the potential for exposure to infectious materials, including body substances, contaminated medical supplies and equipment, contaminated environmental surfaces or contaminated air[1]
   2. Health Canada's Center for Infectious Disease Prevention defines healthcare worker as any individual who has the potential to acquire or transmit infectious agents during the course of his/her own work in healthcare[2]
   3. Includes nurses, nursing assistants, physicians, technicians, therapists, pharmacists, students, contractual staff not employed by facility, emergency medical service personnel, dental personnel, laboratory personnel, autopsy personnel, researchers, volunteers, clerical, dietary and maintenance personnel

G. **Policies and Procedures Needed to Implement an Effective OHP**
   1. Work restrictions—the facility should have a process in place that identifies who has the authority to remove the healthcare worker from duty
   2. Criteria for disease exposure and prophylaxis
   3. Screening procedures
   4. Illness reporting system
   5. Methods of detecting, preventing and controlling disease
   6. Protocols for treatment of occupational injuries and illnesses
   7. Protocols for treatment of nonoccupational illness

H. **Screening for Disease Detection, Prevention and Control**
   1. Determined by
      a. Incidence of disease in local population
      b. Risk of significant exposure in healthcare workers' work-related activities
      c. Cost of screening
      d. Implications of the results of screening

2. Purposes of screening
    a. Preemployment evaluation—medical history, immunization status, pregnancy, compromised immune status, presence of infectious disease
    b. Periodical evaluation—evaluation of illness during employment, communicable disease exposure, changes in health status; percutaneous injury exposure, active infection acquired in the hospital setting
    c. Outbreak and exposure evaluation—evaluation of susceptibility to disease, type and duration of exposure, availability of prophylaxis
3. Components of OHP screening
    a. Medical history—communicable disease history and risk
    b. Health assessment
    c. Laboratory studies
    d. Tuberculosis screening
    e. Immunizations
4. Communicable disease screening by OHP
    a. Tuberculosis
    b. Rubella
    c. Obstetrics and pediatrics—rubella, varicella
    d. Blood/body fluid exposures—hepatitis B vaccine status
5. Employee illness/injury treatment
    a. Percutaneous injuries
    b. Exposure to communicable diseases
    c. Active infections that may or may not have been acquired in the hospital setting
    d. Carrier states associated with transmission of infection
6. Preventive health services
    a. Educational programs to decrease risk or acquisition of infection
    b. Immunization programs
7. Environmental assessment and intervention
    a. Evaluation of percutaneous injury data for areas of high risk or areas needing in-service education
    b. Assessment of ethylene oxide or glutaraldehyde levels of exposure in the central services department and implementation of control measures, if levels are excessive
    c. Determination of high-risk areas for specific diseases (e.g., blood exposures)
8. Occupational health records—confidential unless release form is signed
    a. Communicable disease history
    b. Immune status, if determined by serological testing
    c. Immunization record
    d. Records of exposure to communicable diseases and prophylaxis, if given

I. Transmission of Infection to and from the Healthcare Worker

1. Vaccine preventable diseases
   a. Hepatitis A and B
   b. Influenza
   c. Measles
   d. Mumps
   e. Rubella
   f. Tetanus and diphtheria
   g. Pertussis
   h. Polio
   i. Varicella-zoster (chickenpox)
2. Diseases with postexposure intervention
   a. Tuberculosis
   b. Rubella
   c. Meningitis (*Neisseria meningitidis*)
   d. Hepatitis A, B
   e. Varicella-zoster (chickenpox)
   f. Scabies
   g. Pertussis
   h. Human immunodeficiency virus
3. Diseases with no postexposure intervention
   a. Herpes simplex
   b. Cytomegalovirus
   c. Meningitis other than *N. meningitidis*
   d. Respiratory syncytial virus (RSV)
   e. Rotavirus
   f. Hepatitis C
4. Work restrictions related to communicable disease
   a. Personnel (including department heads) must know illnesses and conditions that should be reported to the occupational health service and may require work restriction
   b. Work restrictions should not penalize employee, or illnesses will not be reported by employee
   c. Personnel who have responsibility to impose work restrictions must have the authority; this must be fully described in policies and procedures
   d. Determination of work restrictions, consider
      (1) Agent
      (2) Mode of transmission
      (3) Method of interruption of transmission

(4) Population at risk and susceptibility
   (5) Educability and compliance of the healthcare worker
   (6) Clinical status (signs and symptoms)
   (7) Degree and type of patients and staff contact

J. Education

1. New healthcare worker employee orientation
2. Annual healthcare worker updates
3. Postexposure counseling
4. HIV/AIDS, hepatitis B or C exposure counseling
5. TB exposure testing recommendations and positive skin test conversions
6. Workers' compensation issues
7. Pregnant worker concerns
8. Community-acquired infections—non–work-related
9. Influenza prevention
10. Measles, mumps, rubella and chickenpox protection and prevention
11. Laboratory, radiology and cardiology results and analysis of testing done by OHP
12. Employee illness guidelines related to fever, respiratory illness, draining lesions, diarrhea, etc.

K. Plan of Action for Detection, Prevention and Control of Diseases That Are a Threat to Healthcare Workers

1. Detection
    a. History of disease
    b. Symptoms
    c. Laboratory studies
    d. Reporting of cases to health department
2. Prevention and control
    a. Isolation precautions for patients
    b. Work restrictions for employees
    c. Appropriate barrier treatment
    d. Prophylaxis of patient and healthcare workers
    e. Education for healthcare worker and patients
    f. Screening tests postexposure
    g. Follow-up to determine secondary cases or delayed outbreak

L. Occupational Blood or Body Fluid Exposure Management

1. Elements of an effective postexposure management program include:
   a. Clearly stated policies and procedures that address confidentiality and how to manage the exposure
   b. Education and training of workers
   c. Resources for rapid access to clinical care, postexposure prophylaxis (PEP) and testing of source patient and worker
   d. Assessment of the injury
2. OSHA's blood-borne pathogens standard[3] provides directives for employers to:
   a. Develop an exposure plan
   b. Provide the hepatitis B vaccine to employees within 10 days of employment
   c. Provide training on potential hazards, personal protective equipment (PPE), engineering controls and work practices
   d. Facilities must maintain a sharps injury log[4]
3. Procedure for exposures should include
   a. Employee should seek first aid—emergency room if injury/exposure involves need for radiograph, sutures, etc., or perform own first aid using soap and water/alcohol to clean site of exposure if skin not intact
   b. Notify immediate supervisor
   c. Obtain baseline laboratory work for HIV and hepatitis B/C
   d. Obtain laboratory work for HIV/hepatitis B/C for source patient following all state and local requirements for consent
   e. Fill out proper reporting forms as soon as possible, during the same work shift as injury
   f. Follow up with occupational health nurse/physician—postexposure testing at his/her recommended intervals; counseling for HIV, hepatitis or high-risk exposure;
   g. Exposure evaluation should include definition of exposure, infectious agent, mode of transmission, degree of contact/duration, use of barriers, susceptibility of healthcare worker, work restrictions.
   h. Postexposure counseling should include:
      (1) Risk of infection
      (2) Signs and symptoms of infection
      (3) Prophylaxis
      (4) Testing
      (5) Side effects of medications
      (6) Interim precautions
      (7) Risk reduction measures

M. Respiratory Protection Program[5,6]

1. Particulate respirator type N95 respirator commonly used to protect workers from a person with suspected or confirmed TB (required by OSHA's respiratory protection standard)
2. OSHA requires employers to designate a program administrator to administer or oversee the respiratory protection program and conduct the required evaluations of program effectiveness
3. Employer must also provide respirators, training and medical evaluations. Respirator must be acceptable to and correctly fit the user
4. OSHA requires that each worker assigned to wear a respirator receive a fit test before the worker is required to wear the respirator in the workplace and a seal check should be performed with each use
5. A qualitative fit test (QLFT) is one that results in a pass or fail test, assesses adequacy of respirator fit
6. A quantitative fit test (QNFT) is an assessment of the adequacy of the respirator fit by measuring the amount of leakage into the respirator
7. A powered air-purifying respirator (PAPR) uses a blower to force the ambient air through air-purifying elements to the inlet covering; a fit test is not required
8. Employers must establish and implement a written respiratory protection program with worksite-specific procedures. Program should be updated as necessary and should include:
   a. Procedures for selecting respirators
   b. Medical evaluations of employees required to use respirators
   c. Fit testing procedures
   d. Procedures for proper use, storing and discarding respirators
   e. Employee training
   f. Procedures for evaluation of the effectiveness of program

N. Occupational Health Hazards: Postexposure Interventions[7]

1. Tuberculosis (*Mycobacterium tuberculosis*)
   a. A TB screening program should include part-time, temporary, contract and full-time employees. Healthcare workers with face-to-face exposure to patients with suspected or confirmed TB should also be included. Also included are workers with the following:
      (1) Entering patient or treatment rooms, whether or not a patient is present
      (2) Participating in aerosol-generating or aerosol-producing procedures
      (3) Participating in suspected or confirmed *M. tuberculosis* specimen processing
      (4) Installing, maintaining or replacing environmental control in areas in which TB patients are encountered

b. Protocol for TB skin testing should be based on the facility TB risk assessment, recent exposures, community population and recent conversions
c. Purified protein derivative (PPD) skin testing before employment (two-step if no documentation of negative PPD test within past year) and at intervals during employment determined by facility incidence of conversion, risk of exposure and state regulations. Interpretation of the tuberculin skin test (TST) depends on measured TST induration in millimeters, the person's risk for being infected with *M. tuberculosis* and risk for progression to active TB. Interpret the TST test according to CDC guidelines
d. Chest radiograph before employment (if there are risk factors identified during the employee interview) and for new positive reactors (should repeat at intervals) when applicable or as required by state regulations
e. Obtain history of symptoms (cough, weight loss, night sweats, etc.)
f. Postexposure skin testing baseline and 10 weeks after exposure; positive converters need chest radiograph, laboratory tests (liver chemistries) and referral for medical evaluation. Consider retesting immunocompromised personnel at least every 6 months because immunocompromised persons may be unable to react sufficiently to the Mantoux test

Figure 4–1. Interpretation of tuberculin skin test (TST) and QuantiFERON®-TB t (QFT) according to the purpose of testing for *Mycobacterium tuberculosis* infection in a healthcare setting[3]

Purpose of testing	TST	QFT
1. Baseline	1. ≥10mm is considered a positive result	1. Positive (only one-step)
2. Serial testing without known exposure	2. Increase of ≥10mm is considered a positive results (TST conversion)	2. Change from negative to positive
3. Known exposure (close contact)	3. ≥5mm is considered a positive results in persons who have a baseline TST result of 0mm; an increase of ≥10mm is considered a positive result in persons with a negative baseline TST result or previous follow-up screening TST result of ≥0mm	3. Change to positive

2. Measles, mumps, rubella
   a. MMR vaccine is a live virus vaccine; do not administer to pregnant personnel or those who might become pregnant in next 30 days

3. Rubella
   a. Employees should have documentation of one dose of live rubella vaccine or laboratory evidence of immunity to rubella
   b. One dose of MMR is recommended for those personnel who were born before 1956 and who do not have serological evidence of immunity
4. Measles
   a. All workers should have documentation of measles immunity
   b. Vaccinate nonimmune or unvaccinated personnel
   c. Persons born on or after 1957 can be considered immune if documentation of physician-diagnosed measles, documentation of two doses of live vaccine or serological evidence of immunity
   d. Personnel born before 1957 considered immune if history of previous measles disease, documentation of one dose of vaccine or serological evidence
   e. Measles vaccine should be given to susceptible workers who have contact with a measles patient within 72 hours of the exposure; also need to be excluded from duty 5 days after first exposure to 21 days after last exposure[1]
5. Mumps
   a. Employees are considered immune if they have documentation of physician-diagnosed mumps, documentation of two doses of live mumps vaccine or serological evidence of immunity
   b. Two doses of MMR vaccine should be given to employees without this documentation
6. Meningococcal meningitis—*N. meningitidis*
   a. Postexposure prophylaxis is advised for healthcare workers having direct intimate contact (mouth- to-mouth, assisting intubation, endotracheal suctioning)
   b. Prophylactic therapy should be given immediately after exposure. Current recommendations include: ciprofloxacin orally (adults only, nonpregnant), cefotaxime intramuscular (children or pregnant females) or rifampin orally (children or adults)
   c. Preexposure vaccination should be offered to laboratory workers who handle soluble preparations of *N. meningitis*
7. Hepatitis B virus (HBV)
   a. At time of hire, the worker's potential for exposure should be determined and vaccine status assessed
   b. Revaccinate nonresponders with an additional three-dose series and retest
   c. An exposure to HBV is defined as the source person being HbsAg positive or status unknown
   d. If exposed person is vaccinated, but the vaccine response is unknown, perform baseline test for anti-HBs

e. Baseline testing is not necessary if exposed person has not been vaccinated or vaccine response is known
   f. If unvaccinated, begin vaccine series at time of exposure and administer hepatitis B immune globulin (HBIG) within 24 hours of exposure if possible
   g. Booster doses of the HBV vaccine are not necessary
8. Hepatitis C virus (HCV)
   a. Average risk for transmission following percutaneous exposure is 1.8%
   b. Postexposure prophylaxis not recommended
   c. Worker who has been exposed to HCV should not donate blood, plasma, organs, tissue or semen
   d. There is no need for modification of sexual practices or special precautions to prevent secondary transmission
   e. Healthcare personnel who have been exposed to an HCV-positive source should have baseline testing for anti-HCV and ALT activity performed, followed by testing for anti-HCV and ALT activity at 4 to 6 months after the exposure. Testing for HCV RNA may be performed 4 to 6 weeks after exposure if desired[8]
   f. No guidelines for therapy during infection—specialist referral
9. HIV
   a. Average risk for transmission is 0.3% for percutaneous exposure, 0.1% for mucous membrane contact, less that 0.1% for nonintact skin contact[9]
   b. Immediately after exposure, the worker and source person should be tested to assess HIV-AB status
   c. Workers should be counseled to undergo baseline and follow-up testing for 6 months after exposure (e.g., 6 weeks, 3 months and 6 months)
   d. HIV PEP and counseling should start as soon as possible postexposure (within hours)
   e. Consider reevaluation of the exposed person within 72 hours
   f. If source HIV-negative, stop PEP
   g. PEP not contraindicated in pregnancy, consult obstetric physician (choosing regimen is more complex)
10. Varicella
   a. A history of varicella in adults is highly predictive of serological immunity; most adults with negative or unknown histories are also seropositive
   b. Healthcare workers are considered immune if they have laboratory evidence of immunity, a history of clinical diagnosed or verified varicella or zoster, or documentation of vaccination
   c. Varicella vaccination should be given to all healthcare workers without evidence of immunity

d. Serotest a vaccinated worker immediately after exposure to assess the presence of antibody
e. Postexposure—serological screening for varicella titer of employees with negative or unknown history of chickenpox, furlough employees with negative or inadequate titer from day 10 through day 21 postexposure or monitor daily for the development of symptoms. If fever, upper respiratory tract symptoms, or rash develop, then exclude from duty and give varicella vaccine; varicella-zoster immune globulin may be given to persons under 15 years of age or immunocompromised hosts over age 15

11. Scabies and pediculosis
    a. Scabies is spread by prolonged skin-to-skin contact with an infested person; contact precaution can reduce spread
    b. Evaluate employees for signs and symptoms and provide appropriate therapy for confirmed or suspected scabies
    c. Pediculosis is caused by infestation with the human head louse, human body louse and pubic, or crab, louse
    d. Treatment should be provided for exposed employees with evidence of infestation
    e. Prophylactic treatment should not be given

12. Pertussis
    a. Highly contagious, healthcare worker immunity is essential
    b. Workers who provide direct patient care should receive one dose of Tdap[10]
    c. Prophylactic treatment is indicated using erythromycin 500 mg four times daily or 1 tablet of trimethoprim-sulfamethoxazole twice daily[1]

13. Influenza
    a. Influenza vaccination is recommended for all healthcare workers annually
    b. OHP must include an annual influenza prevention campaign that is directed towards the vaccination of healthcare workers
    c. Chemoprophylaxis should be offered to patients, residents and workers when necessary (e.g., during an outbreak)

O. **Guidelines for Work Restrictions for Employees with Infectious Diseases**[1]

1. Conjunctivitis—restrict from patient contact and contact with the patient's environment until discharge ceases
2. Cytomegalovirus infection—no restriction
3. Diarrhea
   a. Acute stage—restrict from patient contact or food handling until symptoms resolve
   b. Convalescent stage (*Salmonella* spp.)—restrict from care of high-risk patients until symptoms resolve

4. Diphtheria—exclude from duty until antimicrobial therapy completed and two negative cultures (24 hours apart)
5. Enteroviral infection—restrict from care of infants, neonates and immunocompromised patients until symptoms resolve
6. Hepatitis A—restrict from patient contact or food handling until 7 days after onset of jaundice
7. Hepatitis B—(when considered infectious) restrict personnel who perform exposure-prone invasive procedures from duty until expert review council has been consulted, review state regulations, no restrictions for employees who do not have exposure-prone duties
8. Hepatitis C—no recommendations, refer to facility and state regulations
9. Herpes simplex
    a. Genital—no restriction
    b. Hands (herpetic whitlow)—restrict from patient contact until lesions heal
    c. Orofacial—evaluate for need to restrict from care of high-risk patients until lesions heal
10. HIV—restrict personnel who perform exposure-prone invasive procedures from duty until expert review council has been consulted, refer to state regulations, no restriction for employees who do not perform exposure-prone procedures
11. Measles
    a. Active—exclude from duty until 7 days after the rash appears
    b. Postexposure (susceptible personnel)—exclude from duty from day 5 through day 21 after last exposure and 7 days after rash appears
12. Meningococcal infection—exclude from duty until 24 hours after start of effective therapy
13. Multidrug-resistant organisms
    a. No recommendations for restrictions of healthcare workers colonized with multidrug-resistant organisms unless epidemiologically linked to transmission within the healthcare facility
14. Parvovirus
    a. Restrict pregnant healthcare worker from caring for patients with aplastic crisis, chronic anemia in immunosuppression
    b. Pregnant healthcare worker—antibody screen and refer to obstetrician
15. Pertussis
    a. Active—exclude from duty from beginning of catarrhal state through third week after onset of paroxysms or until 5 days after start of effective antimicrobial therapy
    b. Postexposure (asymptomatic)—no restriction but prophylaxis is recommended
    c. Postexposure (symptomatic)—exclude from duty until 5 days after start of effective antimicrobial therapy

16. Respiratory syncytial virus—personnel with acute respiratory infections should be excluded from caring for high-risk patients
17. Rubella
    a. Active—exclude from duty until 5 days after rash appears
    b. Post exposure (susceptible personnel)—exclude from duty from day 7 after first exposure through day 21 after last exposure
18. Scabies—restrict from patient contact until cleared by medical evaluation after treatment
19. Staphylococcal infection or carriage
    a. Active, draining lesions—restrict from contact with patients or food handling
    b. Carrier state—no restriction unless personnel are epidemiologically linked to transmission of the organism
20. Streptococcal infection, group A—restrict from patient contact or food handling until 24 hours after adequate treatment started
21. Tuberculosis
    a. Active pulmonary disease—exclude from duty until proven noninfectious
    b. PPD converter—no restriction
22. Varicella (chickenpox)
    a. Active disease—exclude from duty until all lesions are dry and crusted
    b. Postexposure (susceptible personnel)—exclude from duty day 10 through day 21 (day 28 if VZIG was given) after last exposure or if varicella occurs, until all lesions are dry and crusted
23. Varicella-zoster (shingles)
    a. Localized in healthy person—cover lesions and restrict from care of high-risk patients until all lesions are dry and crusted
    b. Generalized or localized in immunosuppressed person—restrict from patient contact until all lesions are dry and crusted
    c. Postexposure (susceptible personnel)—restrict from patient contact from day 10 through day 21 (day 28 if VZIG was given) after last exposure or if varicella occurs until all lesions are dry and crusted
    d. Routine vaccination of all persons aged 60 years of older with one dose of zoster vaccine[11]

Table 4–1. Immunobiologicals and Schedules for Healthcare Personnel (Modified from ACIP Recommendations): Immunizing Agents Strongly Recommended for Healthcare Personnel

Generic name	Primary booster dose schedule	Indications	Major precautions and contraindications	Special considerations
Hepatitis B	Three doses of 1 mL IM at 0, 1, and 6 to 12 months Two doses IM at 0, 1, and 6 to 12 months	Occupational exposure healthcare personnel, exposure to blood, exposure to blood products and bodily fluids and secretions	No apparent adverse effects to developing fetuses, not contraindicated in pregnancy; history of anaphylactic reaction to common baker's yeast	No therapeutic or adverse effects on HBV-infected persons; cost-effectiveness of prevaccination screening for susceptibility to HBV depends on costs of vaccination and testing and prevalence of immunity in the group of potential vaccines; healthcare personnel who have ongoing contact with patients or blood should be tested 1–2 mo after completing the vaccination series to determine serological response
Influenza vaccine— -Inactivated vaccine Flu-Mist	One dose 0.5 mL IM annually Intranasal dose of 0.2 mL annually (split between each nostril)	All healthcare personnel should receive the flu vaccine	History of anaphylactic hypersensitivity after egg ingestion	No evidence of maternal or fetal risk when vaccine was given to pregnant women with underlying conditions that render them at high risk for serious influenza complications
Measles live virus vaccine	One dose subcutaneously; 2nd dose healthcare personnel at least 1 mo later	Healthcare personnel born in or after 1957 without documentation of (a) receipt of two doses of live vaccine on or after their first birthday, (b) physician—diagnosed measles, or (c) laboratory evidence of immunity; vaccine should be considered for all personnel, including those born before 1957 that have no proof of immunity	Pregnancy; immunocompromised* state; (including HIV-infected persons with severe immunosuppression) history of anaphylactic reactions after gelatin ingestion or receipt of neomycin; or recent receipt of immune globulin	MMR is the vaccine of choice if recipients are also likely to be susceptible to rubella and/or mumps; persons vaccinated between 1963 and 1967 with (a) a killed measles vaccine alone, (b) killed vaccine followed by live vaccine or (c) a vaccine of unknown type should be revaccinated with two doses of live measles vaccine

Table 4-1. Immunobiologicals and Schedules for Healthcare Personnel (Modified from ACIP Recommendations): Immunizing Agents Strongly Recommended for Healthcare Personnel *(Continued)*

Generic name	Primary booster dose schedule	Indications	Major precautions and contraindications	Special considerations
Mumps live-virus vaccine	One dose subcutaneously; no booster	Healthcare personnel believed to be susceptible can be vaccinated; adults born before 1957 can be considered immune	Pregnancy; immunocompromised* state; history of anaphylactic reaction after gelatin ingestion or receipt of neomycin of immunity; adults born before 1957 can be considered immune, except women of childbearing age	MMR is the vaccine of choice if recipients are also likely to be susceptible to measles and rubella
Rubella live-virus vaccine	One dose subcutaneously; no booster	Healthcare personnel, both male and female, who lack documentation of receipt of live vaccine on or after their 1st birthday, or of laboratory evidence		Pregnancy; immunocompromised* state; history of anaphylactic reaction after gelatin ingestion or receipt of neomycin Women pregnant when vaccinated or who become pregnant within 3 mo of vaccination should be counseled on the theoretic risks to the fetus, the risk of rubella vaccine-associated malformations in these women is negligible; MMR is the vaccine of choice if recipients are also likely to be susceptible to measles or mumps

Table 4–1. Immunobiologicals and Schedules for Healthcare Personnel (Modified from ACIP Recommendations): Immunizing Agents Strongly Recommended for Healthcare Personnel *(Continued)*

Generic name	Primary booster dose schedule	Indications	Major precautions and contraindications	Special considerations
Varicella-zoster live-virus vaccine	Two 0.5 mL doses SC, 4–8 wk apart if ≥13 yr	Healthcare personnel without reliable history of varicella or laboratory evidence of varicella immunity	Pregnancy; immunocompromised* state; history of anaphylactic reaction after receipt of neomycin or gelatin; salicylate use should be avoided for 6 wk after vaccination	Because 71%–93% of persons without a history of varicella are immune, serological testing before vaccination may be cost-effective

IM, intramuscularly; SC, subcutaneously.
* Persons immunocompromised because of immune deficiencies, HIV infection, leukemia, lymphoma, generalized malignancy, or immunosuppressive therapy with corticosteroids, alkylating drugs, antimetabolites or radiation. (Source: *APIC Text of Infection Control and Epidemiology*, 2009).

Table 4–2. Immunobiologics and Schedules for Healthcare Personnel (Modified from ACIP Recommendations): Other Immunizing Agents Available for Healthcare Personnel in Special Circumstances

Generic name	Primary booster dose schedule	Indications	Major precautions and contraindications	Special considerations
Hepatitis A vaccine	1 mL IM at 0, 6 months	Not routinely indicated for United States healthcare personnel; persons who work with HAV-infected primates or HAV in a laboratory setting should be vaccinated	History of anaphylactic reaction to aluminum or the preservative 2-phenoxy ethanol; vaccine safety in pregnant women has not been evaluated, risk to fetus is likely low and should be weighed against the risk for hepatitis A in women at high risk	Healthcare personnel who travel internationally to endemic areas should be evaluated for vaccination
Meningococcal polysaccharide (quadrivalent A, C, W135 and Y) vaccine	One dose in volume and by route specified by manufacturer; need for boosters is unknown	Not routinely indicated for healthcare workers in the United States	Vaccine safety in pregnant women has not been evaluated; vaccine should not be given during pregnancy unless risk of infection is high	May be useful in certain outbreak situations (see text)

Table 4–2. Immunobiologics and Schedules for Healthcare Personnel (Modified from ACIP Recommendations): Other Immunizing Agents Available for Healthcare Personnel in Special Circumstances *(Continued)*

Generic name	Primary booster dose schedule	Indications	Major precautions and contraindications	Special considerations
Polio vaccine	IPV, two doses SC given 4–8 wk apart followed by 3rd dose 6–12 mo after 2nd dose; booster doses may be IPV or OPV	Healthcare personnel in close contact with persons who may be excreting wild virus and laboratory personnel handling specimens that may contain wild poliovirus	History of anaphylactic reaction after receipt of streptomycin or neomycin; because safety of vaccine has not been evaluated in pregnant women, it should not be given during pregnancy	Use only IPV for immunosuppressed persons or personnel who care for immunosuppressed patients; if immediate protection against poliomyelitis is needed, OPV should be used
Pneumococcal polysaccharide vaccine (23 valent)	0.5 mL IM or SC in deltoid	Not routinely indicated; HCWs who smoke or have asthma are considered high risk for pneumococcal disease	Anaphylactic reactions have occurred in persons receiving repeat doses of vaccine more often than recommendations; adverse effects on fetus not observed	Safety in pregnancy has not been evaluated. Previous recipients of vaccine who are at highest risk for infection may be revaccinated $\geq$5 years after first dose
Rabies vaccine	HDCV or PCECV 1 mL IM (deltoid) one each on days 0, 3, 7 and 14. Immunosuppressed individuals require 5th dose on day 28	Personnel who work with rabies virus or infected animals in diagnostic or research activities		The frequency of booster doses should be based on frequency of exposure. See CDC reference for rabies prevention for postexposure recommendations
Tetanus and diphtheria (Td)	3 doses of 0.5mL SC at 0,1–2 and 6 months; booster every 10 yr	All adults; tetanus prophylaxis in wound management	First trimester of pregnancy; history of a neurological reaction or immediate hypersensitivity reaction; individuals with severe local (Arthus-type) reaction after previous dose of Td vaccine should not be given further routine or emergency doses of Td for 10 yr	

Table 4–2. Immunobiologics and Schedules for Healthcare Personnel (Modified from ACIP Recommendations): Other Immunizing Agents Available for Healthcare Personnel in Special Circumstances *(Continued)*

Generic name	Primary booster dose schedule	Indications	Major precautions and contraindications	Special considerations
Typhoid vaccines: IM, subcutaneously and oral	One 0.5 mL dose IM; booster doses of 0.5 mL every 2 yr; (VI capsular polysaccharide) or two 0.5 mL doses SC, 4 or more wk apart; boosters of 0.5 mL SC or 0.1 mL ID every 3 yr if exposure continues or four oral doses on alternate days; (Ty21a) vaccine manufacturer's recommendation is revaccination with the entire four-dose series every 5 yr	Personnel in laboratories who frequently work with *Salmonella typhi*	History of severe local or systemic reaction to a previous dose of typhoid vaccine; TY21a vaccine should not be given to immunocompromised* personnel	Vaccination should not be considered as an alternative to the use of proper procedures when handling specimens and cultures in laboratory
Vaccinia vaccine (smallpox)	One dose administered with a bifurcated needle; boosters every 3 years for persons at continued high risk for exposure to smallpox	Personnel who directly handle cultures of or animals contaminated with recombinant vaccinia viruses or orthopox viruses (monkeypox, cowpox, vaccinia, etc.) that infect human beings; some have been vaccinated for bioterrorism prevention	Pregnancy, presence of history of eczema, or immunocompromised* status in potential vaccinees or their household contacts	Vaccination may be considered for healthcare personnel who have direct contact with contaminated dressings or other infectious material from volunteers in clinical studies involving recombinant vaccinia virus

HDCV, human diploid cell rabies vaccine; *RVA*, rabies vaccine absorbed; *IPV*, inactivated poliovirus vaccine; *OPV*, oral poliovirus vaccine; *ID*, intradermally.
* Persons immunocompromised because of immune deficiencies, HIV infection, leukemia, lymphoma, generalized malignancy, or immunosuppressive therapy with corticosteroids, alkylating drugs, antimetabolites or radiation.
(Source: *APIC Text of Infection Control and Epidemiology, 2009*)

Table 4–3. Immunobiologicals and Schedules for Healthcare Personnel (Modified from ACIP Recommendations): Diseases for Which Postexposure Prophylaxis May Be Indicated for Healthcare Personnel

Generic name	Primary booster dose schedule	Indications	Major precautions and contraindications	Special considerations
Diphtheria penicillin,	Benzathine 1.2 mU IM, single dose, or erythromycin (1 g/day) PO × 7 days	For healthcare personnel exposed to diphtheria or identified as carriers		Also administer one dose Td to previously immunized if no Td has been given in ≥5 yr
Hepatitis A	One IM dose IG 0.02 mL/kg given within 2 wk of exposure in large muscle mass (deltoid, gluteal)	May be indicated for healthcare personnel exposed to feces of infected persons during outbreaks	Persons with IgA deficiency; do not administer within 2 wk after MMR or within 3 wk after varicella vaccine	
Hepatitis B	HBIG 0.06 mL/kg IM as soon as possible (and within 7 days) after exposure (with dose 1 of hepatitis B vaccine given at different body site); if hepatitis B series has not been started, 2nd dose of HBIG should be given 1 mo after 1st	HBV-susceptible healthcare personnel with percutaneous or mucous-membrane exposure to blood known to be HBsAg seropositive		
Meningococcal disease	Rifampin, 600 mg PO every 12 hours for 2 days, or ceftriaxone, 250 mg IM, single dose, or ciprofloxacin, 500 mg PO, single dose	Personnel with direct contact with respiratory secretions from infected persons without the use of proper precautions (e.g., mouth-to-mouth resuscitation, endotracheal intubation, endotracheal tube management, or close examination of oropharynx)	Rifampin and ciprofloxacin not recommended during pregnancy	

Table 4–3. Immunobiologicals and Schedules for Healthcare Personnel (Modified from ACIP Recommendations): Diseases for Which Postexposure Prophylaxis May Be Indicated for Healthcare Personnel *(Continued)*

Generic name	Primary booster dose schedule	Indications	Major precautions and contraindications	Special considerations
Pertussis	Erythromycin, 500 mg qid PO, or trimethoprim-sulfamethoxazole, 1 tablet bid PO, for 14 days after exposure or azithromycin 500 mg day 1 then 250 mg day 2–5	Personnel with direct contact with respiratory secretions or large aerosol droplets from respiratory tract of infected persons		
Rabies	For those never vaccinated, HRIG 20 international units/kg, should be infiltrated around wound, and any remaining volume administered IM at a site distant from vaccine administration	Personnel who have been bitten by human being or animal with rabies or have had scratches, abrasions, open wounds or mucous membranes contaminated with saliva or other potentially infective material (e.g., brain tissue)		Personnel who have previously been vaccinated, give HDCV or RVA vaccine, 1 mL, IM on days 0 and 3; no HRIG is necessary
Varicella-zoster virus	VZIG for persons >50 kg: 125 units/10 kg IM; for persons <50 kg: 625 units	Personnel known or likely to be susceptible to varicella and who have close and prolonged exposure to an infectious healthcare worker or patient, particularly those at high risk for complications, such as pregnant or immunocompromised persons	Rifampin and ciprofloxacin not recommended during pregnancy	Serologic testing may help in assessing whether to administer VZIG; if varicella is prevented by the use of VZIG, vaccine should be offered later

P. **Immunizations Recommended for Healthcare Workers**
   See Tables 6-1, 6-2, and 6-3

Q. **Performance Improvement in Preventing Occupational Exposure**
   1. Purpose
      a. Evaluate the effectiveness of prevention programs
      b. Choose the most effective means of prevention
      c. Prove cost-effectiveness of injury and exposure prevention
   2. Improvement measures to monitor
      a. Monitor reductions or increases in injuries and exposures over time
      b. Identify the causes of injuries and exposure
      c. Analyze variations that occur
      d. Design and implement prevention strategies
      e. Provide education for the healthcare worker regarding the incidence of injuries and exposures and preventive measures
      f. Track the effectiveness of prevention strategies by comparing injury and exposure rates to the previous rates
      g. Provide feedback to the healthcare workers involved in the effectiveness of the prevention strategies
      h. Monitor actions involving injury
      i. Monitor devices used during injury
   3. Calculation of rates of reported injuries and exposures for measuring performance improvement
      a. Total number of percutaneous injuries (1 year) divided by the number of occupied beds/average daily census
      b. Total number of percutaneous injuries by nurses (1 year) divided by total number of full-time equivalent nurses employed that year
      c. Number of percutaneous injuries from device type in 1 year divided by number of that device type used or purchased in same year

Practice Questions for Chapter Four

Chapter Four:

Employee Occupational Health

1. During an in-service program on the hepatitis B vaccine, the IP is asked why some healthcare workers who received the hepatitis B vaccine soon after its release did not develop antibody. What is the IP's MOST likely explanation for why this occurred?
   a. The vaccine may have been injected into the buttocks rather than the deltoid
   b. Healthcare workers tend to be less responsive to hepatitis B vaccine because of environmental exposure to blood
   c. The vaccine has been reformulated several times in the past decade, causing it to improve in its effect
   d. Antibody levels wane with time

2. The IP has just reviewed the current public health recommendations concerning influenza vaccines before developing an educational program for employees. The report indicates that the MOST important problem in developing a long-term vaccine for influenza is:
   a. Potential toxicity of the vaccine if the dosage is increased
   b. Lack of potency
   c. Antigenic drift of the viruses
   d. Short storage life of the vaccine

3. The employee health nurse has asked the IP to assist with personnel TB skin testing. Which of the following represents a known TB skin test conversion in a healthcare worker?
   a. Prior tuberculin test results are not available, but the current result is 16 mm after 48 hours
   b. Tuberculin skin test reaction 1 year ago was 9 mm, and the current results are 13 mm
   c. A prior tuberculin reaction was not measured, but the employee states it was dime-sized. The current result is 11 mm
   d. Tuberculin reaction 1 year ago was 3 mm, and the current result is 18 mm

4. A new employee is hired and refuses a chest radiograph or skin test for TB on the grounds that she is pregnant. The nursing director is pressuring you to allow her to start work on Monday. She has no documentation of a prior TB skin test. What should you as the employee health/IP do?
   a. Get written approval from administration and risk management for the employee to work
   b. Tell her director that she cannot be hired until after her delivery
   c. Talk with the director of human resources about making an exception to the rule
   d. Tell the employee she must bring in documentation from her obstetrician that she should neither be x-rayed nor receive a TST

5. The IP is also responsible for employee health. Administration has instructed the IP to evaluate the facility for varicella immunity and then begin a varicella vaccine program. Which of the following actions would be taken LAST?
   a. Develop a policy outlining what constitutes immunity to varicella (e.g., history of chickenpox, positive IgG titer, history of varicella vaccine)
   b. Obtain a freezer for storage of the vaccine in the employee health department
   c. Review the literature related to the varicella vaccine
   d. Develop a mechanism to survey all the employees for history of varicella

6. You are the director of infection prevention and control in a large teaching hospital.

   You learn the hemodialysis unit coordinator has known that one of his nurses has infectious hepatitis B. He does not want to move that person out of the department because the nurse will be retiring in a year. He thinks the nurse's age would hinder learning new skills. The ultimate conclusion to this issue should be:
   a. The nurse will need to retire, and the coordinator should be reprimanded
   b. The nurse will need to take a medical leave of absence
   c. The nurse should be offered another position in another department
   d. The nurse can work in this department but not perform exposure-prone invasive procedures until expert review council has been consulted

7. You are called to the ICU to review the chart of a 43-year-old man with suspected bacterial meningitis. The Gram stain of the patient's CSF shows many gram-negative diplococci. The emergency room physician has written a prescription for "Cipro 500 mg PO for all employees with direct, intimate contact." In talking with employees, you learn that one exposed employee is pregnant. You would recommend:
   a. The pregnant employee should be given pharmaceutical information, with benefits and risks explained, so she can make her own decision
   b. All employees must sign a release of responsibility before receiving medication
   c. The pregnant employee should go to her obstetrician for treatment
   d. The pregnant employee should be offered ceftriaxone 250 mg IM but should call her obstetrician for permission first

8. An employee reports to you that she has walked a man in the hall who now has shingles. She did not wear gloves and cannot remember washing her hands right away. She states that her mother says she has never had chickenpox. You advise her to:
   a. See the employee health nurse for a varicella titer and recommendations
   b. Go to her physician for the varicella vaccine right away
   c. Go to the employee health nurse because this is a Workers' Compensation issue and she will be missing some work; then call her supervisor
   d. Not worry because she probably had chickenpox and just did not break out with many lesions

9. A 39-year-old man is admitted with a high fever and disorientation. He has been suffering with an ear infection for 2 weeks. At this point, before the results of the spinal tap are known, which of the following statements are true?
   (1) He could possibly have meningitis from *Streptococcus pneumoniae*
   (2) Employees and family members should be treated prophylactically after the Gram stain report is known
   (3) The public health department should be notified to treat the family contacts prophylactically
   (4) He should be treated by an infectious disease physician because of the infectious risk to the employees
   (5) Employees and family contacts may not need any prophylactic treatment
      a. 1, 5
      b. 1, 2
      c. 2, 3
      d. 3, 4

10. In evaluating a new labor and delivery/nursery employee's medical history, which of the following would be MOST important to provide protection to newborns?
    (1) Measles, mumps, rubella immune status
    (2) Hepatitis B immunity
    (3) Chickenpox or shingles history
    (4) Tetanus/diphtheria immunization status
    (5) Absence of any skin lesions, skin infections
       a. 1, 2, 3
       b. 1, 3, 5
       c. 1, 4, 5
       d. 1, 3, 4

11. For a labor and delivery/nursery employee, which one of the following would be MOST important to provide protection to the nurse from infectious disease?
    a. Measles, mumps, rubella immune status
    b. Hepatitis B immunity
    c. Chickenpox or shingles history
    d. Tetanus/diphtheria immunization status

12. Which of the following diseases are preventable by immunization?
    (1) Diphtheria
    (2) Varicella
    (3) Pertussis
    (4) Cytomegalovirus
       a. 1, 2, 3
       b. 2, 3, 4
       c. 1, 3, 4
       d. 1, 2, 3, 4

13. A young man is admitted after a car accident and placed on a ventilator overnight because of severe chest contusions. While on the ventilator, a sputum specimen is obtained by suctioning. After the ventilator is discontinued, he is afebrile and not on oxygen. Chest radiography showed early atelectasis, which is now clearing. Sputum culture report from admission shows *Neisseria meningitidis*. What should be done?
    a. Rifampin or cipro prophylaxis for family members and staff with close contact
    b. Rifampin or cipro prophylaxis for staff or physicians who assisted with intubation or suctioning while he was on the ventilator
    c. Droplet Precautions for 24 hours and no one treated prophylactically
    d. Standard Precautions with no one treated prophylactically

Questions 14–16 You are called to the ICU to examine a patient with a rash who was admitted earlier because of seizures. He has been a resident of the jail for the past 2 months. The young man is sedated and unable to tell you anything about the rash. You are told by the nurses that he has a rash only on his legs from the knees down.

14. The surgeon has diagnosed scabies and ordered lindane lotion to the patient's legs and a consult with a dermatologist. The MOST urgent recommendation you should make is:
    a. The charge nurse should make a list of all nurses and technicians exposed to this patient to send to the employee health nurse for treatment
    b. The lindane lotion should not be used, and the attending physician should be advised of drug precautions
    c. The nurses can use the lindane lotion but should monitor the patient closely for any problems
    d. All treatment should be held until the dermatologist can see and evaluate the patient's rash

15. The dermatologist performs a skin biopsy and orders hydrocortisone cream to the legs. The MOST likely cause of the rash is:
    a. Fungal infection
    b. Dry skin dermatitis
    c. Dermatitis from previous scabies infection
    d. Bacterial dermatitis

16. The nurses who have been exposed to the patient should be treated with:
    a. Lindane lotion
    b. Permethrin lotion
    c. Hydrocortisone cream
    d. No treatment necessary

17. When determining employee work restrictions, the IP should consider:
    1. Mode of transmission
    2. Clinical status of employee
    3. Laboratory testing requirements
    4. Degree and type of patient contact
        a. 1, 2, 3
        b. 1, 2, 4
        c. 2, 3, 4
        d. 1, 3,4

18. During an in-service program for new employees, the IP describes how hepatitis B and HIV are transmitted. A major difference in the epidemiology of the two diseases is:
    a. Presence of the causative agent in various body fluids
    b. The ability of the diseases to be transmitted during sexual intercourse
    c. The ease of transmission through needle punctures
    d. The potential for airborne transmission

19. Which infectious disease exposure requires prophylactic treatment and urgent counseling?
    a. Mumps
    b. CMV
    c. RSV
    d. Syphilis

20. As the IP you are consulted by the employee health nurse to assist in counseling an HIV-positive employee who is worried about having exposures to infections. The employee has recently lost a friend to AIDS-related opportunistic infections. The employee is a registered nurse working in surgery. What topics are MOST important to include in the counseling?
    (1) Statistics about healthcare providers with HIV infection
    (2) Facts about transmission of HIV
    (3) Measures to prevent transmission of infectious organisms
    (4) Barriers to wear for common organism transmission prevention
    (5) Monitoring and maintaining good immunity with HIV infection
    a. 3, 4, 5
    b. 1, 2, 5
    c. 2, 3, 4
    d. 1, 2, 3

21. A pregnant employee is worried about her exposure to a patient with shingles. She tells you that she has walked him in the hall every day for the past week. All of the following questions are important EXCEPT which one?
    a. When is the baby due?
    b. Has she ever had chickenpox?
    c. Has she contacted her obstetrician about her concerns?
    d. Where were the lesions located?

22. The laboratory notifies you that a patient on the nursing unit has a positive hepatitis A antibody IgM. Which of the following is true?
    a. The nurses should be immunized with immune globulin
    b. The patient is infectious
    c. The patient is immune but has had hepatitis A in the recent past
    d. The patient has had hepatitis A sometime in his life, time unknown

23. You are the employee health nurse and IP for a small health department. Which of the following are MOST important to include in a brief educational program?
    a. Hand-washing, isolation precautions, exposure protocols, incident reporting and sick protocols
    b. Hand-washing, ETO and glutaraldehyde exposure limits, Workers' Compensation reports and incident reporting
    c. Hand-washing, isolation protocols for each disease, employee health guidelines and policies and exposure procedures
    d. Signs and symptoms of diseases commonly seen, hand-washing, isolation procedures and exposure procedure

24. Which of the following employee infections would require the employee (nurse) to be sent home?
    a. Sinus infection being treated by antibiotic
    b. Small vesicular lesion on the fingertip, which is painful
    c. Shingles, which has been treated with an antiviral for past 4 days
    d. Dry, crusted lesion on right arm with no new drainage

25. You are the IP and employee health nurse for a large outpatient surgical center. You are developing a screening tool to use when interviewing potential employees. What testing, related to infection prevention and control, should be performed?
    a. Chest radiograph
    b. Drug testing
    c. Hepatitis B surface antigen/antibody
    d. Nasal culturing

26. You meet with an upset employee who has just found out that she has a positive PPD. She has been HIV-positive for 8 years. The employee admits to you that as a child she also had a reactive skin test. She was not tested again until last year when she tested negative. What is your BEST explanation for this?
    a. She may have had low immunity last year and failed to show response to the skin test
    b. Her childhood test was probably inaccurate, and this represents a new conversion
    c. Her recent positive test may have been a "boosted" reaction
    d. The recent testing is probably inaccurate because of the HIV disease

27. She comes to visit you 3 weeks after her TB medication is started. She is having difficulty taking her medicines, and is experiencing bouts of nausea and vomiting. Her physician has placed her on four drugs despite a negative chest radiograph. Your advice should include all EXCEPT which statement?
    a. She must let her physician know immediately that she is vomiting
    b. She should keep you informed of her medication success
    c. Chest radiograph findings may not be reliable for diagnosis in HIV infection
    d. She should hold her TB meds until her next doctor visit because the HIV medications are much more important

28. An employee receives a needle-stick injury while working in the operating room. Place the following steps in order of importance:
    1. Obtain baseline laboratory tests for HIV and hepatitis B and C
    2. Seek first aid
    3. Notify immediate supervisor
    4. Fill out proper reporting forms
    a. 1, 2, 3, 4
    b. 2, 1, 3, 4
    c. 2, 3, 1, 4
    d. 3, 2, 4, 1

29. An employee who has received all three doses of hepatitis B vaccine and who has never had hepatitis B virus infection would be expected to have which of the following serological marker(s)?
    a. HBcAb
    b. HBsAb
    c. HBeAb
    d. HBeAb and HBsAb

30. You are the IP in a small county health department. You are interviewing a nurse for a position in the clinic. She said she does not need a PPD skin test because she can bring in a copy of her test done 2 months ago at her previous home health position. The LEAST correct response is:
    a. TB could have been acquired in the past 2 months
    b. She should bring in a copy of the test signed by her previous employer
    c. She still needs to be tested before employment
    d. She can get a chest radiograph and skip the PPD test until next year

Answers for Practice Questions Chapter Six

1. a	9. a	17. b	25. c
2. c	10. b	18. c	26. a
3. d	11. b	19. d	27. d
4. d	12. a	20. a	28. c
5. b	13. d	21. a	29. b
6. d	14. d	22. b	30. d
7. d	15. b	23. a	
8. a	16. d	24. b	

References

1. Centers for Disease Control and Prevention. Guidelines for infection control in healthcare personnel, 1998. *Am J Infect Control* 1998;26:289–354.

2. Division of Nosocomial and Occupational Infections, Bureau of Infectious Disease, Centre for Infectious Disease Prevention and Control. Prevention and Control of Occupational Infections in HealthCare: Infection Control Guidelines. Ottawa, Ontario, Canada: Health Canada, 2002:28S1.

3. U.S. Department of Labor. 29CFR Part 1910.1030. Occupational exposure to bloodborne pathogens: final rule. *Fed Registr* 1991;56:64174–64182.

4. U.S. Department of Labor. 29CFR Part 1910.1030. Occupational exposure to bloodborne pathogens; needlesticks and other sharps injuries: final rule. *Fed Registr* 2001;55:5317–5325.

5. Fairfax RE. The OSHA interpretation of respiratory protection requirements with regards to tuberculosis (TB) exposure. U.S Department of Labor, Standard Interpretation, February 5, 1999. Available at: http://www.osha.gov/pls/oshaweb/owadisp.show_document?p_table=INTERPRETATIONS&p_id=22062. Accessed November 9, 2010.

6. U.S. Department of Labor. OSHA's Respiratory Protection Standard 29 CFR 1910.134. Available at: http://www.osha.gov/dte/library/respirators/presentation/index.html. Accessed November 9, 2010.

7. Centers for Disease Control and Prevention. Guidelines for preventing the transmission of Mycobacterium tuberculosis in health-care settings, 2005. *MMWR* 2005;54:1–144.

8. Centers for Disease Control and Prevention. Updated U.S. Public Health Service guidelines for the management of occupational exposures to HBV, HCV, and HIV and recommendations for postexposure prophylaxis. *MMWR Recomm Rep* 2001;50(RR-11):1–52.

9. Centers for Disease Control and Prevention. Updated U.S. Public Health Service guidelines for the management of occupational exposures to HBV, HCV, and HIV and recommendations for postexposure prophylaxis. *MMWR* 2001;50:1–52.

10. Centers for Disease Control and Prevention. Preventing tetanus, diphtheria, and pertussis among adults: use of tetanus toxoid, reduced diphtheria toxoid, and acellular pertussis vaccine. Recommendations of the

Advisory Committee on Immunization Practices and Recommendations of ACIP, supported by the Healthcare Infection Control Practices Advisory Committee (HICPAC), for use of Tdap among healthcare personnel. *MMWR* 2006;55:1–53.

11. Centers for Disease Control and Prevention. Prevention of herpes zoster: recommendations of the Advisory Committee on Immunization Practices (ACIP). *MMWR* 2008;57:1–30.

CHAPTER FIVE

MANAGEMENT AND COMMUNICATION

CONTENTS

Article	Page
CBIC Content Outline for Management and Communication	280
Chapter Five: Management and Communication	281
I. The Infection Prevention and Control Program	281
II. Communication and Feedback	286
III. Quality/Performance Improvement	287
Practice Questions for Chapter Five	292
References	308

CBIC CONTENT OUTLINE

Management and Communication (16 Questions)

A. Planning

1. Conduct an infection risk assessment of the organization
2. Develop, evaluate and revise a mission and vision statement, goals, measurable objectives and action plans for the infection prevention and control program
3. Recommend specific equipment, personnel and resources for the infection prevention and control program
4. Participate in cost-benefit assessments, efficacy studies and product evaluations
5. Recommend changes in practice based on clinical outcomes and financial implications

B. Communication and Feedback

1. Provide infection prevention and control findings, recommendations, annual reports and policies and procedures to appropriate individuals, committees, departments and units
2. Communicate with internal and external customers (e.g., related to infection prevention and control issues of continuity of care, reporting communicable disease)
3. Collaborate with risk management/quality management personnel in the identification and review of adverse and sentinel events
4. Evaluate accreditation/regulatory issues and facilitate compliance

C. Quality/Performance Improvement

1. Participate in quality/performance improvement and patient safety cactivities related to infection prevention and control
2. Demonstrate quality/performance improvement projects through the use of graphic tools (e.g., "fishbone" diagram, Pareto charts, flow charts)

Chapter Five: Management and Communication

I. **The Infection Prevention and Control Program**

   A. **Infection Prevention and Control Team**
   1. Core of team—infection preventionist (IP), the infection prevention and control committee chair and the healthcare epidemiologist
   2. One person should be designated as having responsibility for the program[1,2]
   3. All members should be qualified and guided by sound principles and current information

   B. **Infection Prevention and Control Committee (IPC)**
   1. Function—the central decision and policymaking body for all infection prevention and control issues/policies
   2. Reporting—IPC chair reports to either the medical staff or administration
   3. Purpose—acts as the advocate for prevention and control of infections in the facility; formulates and monitors patient care policies; educates staff; provides political support that empowers the team[3,4]
   4. Membership—should be multidisciplinary; including members of administration, clinical and ancillary staff (e.g., IP team, employee health, pharmacy, microbiology, risk management, perioperative services, respiratory therapy, nursing, housekeeping)
   5. Goals:
      a. Refines and ratifies the ideas of the IP team
      b. Disseminate surveillance data and policy decisions
   6. IPC not requirement of The Joint Commission (TJC), but function is required; many states require IPC

   C. **Infection Preventionist Professionals**
   1. Role and responsibilities[1,2,5,6]
      a. Collection and analysis of data
      b. Evaluation of products and procedures
      c. Development and review of policies
      d. Consultation on infection risk assessment, prevention and control strategies; includes activities related to occupational health, construction and disaster planning
      e. Education efforts directed at interventions to reduce infection risks
      f. Implementation of changes mandated by regulatory, accrediting and licensing agencies; includes reporting communicable diseases to health departments
      g. Application of epidemiological principles, including activities directed at improving patient outcomes
      h. Provision of high-quality services in a cost-effective manner
      i. Participation in research projects

2. Many IPs work less than full-time on infection prevention[7]; they may also be involved in such areas as:
   a. Employee health
   b. Quality management/performance improvement
   c. Risk management
3. IP roles may be filled by two key positions:
   a. Infection prevention professional—usually has a background in nursing, medical technology, infectious disease or microbiology
   b. Hospital epidemiologist—physician or individual with master's degree in public health who has special training in hospital epidemiology or infectious disease may serve at the IPC chair or IP advisor; training is offered at locations throughout the United States sponsored by the Society for Healthcare Epidemiology of America (SHEA), American Hospital Association (AHA), Centers for Disease Control and Prevention (CDC) and many universities
4. Staffing
   a. The CDC (1969) and Study on the Efficacy of Nosocomial Infection Control (SENIC) study results recommend one full-time IP for every 250 occupied beds[8,9]
   b. University health system consortium indicates one full-time IP for every 30 to 40 ICU beds[10,11]
   c. APIC's DELPHI study noted that staffing must consider the number of occupied beds, scope of the program, complexity of the healthcare facility, characteristics of the patient population and unique needs of the facility; recommends ration of 8 to 1 IP for every 100 occupied acute care beds[12]

D. **Infection Prevention and Control Program**
   1. The three principal goals for infection prevention and control programs are to:
      a. Protect the patient
      b. Protect the healthcare worker, visitors, and others in the healthcare environment
      c. Accomplish the previous two goals in a cost-effective manner whenever possible
   2. The functions of the infection prevention programs are:
      a. To obtain and manage critical data and information, including surveillance for infections
      b. To develop and recommend policies and procedures
      c. To intervene directly to prevent the transmission of infectious diseases
      d. To educate and train healthcare workers, patients, and nonmedical caregivers
   3. Increase effectiveness
      a. Influence of the IP is based on visibility, provision of resources to the staff, use of scientific evidence to make recommendations

b. Document the impact of the program with a cost-benefit analysis. Targeted surveillance should be tied to specific interventions to decrease HAIs. Appropriate interventions to decrease infections would then result in documentation of cost savings.[13-15]
4. Annual risk assessment—perform to determine goals and objectives for the IP program
   a. Steps to setting priorities and realistic strategies[16]
      (1) Establishing a reliable, focused surveillance system
      (2) Streamlining data management activities
      (3) Analyzing healthcare-associated infection (HAI) rates
      (4) Aiming for zero HAIs
      (5) Educating staff regarding prevention techniques
      (6) Identifying opportunities for performance improvement
      (7) Taking a leadership role on performance improvement teams
      (8) Developing and implementing action plans that outline the steps needed to accomplish each objective[17,18]
5. Assess quality of the infection prevention program by evaluating customer satisfaction,[19] appropriateness, efficacy, timeliness, availability, effectiveness and efficiency
6. Infection prevention and control program reporting relationships—depending on the needs of the institution, the IP may report to or be integrated with
   a. Administration
   b. Nursing services
   c. Quality management/performance improvement
   d. State agencies (for reportable diseases or hospital infection rates), local health department
   e. Risk management
      (1) Assist with investigation of patient claims or sentinel events related to HAI
      (2) Report cases with potential for legal action; incidents; product recalls
   f. Safety
   g. Human resources
   h. Employee health
      (1) Consult regarding Workers' Compensation related to infections or exposures
      (2) Consult regarding employee infections and illnesses
      (3) Integrate infection prevention and control related employee health policies
      (4) Assist EH with surveillance of employee illnesses/exposures (required by TJC standard)
7. Infection prevention and control surveillance programs should be influenced by
   a. Mandated reporting requirements
   b. Procedures, service lines, surgeries, etc., performed by facility (high volume, high risk, high cost, etc.)

  c. New equipment, instruments, procedures, etc., with infection prevention and infection control related risks, concerns or benefits
  d. Patient demographics
    (1) Diseases common to patient population
    (2) Risk factors common to patient population
    (3) Socioeconomic status of community
8. Infection prevention and control policies and procedures
  a. General policies are applicable to staff in the whole facility; form the basis of the infection prevention and control manual
  b. Specific policies should be developed for each unit/area
  c. Policies must be supported scientifically and address infection prevention and control needs for the institution
  d. Application of infection prevention and control practices occurs primarily when providers of direct patient care consistently implement these policies to benefit patients and protect staff
  e. Education of staff is crucial to efficient implementation of infection prevention and control policies and quality of patient care practices related to infection prevention[20]
9. Administrative support
  a. Important that administrative leaders of the organization approve and support the infection prevention and control activities
  b. IP professionals should schedule regular meetings with administrator to whom they are responsible; keep administration well informed of the infection prevention and control activities; IP professionals should have input in the planning and future of the program
  c. Annual goals and objectives should be developed based on the goals of the organization
  d. Staff and data systems needs should be defined by the specific requirements of the infection risk reduction process of the organization
  e. Annual evaluation of the infection prevention and control program is important to outline the achievements and activities of the program and describe support requirements; value of the IP program should be emphasized, as well as patient outcomes and cost savings
10. Vision/mission/values
  a. Decision makers need to be informed of the value of the infection prevention and control program; one way to explain the importance of the program to others is through a mission statement and a description of the vision for the program
  b. What? Why? How? These governing ideas answer three critical questions:
    (1) Vision is the what—the picture of the future that the infection prevention and control program seeks to create; vision is long term

(2) Mission is the why—the answer to the question: "Why does the program exist?"—a vision is needed to make the mission more concrete and tangible

(3) Core values answer the question, "How does the infection prevention and control program want to act, consistent with our mission, along the path toward achieving our vision?"—values describe how the program functions on a day-to-day basis, while pursuing the vision

    c. Vision paints a picture of where the infection prevention and control program wants the organization to go and wants it to be. Vision needs to:
       (1) Focus on strategic advantages—begin by identifying the program's strategic advantage in the organization
       (2) Add value to others

    d. Mission statement defines the common purpose, focus and context for all departmental activities; mission statements enable a group to set boundaries for their activities, to know what is and what is not within their jurisdiction and to understand where they fit in the organization's overall improvement efforts; mission should support the overall institutional mission

11. Customer identification
    a. Customer is anyone to whom the infection prevention and control program provides service; includes patients, patients' families, physicians, nurses, visitors and all employees at facility
    b. Distinction between external and internal customers is based on amount of influence the infection prevention and control program has on the customer:
       (1) Internal—nurses, physicians, administrators, patients, patients' families, facility employees
       (2) External—visitors, community, IP professionals at other facilities, regulatory agency personnel
    c. Identification of customer needs—all work processes should be studied and constantly improved so that the final product or service exceeds customer expectations

12. IP professional as customer/supplier
    a. For any transaction involving a product, service or information, the person or organization being supplied something is the customer; the IP professional is the supplier; roles may reverse for different transactions

13. Multidisciplinary activities
    a. Collaborative teams are often most effective in identifying processes or problems needing improvement and working together to find solutions
    b. Teams should include individuals from multiple functional areas integral to the specific issue being studied

c. Flowcharting the process at a macro level is one way to determine which areas should be involved in the team

II. Communication and Feedback

A. Communication with IPC Chairperson

1. Emergency situations, problems and outbreaks
2. Education about emerging diseases and conditions
3. Employee health issues
4. Surveillance results
5. Surveillance and infection prevention and control program proposals
6. Healthcare practices and procedures that need improvement
7. Community concerns
8. Topics for discussion at IPC
9. Construction or renovation issues or problems
10. Advice from infection prevention and control chair regarding actions to take
11. Notification of sentinel event because of infection

B. Communication with Facility Management

1. Resources with costs needed for infection prevention and control program
2. Emergency situations, problems and outbreaks
3. Employee situations affecting several departments
4. Construction or renovation issues or problems
5. Surveillance rates and IPC minutes
6. Changing legislation and regulations
7. Notification of sentinel event because of infection
8. Develop reports to be presented to the facility board

C. Communication with Medical Staff

1. Surveillance rates and IPC minutes
2. Procedural issues involving physicians
3. Emergency situations
4. Changing legislation and regulations
5. Recommendations to change practices

D. Communication with Nursing

1. Changing legislation and regulations
2. Surveillance rates
3. Emergency situations, problems and outbreaks

4. Employee practices and procedures that need improvement
5. Education about emerging diseases and conditions and high-risk practices
6. Product recall notification
7. Recommendations to change practices
8. Assistance in root cause analysis

E. Communication with Other Clinical Departments and Support Staff

1. Education related to infection prevention practices
2. Education related to infectious diseases and high-risk practices
3. Advice from staff related to improving practices
4. Product recall notification
5. Assistance in root cause analysis

F. Communications with Risk Management

1. Information about product recalls
2. Patient names from exposure risk/incident reports
3. Notification of inappropriate actions that place patients at risk for an infection
4. Follow-up results from patients with infection exposure risks
5. Notification of patient needing root cause analysis performed because of infection-related death or disability

III. Quality/Performance Improvement

A. Quality Concepts

1. Strategic plan[21]—determines the direction an organization will go in the future and what is required to meet goal, mission or vision; includes:
   a. An analysis of the organization
   b. Forming conclusions about what an organization must do as a result of issues facing the organization
   c. Action planning (include the tactic to accomplish goals, who will carry out the action, the timeline, resources and evaluation criteria)
   d. The Joint Commission requirements of a detailed strategic plan
      (1) Prioritizes the identified risk for acquiring and transmitting infections
      (2) Sets goals that include limiting unprotected exposures to pathogens; the transmission of infections associated with procedures; the transmission of infections associated with the use of medical equipment, devices and supplies
      (3) Describes activities, including surveillance to minimize, to reduce or eliminate the risk for infection
      (4) Describes the process to evaluate the infection prevention control plan

B. Performance Improvement Teams[22]

1. Valuable tool to deploy the quality-focused culture or process
2. Multidisciplinary team includes a leader, facilitator and team members with fundamental knowledge of the process

C. Gap Analysis[23]

1. Technique to determine the steps necessary to take to move from a current state to a desired future state, based on identified gaps in processes

D. Root Cause Analysis (RCA)[24,25]

1. Takes a retrospective look at adverse outcomes and determines what happened, why it happened and what the organization can do to prevent reoccurrence
2. Used to investigate major incidents, sentinel events and errors
3. Avoids individual blame, considers human factor engineering and analyzes redesign for a safer system
4. Team collects data through structured interviews, document reviews and field observations
5. Contributing factors categorized as associated with clinical practice; regulatory, policy or accreditation factors; operational or management factors; and staff tasks and patient characteristics
6. Uses a tree diagram to identify areas of responsibility
7. At conclusion, team summarizes and identifies causes and begins to strategize about process redesign

Table 5-1. Sample GAP Analyses

Duty Number	Description	Evidence	Gap/Compliance Action
1	To protect patients, staff, and others from HAIs	Joint Commission Standard IP.01.05.01 2009 EP:7	Yes
2	Assess risk of acquiring HAIs and take action to reduce or control such risks	Joint Commission Standard IP.01.03.01 2009 EP:5	No; Review risk assessment quarterly and communicate to infection prevention program committee

Source: APIC Text 2009.

E. **Failure Mode Effect Analysis (FMEA)**[26]
   1. Proactive, preventive approach to identify potential failures and opportunities for error
   2. Components of healthcare FMEA
      a. Determine a process or topic to study; should carry risk for harm
      b. Convene a team of process or content experts
      c. Develop a flow diagram to clearly identify steps of the process and any subprocesses
      d. Brainstorm possible reasons for failure; rate these based on severity and probability of occurrence
      e. Determine appropriate actions to eliminate the failure or redesign the process
      f. Identify outcome measures to test the redesigned process

F. **Strengths, Weaknesses, Opportunities, Threats (SWOT) Analysis**[26]
   1. Investigate public health issues and improve healthcare outcomes
   2. Points out what the organization should plan for and how to use resources to guide efforts

G. **Multivoting (nominal voting)**[28]
   1. Process of prioritizing a large list of topics to a final selection

H. **Goal-Directed Checklists**[29]
   1. Contain multiple evidence-based criteria
   2. Help with memory recall and make expected steps explicit

I. **Statistical Process Control (See Chapter 2)**

J. **Six Sigma and the Lean Approach**[30]
   1. Six Sigma concentrates on precision and accuracy that leads to data-driven decisions
   2. Lean Six Sigma speaks to the speed and efficiency and the elimination of "waste"
   3. Value stream mapping used to visualize flow of materials and information and identify bottlenecks, barriers and waste
   4. DMAIC format used to create a data-driven improvement strategy
      a. Define the customer, project boundaries and improvement process
      b. Measure the performance of the process involved
      c. Analyze the data collected and map the process to determine root causes and improvement opportunities

d. Improve the target process by designing creative solutions to fix and prevent problems
e. Control the improvements to keep the process on the new course

K. Plan, Do, Study, Act (PDSA)[31]
1. Plan—identify responsibilities of the program, resources, risks and goals
2. Do—implement strategies specified in the plan to achieve goals
3. Study—collect and display data about goal achievement
4. Act—continual change in order to achieve goals and stay abreast of new developments

L. Customer Satisfaction
1. Internal customers—staff receive and analyze surveillance data, review program policies and receive ongoing education about infection prevention
2. External customers—individuals or groups outside of the immediate organization (patients, family members, community); expect evidence-based practice and compliance with rules, regulations and guidelines

M. Performance Measures
1. Fundamental concepts
   a. Quality of measures
      (1) Valid—the extent to which a measure accurately reflects the concept or construct it is intended to measure[32]
      (2) Reliable—ability of an indicator to accurately and consistently identify the events it was designed to identify[32]
   b. Outcome measure—indicates the result of the performance of a function or process (e.g., SSI, VAP)
   c. Process measure—focus on a process or the steps in a process that lead to specific outcomes (e.g., compliance with aseptic technique for dressing change)

N. Determining the Patient Population to Measure
1. Risk potential—when individual patient characteristics increase the likelihood of the outcome of interest, it is necessary to adjust the metrics to control these risks (e.g., American Society of Anesthesiologists [ASA] score, wound contamination classification, duration of surgical procedure)
2. Sample size:
   a. When the volume of patients in the selected population is large, a sample approach to data collection may be an acceptable way to minimize resources and still obtain valid data

    b. Common sampling methods include general random samples and stratified random samples (e.g., every third surgery)
    c. Small sample sizes are problematic, data analyses and conclusions are limited; may require measurement of the entire population at risk
 3. Data analysis—use risk-adjustment and stratification when necessary
 4. Evaluate existing performance measures—be clear about the purpose and how data will be used; determine whether the measure adequately defines the event and patient population of interest to the organization
 5. Developing performance measures[33]
    a. Developing unit-specific policies and procedures
    b. Becoming familiar with regulatory and accrediting standards and requirements
    c. Collect and report data in a timely manner
    d. Ensure accuracy and completeness of data collection
    e. Increase feasibility and ease of data collection
 6. Measurement tools include:
    a. Check sheets
    b. Run charts—graph that displays observed data in a time sequence; analyzed to find anomalies in data that suggest shifts in a process over time or special factors that may be influencing the variability of a process
    c. Histograms—graphical representation, showing a visual impression of the distribution of data
    d. Statistical process control charts—used to determine whether or not a process is in a state of statistical control (Chapter 2)
    e. Cause-and-effect or fishbone diagram—show the causes of a certain event; commonly used to identify potential factors causing an overall effect; takes an event or piece of information and works backward to determine causes; causes usually grouped into major categories to identify these sources of variation (e.g., people, method, environment)
    f. Pareto chart—contains both bars and a line graph, with individual values represented in descending order by bars; the cumulative total is represented by the line; used to highlight the most important among a set of factors

O. **Using Data to Drive Improvement**
 1. Internal tracking versus external comparisons—to compare data between institutions requires data collected by the same methodologies, including training of data collectors, definitions used and resources used to make determinations
 2. Relation to quality improvement and patient safety—there must be a link between the collection of infection data and the organization's continuous improvement strategy

Practice Questions for Chapter Five

Chapter Five:

Management and Communication Questions

1. You notice a rise in the number of ventilator-associated pneumonias (VAPs) in the medical intensive care unit (MICU). Your actions in order of priority are:
   (1) Calculate rates based on ventilator days in the unit and compare with National Healthcare Safety Network (NHSN) rates for similar units
   (2) Communicate the number of VAPs to the medical and hospital staff
   (3) Obtain the total numbers of ventilator days during the time period specified.
   (4) Consult with the epidemiologist for significance of the data
   (5) Work with MICU team to develop interventions to reduce infections
   a. 4, 5, 3, 1, 2
   b. 5, 1, 4, 3, 2
   c. 3, 1, 4, 5, 2
   d. 3, 1, 4, 2, 5

2. Because of an increase in acuity in the intensive care unit (ICU), the number of ventilator days has doubled. Your VAP rate has increased compared with prior rates. Your first action would be:
   a. Communicate the infection rates to the medical and hospital staff
   b. Continue to collect and trend data
   c. Stratify risk factors; then develop charts and tables showing infections/acuity rate
   d. Assemble a team to reduce the numbers of VAPs

3. Your program has selected reduction in the VAP rate as its performance improvement activity for the year. In your annual evaluation, you note that the rate has consistently been at or just below the NHSN 50th percentile for the past year compared with above the NHSN 50th percentile for the previous year. You recommend:
   a. Assembling a team to analyze the problem and develop interventions to reduce the rate to 10% below the NHSN 50th percentile because of the high mortality associated with infection
   b. Changing the focus for the year to central line-related infections because that rate has been consistently above the NHSN 50th percentile and also has a high associated mortality
   c. Changing the focus for the year to Foley-related urinary tract infections (UTIs) because there is a new catheter available with a guarantee that its use will reduce infection rates
   d. Developing a team to study preventive measures for VAP that can be implemented before the study is started

4. The manager for cardiopulmonary services indicates that the department would like to increase the length of time for changes of ventilator tubing from every 7 days to every 14 days. You would:
   (1) Search the literature for studies documenting no increase in adverse patient outcomes with the change
   (2) Review the abstracts published from the APIC conferences for information pertaining to the issue
   (3) Check practice patterns with your peers in other hospitals
   (4) Evaluate the potential cost savings
   (5) Compromise with the manager with a change to every 10 days
   a. 1, 2, 3
   b. 1, 3, 4
   c. 1, 2, 4
   d. 1, 3, 5

5. When developing an infection prevention and control program, one of the first steps would be:
   a. Developing policies and procedures
   b. Collecting resource materials, such as regulatory or accrediting standards
   c. Developing protocols for employee health
   d. Collecting material relating to antibiotic usage in community hospitals

6. IP managers are individuals who plan, organize, direct, control and coordinate activities in order to move the organization toward:
   a. Higher profits
   b. Greater social influence
   c. Desired objectives
   d. Economic stability

7. While performing the infection prevention and control program assessment, it is noted that program mission, goals and objectives have not been developed. A special departmental staff meeting is held to accomplish this task. Which of the following best describes a mission statement for an infection prevention and control program?
   a. The statement tells what the program will do
   b. The statement tells why the program exists
   c. The statement tells what the future of the program will be
   d. The statement tells who is responsible for the program

8. In developing the program goals, all the following could be considered a program goal EXCEPT:
   a. Protect the patient
   b. Protect the healthcare worker
   c. Perform surveillance in the ICU over 6 months
   d. Provide cost-effective infection prevention and control

9. Strategic planning includes all of the following steps EXCEPT:
   a. An analysis of the organization
   b. Forming conclusions about what an organization must do
   c. Action planning
   d. Defining the common purpose for all departmental activities

10. Which of the following is the MOST important reason for having an infection prevention and control committee?
    a. The IPC function is required by The Joint Commission
    b. The IPC is a vehicle for communication and consensus building
    c. The IPC is necessary to justify the IP's position
    d. The IPC can replace the organization's safety committee

11. Your infection control staff verbalizes frustrations with employee compliance with isolation precautions at both acute and long-term care facilities. Monitoring actions have been performed in the past and reported to the infection prevention and control committee (IPC). As the manager, what would be your FIRST step to address this problem?
    a. Review the monitoring results to familiarize yourself with the data
    b. Prepare a written report to administration
    c. Meet with unit managers, discuss concerns and invite their input in improving isolation practices
    d. Develop an action plan and present it to the IPC

12. The department has received reports of diarrhea among patients following flexible sigmoidoscopy procedures at an ambulatory clinic. A visit to the clinic notes poor housekeeping practices, no written procedures for cleaning of endoscopes, questionable practices with endoscopy and recent staff turnover. In addressing this problem, the first action the IP should take is:
    a. Meet with administration and discuss the new regulations
    b. Inform the IPC and safety committee of the regulation
    c. Review the policies and procedures for sharps
    d. Discuss findings with clinic administration

13. The IP could contribute to the risk management program by all EXCEPT which of the following?
    a. Monitoring compliance with existing policies and procedures
    b. Presenting educational programs
    c. Advising patients of the risks associated with hospitalization
    d. Serving as a consultant on the safety of the hospital environment

14. The human resources department requested that your infection prevention staff competencies be submitted in 1 month. You discover that no competencies have been developed for your IP staff. Which of the following would NOT be considered in developing competencies for infection prevention and control?
    a. Leadership
    b. Problem solving
    c. Surveillance and analysis
    d. Attendance

15. You are facilitating a group aimed at decreasing surgical site infection rates. Which of the following methodologies would be most helpful to determine the steps to take to move toward lower rates?
    a. Gap analysis
    b. Root cause analysis
    c. Failure mode effect analysis
    d. Multivoting

16. Which surveillance study measures quality improvement related to outcome?
    a. Monitoring compliance with isolation measures
    b. Observing handwashing in a critical care unit
    c. Calculating a ventilator-associated pneumonia rate for the ICU
    d. Measuring the rates of compliance to a needleless IV system

17. A new handwashing soap is being placed in each department. The soap was purchased without your involvement. Use of the soap will save your facility a lot of money over a year's time. What statement is LEAST accurate when describing actions you should take?
    a. The soap should be used for several months while evaluations are done of: employee usage and approval, allergic reactions, dermatitis, effectiveness, and nosocomial infection rates
    b. The MSDS sheet should be checked immediately for FDA registration, chemical ingredients, manufacturer's recommendations, etc.
    c. Check with other area facilities regarding use of this product
    d. The soap should be used despite concerns about the effectiveness because of the significant cost savings

18. The safety committee has asked you to evaluate and recommend a safety syringe. You want to develop a team to look at several products. You have been told to keep the team small. Besides you, the following persons should be included on the team:
    (1) Nursing educational instructor
    (2) Administrator
    (3) Safety officer
    (4) Employee health nurse
    (5) Purchasing manager
    (6) Several nursing managers
    a. 3, 4, 5, 6
    b. 2, 3, 4, 5
    c. 1, 3, 5, 6
    d. 1, 2, 3, 5

19. Infection prevention and control in ancillary and clinical departments routinely involves all of the following EXCEPT:
    a. Evaluate patient care procedures to give input on infection prevention and control techniques
    b. Consult with surgery and sterile processing regarding any purchase of equipment and supplies used for sterilization
    c. Oversee all food preparation and department cleaning activities
    d. Consult with environmental services on changes in cleaning products

20. You are developing a new policy for employee illness and sick leave. When implementing the policy, the FIRST action will be to:
    a. Obtain approval from administration
    b. Survey the nursing department managers for their support
    c. Send a memo to all departments, summarizing the changes in policy
    d. Send a copy of the policy to each department director so they can educate their staffs

21. The first step in preparing a strategic plan for an infection prevention and control program is to:
    a. Formulate a mission and vision statement
    b. Develop a surveillance plan
    c. Develop an infection prevention and control manual
    d. Conduct blood-borne pathogen in-service training

22. Organizational characteristics that influence the effectiveness of the infection prevention and control program include all EXCEPT:
    a. Staffing ratios (employees : patients)
    b. Administrative support
    c. Educational level of the IP
    d. Population of patients served

23. You are preparing a report for the infection prevention and control committee to summarize the year's surveillance and accomplishments. This annual report should contain all of the following EXCEPT:
    a. Review of the surgical site infection by type of surgery, rates and risk factors
    b. Analysis of the IP's work with time documented for each project and area
    c. Surgeon-specific surgical site infection rates for the year
    d. Device-associated infection rates for the year

24. You are choosing focus surveillance projects for the next year. You want one study to include a focus on a fungal infection. Which surveillance project would be most valuable?
    a. Aspergillosis during renovation of the healthcare facility
    b. *Candida* infections in patients with cancer
    c. Fungal infections in patients with acquired immunodeficiency syndrome (AIDS)
    d. Thrush infections in babies

25. Which of the following policies would be MOST important for the infection prevention and control function?
    a. Nosocomial infection definitions
    b. Procedure for conducting surveillance
    c. Procedure for cleaning and disinfecting the operating rooms
    d. Protocol for employee exposure follow-up

26. The DMAIC format includes all of these except:
    a. Define the customer, project boundaries and improvement process
    b. Measure the performance of the process involved
    c. Improve the target process by designing creative solutions to fix and prevent problems
    d. Control the improvements only until problems are no longer prevalent

27. What is the most common method of evaluating major incidents, sentinel events and medical errors?
    a. Statistical process control
    b. Strengths, weaknesses, opportunities, threats analysis
    c. Root cause analysis
    d. Plan, do, study, act

28. Which of the following is NOT a step that should be taken when developing a performance measure about BSI prevention?
    a. Use the NHSN criteria to define BSI
    b. Feedback information about each BSI as it is identified
    c. To increase ease of data collection, rely on the ICU to report BSI for you to investigate
    d. Consistently use the same area of nursing documentation to identify if potential cases have a central line in place

29. Infection prevention policies
    a. Should be developed for each unit/area separately
    b. Should be supported scientifically
    c. Do not need to be supported with education of staff
    d. Are generally applied by administration and support staff

30. You are a seasoned IP who wishes to increase the influence of your program. Which of the following steps should you take?
    (1) Increase your rounds to patient care areas
    (2) Do a cost-benefit analysis focusing on your success from the past year
    (3) Perform a literature search to answer several questions you have received lately about discontinuation of contact isolation
    (4) Take a class on performing root cause analysis
        a. All of the above
        b. 2 and 4
        c. 1 and 2
        d. 1, 2, and 3

31. You are new to a facility but feel sure you will become accustomed to the job quickly. One of the first areas you need to learn about is:
    a. Structure and function of the committees that interact with infection prevention and control
    b. Salary levels of all personnel on your level of responsibility
    c. State laws that govern your department
    d. Policies that refer to the functions of the facility

32. Obtaining support for a change in practice from healthcare providers may be met with resistance when:
    a. It concerns people who do not share in the benefit of the change
    b. It concerns people who do share in the benefit of the change
    c. It does not threaten the security of those involved in the change
    d. It offers greater job satisfaction to all involved

33. At the end of your first year on the job, you review your accomplishments and decide you did not accomplish as much as you had planned. The quickest and easiest way to improve your time management would be to:
    a. Take a time management training course
    b. Look for ways to organize your office
    c. Review your crisis management skill
    d. Look for ways to reduce distractions and address time-wasters

34. A decrease in surgical site infections is an example of the following quality care measurement?
    a. Structure criteria
    b. Process criteria
    c. Outcome criteria
    d. Clinical indicators

35. You must develop goals for the infection prevention and control program. An example of a program goal statement is:
    a. Improve patient care by the reduction of healthcare-associated infection
    b. Improve patient care by the 25% reduction of healthcare-associated infections by the nursing staff
    c. Improve patient care by targeting zero UTIs in the ICU after implementation of a recommended strategies to reduce infections.
    d. Improve patient care by the 50% reduction of healthcare-associated infections by the nursing staff

36. A correctly written committee objective is:
    a. The IPC will develop an antibiotics program
    b. The IPC will meet TJC requirements for implementation of an antibiotics program
    c. The IPC will develop an antibiotics program, within the next 5 months, to meet TJC standards
    d. Improve patient care by the reduction of healthcare-associated infections

37. In selecting committee members, which of the following personal characteristics should be MOST important in influencing your choices:
    a. Individuals who are usually on time for meetings
    b. Individuals who have a strong interest in infection prevention and control
    c. Individuals who have decision-making power
    d. Individuals who will be faithful in attending meetings

38. As an IP, you realize that hospital administration can BEST support the infection control committee by:
    a. Information dissemination
    b. Requiring a tuberculin skin test for all new employees
    c. Emotional support
    d. Financial and political support

39. A policy that is LEAST likely to reduce infection risk to personnel is:
    a. Defined eating, drinking and smoking areas
    b. Compliance with employee immunization programs
    c. Attendance at educational programs on infection prevention and control principles
    d. Wearing protective barriers only for selected high-risk patients

40. You have prepared an agenda allowing a specific amount of time for each item. At the meeting, one of the members is overly talkative and you are afraid that important items will need to be tabled until the next meeting. You can gain control of the meeting by:
    a. Ignoring the person and changing the subject to the next topic on the agenda
    b. Letting the group take care of itself, allowing the conversation to finish before moving on
    c. Calling the person by name and asking them a difficult question; the person will be embarrassed and stop talking
    d. Interrupting with, "That's an interesting point, but we have several important things to discuss today"

41. One of the surgeon committee members strongly opposed a new policy that would allow certified nurses to insert peripheral central catheters. Although the literature supports that this would be cost-saving for the patient with a much lower morbidity rate, you believe the surgeon perceives he may experience a loss of income and/or control. You would resolve the conflict by which of the following:
    a. Agreeing with him, because surgeons are usually right
    b. Telling him he has no choice and that a change will be made
    c. Listening to his point of view, even if it takes up the entire meeting
    d. Tabling the policy to the next meeting and allowing the surgeon to express his opinion after the meeting

42. A program or system for monitoring and providing a safe environment for the employee and quality care for patients to reduce liability is:
    a. Quality/performance improvement
    b. Utilization management
    c. Risk management
    d. Prospective payment system

43. An effective infection prevention and control plan will provide:
    a. Program goals and objectives
    b. Authorities of the committee members
    c. Responsibilities of employee health department
    d. Adequate budget

44. Failure of multidisciplinary teams occurs when:
    a. There is acceptance of the solution
    b. A clean mission statement is provided
    c. Resources are provided
    d. There is confusion about their roles

45. You have been asked to consult with a physician's office on the disposal of infectious waste. Which of the following steps would you initiate first?
    a. Develop an overall plan for waste disposal
    b. Make sure the office has red bags for trash
    c. Assess local infectious waste regulations
    d. Conduct an in-service program on waste disposal for the office workers

46. Protocols for a reuse program for disposable devices would include all of the following EXCEPT:
    a. Establishment of feasibility
    b. Assessment of new technology
    c. Recommendations of the user department
    d. Validation of the effectiveness of the processing procedures

47. One of the BEST ways to develop your communication skills with co-workers in your facility is to:
    a. Take a Dale Carnegie course
    b. Practice giving speeches
    c. Develop your listening skills
    d. Join a social club where many of the others are members

48. Rapport with personnel can BEST be improved by:
    a. Being consistent
    b. Being agreeable
    c. Being a good leader
    d. Being independent

49. The quality/performance improvement director at your facility has asked you to select some performance measures for outcome of care in patients. You will choose one related to nosocomial infections. A critical step in determining the selection of nosocomial infection indicators for use in hospitalized patients is:
    a. Reviewing current performance measures in use in U.S. hospitals for interhospital comparison
    b. Surveying other hospitals in your city to determine the performance measures they have chosen
    c. Developing performance measures based primarily on economic costs of the related nosocomial infection
    d. Developing indicators that measure processes

50. Changes in outcome indicator rates may occur as a result of:
    (1) Changes unrelated to changes in quality
    (2) Changes related to changes in quality
    (3) Changes in case mix or systems of case finding
    (4) Variables that are not adjusted for
    (5) Variables that occurred in every case studied
       a. 1, 2, 3, 4
       b. 2, 3, 4
       c. 3, 4, 5
       d. 1, 3, 4, 5

51. In reviewing a process, you note that many different factors can affect the outcome data. Which of the following takes an event or piece of information and works backward to determine causes?
    a. Fishbone diagram
    b. Control chart
    c. Histogram
    d. Scatter diagram

52. Over the past 6 months, you have been following all the infections in the ICU. In your surveillance, you note an increasing time period between the time an antibiotic is ordered and the time it is first administered. Which action would follow the quality/performance improvement process?
    a. Continue to monitor it another 6 months and report results to the director
    b. Develop an interdisciplinary team to look at the process and recommend possible improvements
    c. Have administration send the director a memorandum
    d. Send an incident report to management and a copy to the department director

53. Important concepts in quality/performance improvement include:
    (1) Breaking down barriers between departments
    (2) Knowing your customers' needs
    (3) Not fixing processes that are not broken
    (4) Determining the cause of a problem by observation before working to resolve it

    a. 1, 2
    b. 2, 3
    c. 1, 4
    d. 3, 4

Questions 54–56: Your healthcare facility is planning on incorporating a dental clinic, and you have been asked to help set up an effective infection prevention and control program in the dental office. Areas of concern are training, employee health, selection of disinfectants, proper sterilization, waste management and development of a procedure book. Besides the dentist, there are four employees: an office manager, a hygienist and two dental assistants.

54. The first step in the consulting process is:
    a. Evaluate the infection prevention and control program by visiting the clinic, reviewing the present policy manual and obtaining the training records of the employees
    b. Plan a corrective action program for implementation
    c. Provide educational materials for the staff
    d. Prepare a report that outlines responsibilities of each employee of the clinic

55. You have made a site visit and assessed the current infection prevention and control program. The MOST important factor to consider in planning corrective action is:
    a. Cost effectiveness
    b. Feasibility
    c. Assignment to a person(s) for completion
    d. Office equipment

56. As the consultant, you determine that the disinfection and sterilization of instruments used in the dental operation does not comply with accepted standards. Further assessment reveals that the problem is not related to disinfecting agents or sterilization equipment but is related to lack of knowledge and, as a result, to incorrect procedures on the part of dental assistants involved in the process. One of the critical concepts for the consultant to remember while attempting to impart knowledge that will lead to a change in staff members' behavior is:
    a. Continual repetition of the concepts involved in sterilization will ensure correct behavior in the dental technicians
    b. Teaching regarding disinfection/sterilization is not necessary if policies are formulated correctly
    c. Changes in procedures are more likely to be accepted by the dental technicians than by the dentist
    d. Changes in procedures will be more readily accepted if the dental assistants are provided with educational materials and involved in developing the new procedures

57. You are starting a new job as an IP in a large acute care facility that has 35 ambulatory care centers. As preparation, you would review all of the following EXCEPT:
    a. Policies and procedures for the acute care facility and ambulatory care centers
    b. Organizational goals and objectives for the healthcare system
    c. Surveillance data for all areas of care at the facility
    d. Minutes from all meetings the previous IP attended

58. Faced with increasing pressure from a cost-conscious administration to reduce infection prevention and control related expenses, you should:
    a. Reaffirm your past decisions on procedures that have proved to be effective infection prevention and control measures
    b. Look for new data that could support less costly alternatives without compromising patient care
    c. Decrease your time in the patient care areas to allow time for paperwork justification
    d. Eliminate time-consuming educational activities

59. In your role as IP you discover the various relationships that form within the hospital organization. Many of these relationships develop into an informal organizational structure. You should:
    a. Not be concerned with the informal organization because it is not formally recognized by the hospital
    b. Listen to the informal organization because it may be the first to note a problem area
    c. Use the informal organization to disperse information because of its reliability
    d. Use the informal organization as a prime information source

60. External characteristics of the IP that influence and motivate the practice of healthcare providers include all of the following EXCEPT:
    a. Visibility and availability of the IP
    b. Assertiveness and diplomacy of the IP
    c. Use of education and management strategies to bring about change
    d. Personal beliefs and motivations

61. An infection prevention and control problem has surfaced on one of the nursing units. You feel that it is significant, but you are not sure that the IPC will share your concern. Which of the following would be an INAPPROPRIATE action to prepare for the meeting?
    a. Be prepared with the facts
    b. Give an emotional plea for support
    c. Talk to sympathetic committee members prior to the meeting to enlist their support
    d. Have visual materials such as charts or graphs to clearly define the problem

62. In the decision-making process, it is best to find a solution that:
    a. Will ensure administrative support
    b. Can be accomplished in a usual time frame
    c. Relies on a single source of information
    d. Minimizes personal risk

Answers for Practice Questions Chapter Five

1.	c	22.	c	43.	a
2.	c	23.	c	44.	d
3.	b	24.	a	45.	c
4.	a	25.	a	46.	c
5.	b	26.	d	47.	c
6.	c	27.	c	48.	a
7.	b	28.	c	49.	a
8.	c	29.	b	50.	a
9.	d	30.	b	51.	a
10.	b	31.	a	52.	b
11.	a	32.	a	53.	a
12.	d	33.	d	54.	a
13.	c	34.	c	55.	b
14.	d	35.	c	56.	d
15.	a	36.	c	57.	d
16.	c	37.	c	58.	b
17.	d	38.	d	59.	b
18.	c	39.	d	60.	d
19.	c	40.	d	61.	b
20.	a	41.	d	62.	a
21.	a	42.	c		

References

1. Scheckler WE, Brimhall D, Buck AS, et al. Requirements for infrastructure and essential activities of infection control and epidemiology in hospitals: A consensus panel report. *Am J Infect Control* 1998;26:47–60.

2. Friedman C, Barnette M, Buck AS, et al. Requirements for infrastructure and essential activities of infection control and epidemiology in out-of-hospital settings: a consensus panel report. *Am J Infect Control* 1999;27:418–430.

3. Wiblin RT, Wenzel RP. The infection control committee. *Infect Control Hosp Epidemiol* 1996;17:44–46.

4. Wenzel RP. Leadership and management for health-care epidemiology. In Wenzel RP, Ed. *Prevention and control of nosocomial infections*. 4th ed. Philadelphia: Lippincott Williams & Wilkins, 2003:609–616.

5. Friedman C, Curchoe R, Foster M, et al. APIC/CHICA-Canada infection control and epidemiology: Professional and practice standards. *Am J Infect Control* 2008;36:385–389.

6. Osguthorpe SG, Ormond L. Management constraints in infection control. *Crit Care Nurs Clin* 1995;7:703–712.

7. Smith PW, Bennett G, Bradley S, et al. SHEA/APIC Guideline: Infection Prevention and Control in the Long-Term Care Facility. *Am J Infect Control* 2008;36:504–535.

8. Haley RW, Quade D, Freeman HE, et al. Study on the efficacy of nosocomial infection control (SENIC Project): Summary of study design. *Am J Epidemiol* 1980;111:472–485.

9. Eickhoff TC, Brachman PS, Bennett JV, et al. Surveillance of nosocomial infections in community hospitals. I. Surveillance methods, effectiveness, and initial results. *J Infect Dis* 1969;120:305–317.

10. Friedman C, Chenoweth C. A survey of infection control professionals staffing patterns at University HealthSystem Consortium institutions. *Am J Infect Control* 1998;26:239–244.

11. Friedman C, Chenoweth C. Infection control staffing patterns. *Am J Infect Control* 2001;29:130–132.

12. O'Boyle C, Jackson M, Henly SJ. Staffing requirements for infection control programs in US health care facilities: Delphi project. *Am J Infect Control* 2002;30:321–333.

13. Fraser VJ, Olsen MA. The business of health care epidemiology: Creating a vision for service excellence. *Am J Infect Control* 2002;30:77–85.

14. Pronovost P, Needham D, Berenholz S, et al. An Intervention to Decrease Catheter-Related Bloodstream Infections in the ICU. *N Engl J Med* 2006;355:2725–2732.

15. APIC Targeting Zero. Available at:

    http://www.apic.org/AM/Template.cfm?Section=Targeting_Zero2&Template=/CM/HTMLDisplay.cfm&ContentID=14855. Accessed January 16, 2011.

16. Murphy DM. From expert data collectors to interventionists: Changing the focus of infection control professionals. *Am J Infect Control* 2002;30:120–132.

17. Bennett G, Baker O. Developing an integrated quality improvement program. *Am J Infect Control* 1990;18:118–125.

18. Haley RW. Surveillance by objective: a new priority-directed approach to the control of nosocomial infections. *Am J Infect Control* 1985;13:78–89.

19. Friedman C, Baker CA, Mowry-Hanley J, et al. Use of the total quality process in an infection control program: A surprising customer-needs assessment. *Am J Infect Control* 1993;21:155–159.

20. Haley RW. The development of infection surveillance and control programs. In: Bennett JV, Brachman JS, eds. *Hospital Infections*, 4th ed. Philadelphia: Lippincott-Raven, 1998.

21. McNamara C. Basic *Description of Strategic Planning (Including Key Terms to Know)*. Adapted from the Field Guide to Nonprofit Strategic Planning and Facilitation. Referenced from Strategic Planning. Available online at: http://managementhelp.org/plan_dec/str_plan/basics.htm. Accessed November 16, 2010.

22. Brown DS, Aydin CE, Donaldson N. Quartile dashboards: translating large data sets into performance improvement priorities. *J Healthc Qual* 2008;30(6):18–30.

23. Agency for Healthcare Research and Quality. Closing the Quality Gap: A Critical Analysis of Quality Improvement Strategies. Available online at: http://www.ahrq.gov/clinic/epc/qgapfact.htm. Accessed March 25, 2009.

24. Department of Veteran Affairs, National Center for Patient Safety. Root Cause Analysis. Available online at: http://www.patientsafety.gov/rca.html. Accessed March 16, 2009.

25. Wald H, Shojania KG. Root cause analysis. In: Shojania KG, Duncan BW, McDonald KM, et al, eds. *Making Health Care Safer: A Critical Analysis of Patient Safety Practices*. Evidence Report/Technology Assessment No. 43 from the Agency for Healthcare Research and Quality: AHRQ Publication No. 01-E058; 2001.

26. Institute for Healthcare Improvement. Failure Modes and Effects Analysis Tool. Available online at: http://www.ihi.org/ihi/workspace/tools/fmea/. Accessed November 16, 2010.

27. *Business SWOT Analysis*. Available online at:. http://www.mindtools.com/pages/article/newTMC_05.htm. Accessed November 16, 2010.

28. Tague NR, ed. Multivoting. In: *The Quality Toolbox*. 2nd ed. Milwaukee, WI: American Society of Quality, Quality Press; 2004:359.

29. Khorfan F. Quality toolbox daily goals checklist: a goal-driven method to eliminate nosocomial infection in the intensive care unit. *J Healthc Qual* 2008;30(6):13–17.

30. Six Sigma. Available online at: http://www.isixsigma.com/sixsigma/six_sigma.asp. Accessed November 16, 2010.

31. Institute for Healthcare Improvement. Testing for Change. Available online at: http://www.ihi.org/IHI/Topics/Improvement/ImprovementMethods/HowToImprove/testingchanges.htm. Accessed November 16, 2010.

32. Joint Commission. *Managing Performance Measurement Data in Health Care*. Oak Brook, IL: Joint Commission; 2008:118.

33. The Joint Commission. Attributes of core performance measures and associated evaluation criteria. The Joint Commission Web site.

    Available online at: http://www.jointcommission.org/NR/rdonlyres/7DF24897-A700-4013-A0BD-154881FB2321/0/AttributesofCorePerformanceMeasuresandAssociatedEvaluationCriteria.pdf. Accessed November 16, 2010.

CHAPTER SIX

EDUCATION AND RESEARCH

CONTENTS

Article	Page
CBIC Content Outline for Education and Research	312
Section A: Education	313
I. Basic Principles in Teaching and Learning	313
II. Educational Program Development	314
Section B: Research	318
I. Critiquing Published Research Studies	318
II. Incorporating Research Findings into Practice	320
Practice Questions for Chapter Six	322
References	337

CBIC CONTENT OUTLINE (14 QUESTIONS)

SECTION A: EDUCATION

1. Assess the educational needs of healthcare workers pertaining to infection prevention, develop goals and measurable objectives and prepare lesson plans for educational offerings
2. Apply principles of adult learning to educational strategies and delivery of educational sessions
3. Prepare, present or coordinate educational workshops, lectures, discussion or one-on-one instruction on a variety of infection prevention and control topics
4. Evaluate the effectiveness of education and learner outcomes (e.g., behavior modification, compliance rate)
5. Instruct patients/families and other visitors about methods to prevent and control infections

SECTION B: RESEARCH

1. Apply critical reading skills to evaluate research findings
2. Incorporate research findings into practice through education and consultation

Chapter Six: Education and Research

SECTION A: EDUCATION

I. Basic Principles in Teaching and Learning

A. Major Goals in Teaching: Improve Job Skills and Competence Through:

1. Increased competence in identifying problems
2. Increasing critical thinking
3. Managing existing systems
4. Coping effectively with stress[1]

B. Learning Domain

1. Cognitive: recall, application and analytic levels of knowledge; involves the development of intellectual abilities
2. Affective—learning embraces new attitudes, values, beliefs and ways of feeling; self-esteem and desire to learn grows in caring, respectful relationships
3. Psychomotor: learning new skills or new ways of acting or doing

C. Stages of the Learning Process

1. Awareness—learner perceives a need to think, feel or act differently
2. Information gathering—learner is innately curious and seeks to understand and clarify new ways of behaving
3. Intellectual insight—learner weighs advantages and disadvantages; has mental "trial runs" (cognitive learning)
4. Emotional insight—learner practices new behavior in real situations; usually a time of conflict, trying to get the change to "feel right" (affective learning)
5. New learned behavior—new behavior becomes a part of the learner's way of thinking, feeling and behaving (integrated knowledge)

D. Adult Learning

1. Is a response to current situations
2. Tends to be problem-centered
3. Adults have a readiness to learn and prefer practical (over academic) knowledge
4. Retention increases when immediate application follows instruction[2]
5. Adults attach greater value to personal experience
6. Motivated by job needs, such as the need for new skills or desire for promotion and increased salary[3]

7. Adults need to be perceived by others as self-directional and expect to be treated with respect

E. Overcoming Roadblocks to Learning
1. Experienced educators and well-designed curriculum
2. Consider needs of both younger and more mature adults
3. Educators should assume a facilitator role, limit lectures and include interactive approaches (60/40 rule of active/passive learning)[4]
4. Mix activities and presentation methods[3]
5. Provide a safe, low-risk, nonthreatening learning environment to increase class interaction
6. Educator should provide coaching rather than criticism; consider letting learners evaluate themselves

II. Educational Program Development

A. Program Content
1. Needs assessment to identify deficiencies in knowledge, skills or attitude[5,6]
2. Improve learning transfer by including topics that are relevant, practical and doable
3. Ensure content includes education of patients, families and visitors about methods to prevent and control infections

B. Healthcare Worker Competency Statements[7]
1. Describe the role of microorganisms in disease
2. Describe how microorganism are transmitted in healthcare setting
3. Demonstrate standard and transmission-based precautions for all patient contact in healthcare settings
4. Describe occupational health practices that protect the healthcare worker from acquiring infection
5. Describe occupational health practices that prevent the healthcare worker from transmitting infection to a patient
6. Demonstrate ability to problem-solve and apply knowledge to recognize, contain and prevent infection transmission
7. Describe the importance of healthcare preparedness for natural or human-made infection disease disasters

C. Methods for Assessing Educational Needs
1. Learner self-assessment—learner develops a self-achievement model and compares the present situation to the standard

2. Focus group discussion—learning needs are assessed in small groups with members assisting each other to clarify needs
3. Interest finder surveys—data-gathering tools, such as checklist or questionnaires
4. Test development—tests can be used as diagnostic tools to identify areas of learning deficiencies
5. Personal interviews—educator consults with random or selected individuals to determine learning needs
6. Job analysis and performance reviews—methods provide specific, precise information about work and performance[5]
7. Observational studies—direct observation of personnel working
8. Review of internal reports—incident reports, occupational injury and illness reports, and performance improvement studies

D. Goals and Objectives

1. Goals are statements that communicate the intent of the curriculum and provide direction for planning the educational session; expectations are clearly defined in terms of time and available resources
2. Educator must determine the specific actions the learner will perform as a result of the instruction, known as instructional objectives
3. Objectives—specific actions the learner will perform as a result of instruction; characteristics include:
   a. Be specific—use clear language to define the final goal or purpose
   b. Be measurable—use action verbs to describe what the learner is expected to do; (e.g., improve test scores by 50% within 3 months)
   c. Be achievable—choose verbs that most accurately indicate the domain of expected learning: cognitive or reasoning skills, affective skills or new ways of feeling, and the psychomotor domain of performance, acting, and doing
   d. Be relevant to material presented—recognize that behavioral changes are defined in terms of knowledge, skills or attitudes; use appropriate verbs that correspond to the desired learning domain to meet the learning need
   e. Have a separate outcome—the outcome may require time to be evident

E. Bloom's Taxonomy Cognitive Levels[8]

A common model of increasingly more complex thinking. The three lowest levels are knowledge, comprehension and application; the three highest levels are analysis, synthesis and evaluation. Each level builds on the level below.
1. Recall—measure learner recognition of specific factual information; learner performs by rote

2. Comprehension—requires learner to understand the meaning, interpretation and translation of a problem, learner should be able to explain; predict or paraphrase the objective
3. Application—require learner to comprehend and manipulate data or concepts; the learner must be able to interpret, demonstrate or illustrate the objectives
4. Analysis—require learner to contrast, criticize, differentiate or solve
5. Synthesis—builds a structure from a pattern of diverse elements; learner should be able to categorize, compile, devise, explain, plan, rewrite or summarize
6. Evaluation—learner must be able to make judgments; learner should be able to apprise, compare and contrast, defend, describe, evaluate or justify

F. Engaging the Learner
1. Education leadership theory created by Hersey and Blanchard (formerly life-cycle or situation leadership); pairs a readiness level with a corresponding leadership style[9,10]
    a. Readiness levels
        (1) 1—unable and unwilling or insecure
        (2) 2—unable but willing or confident
        (3) 3—able but unwilling or insecure
        (4) 4—able and willing or confident
    b. Leadership style
        (1) 1—high task, low relationship; an autocratic style wherein the leader provides specific direction regarding what is to be done, when and by whom; the educator determines the process and the content of the decision making
        (2) 2—high task, high relationship; a democratic style wherein the leader participates in the group as a contributor and as a facilitator; educator provides direction but encourages the members to work with each other and the educator for goals
        (3) 3—high relationship, low task; an encouraging and socializing style where the leader promotes cohesion and collaboration but does not interfere or influence decision making; educator serves to encourage and clarify
        (4) 4—low relationship, low task; hands-off style where the educator allows the members to determine the direction of the learning
2. Learning pyramid: educational method correlated with predicted learner retention rates
    a. Lecture 5%
    b. Reading 10%
    c. Audiovisual 20%
    d. Demonstration 30%
    e. Group discussion 50%

f. Practice by doing 75%
g. Teach others 90%

G. Principles of Effective Program Development
1. Learning environment
   a. Provide an atmosphere of mutual respect that is friendly, informal and supportive[11,12]
   b. Create an environment that is comfortable and conducive to learning (private, good seating and lighting, etc.)
   c. Eliminate distractions and try to control noise
   d. Provide working and ready-to-use audiovisual equipment
2. Common classroom settings
   a. Horseshoe—allows face-to-face participation
   b. Team style—arranging small tables and chairs to facilitate group discussion
   c. Conference table—circle or square, facilitator at "head" of table
   d. Chevron or fishbone—repeated V arrangement, creating closeness of participants and visibility of the educator
   e. Stadium or auditorium—tends to limit active training
3. Enhancing the learning experience
   a. Start with an exercise that focuses on the learner and makes it personally relevant
   b. Define terms and use examples to underscore major points
   c. Repetition of the same point in different ways
   d. Summarize and review major points at the end

H. Evaluation[5,13,14]
1. Should include appropriateness of program design, adequacy of teaching and resources, knowledge, skills and attitudes learned by the participants
2. Need a representative sample of data from the learner population
   a. Types
      (1) Formative—conducted during the education session to provide immediate feedback and allow appropriate changes to be made
      (2) Summative—occurs after the program is completed to determine impact and overall effectiveness; evaluate change and growth
3. Methods
   a. Pretest and posttest
   b. Direct observation of practice
   c. Exit questionnaires
   d. One-on-one interviews
   e. Supervisor observation

I. Innovative Instructional Methods

1. Lectures
   a. Symposium—three to six lectures, include open discussion by audience
   b. Forum—one or more speakers engage in free and open discussion
   c. Panel—usually four to seven resource people present facts and ideas in an orderly fashion (e.g., controversial topics)
2. Computer-based training—self-paced, learner-friendly and nonjudgmental; provides positive reinforcement; mistakes are private; can be done on learner's schedule; immediate feedback to learner; graphics reduce boredom; but value is limited with evaluation of psychomotor skills or persons with reduced reading/comprehension ability or inadequate computer skills[13]
3. Games—quizzes or word searches
4. Mass training—personalized education materials using an organization intranet for wide-scale institutional education
5. Train-the-trainer—leaders guides are used to train those responsible for implementing the program and providing further training to others
6. Role play or reenactment—dramatic teaching strategy uses situational learning experience and the technique of simulation to enable all the learners to experience situation[5]
7. Case studies—uses a variety of learning skills (e.g., study of famous outbreaks or epidemics)
8. Mentoring programs—low-cost way to cross-train employees; most mentors are volunteers; link experienced workers with those needing training[15,16]
9. Simulation—provides learning experiences similar to real situations
10. Educational cart—contains different types of information about a topic
11. DVDs, CDs and videotapes
12. Self-instructional modules—self-paced approach to allow learner to gain new information
13. Distance learning—audio, graphic and video-conferencing systems allow for exchange of information from one location to another through electronic communications[17,18]

SECTION B: RESEARCH

I. Critiquing Published Research Studies

A. Components of a Well-Performed Research Study

1. Abstract—brief summary of the study; may be included in Internet databases; may be at the end as "Summary"; states purposes, methods, main findings and main conclusions

2. Introduction—background information, justification and purpose of the research; briefly mentions previous research, relevance of present study to existing problems; relationship to other current research; should clearly state the research question(s)
3. Method—description of population studied; how participants were selected; information on sample size; methods used to obtain and analyze data; other facts pertinent to completion of the study (e.g., selection, assignment to groups)
4. Results—presentation of data obtained in tables, graphs, charts; statistical analysis of data along with p values or confidence intervals; answer to research questions given in the introduction
5. Discussion—brief summary of the entire research process with interpretation of data from the results; conclusions from the data, limitations of the data or study design and suggestions for applications of the findings or future research
6. References—site sources used for the body of the article

B. Factors in a Critical Review of a Published Study

1. Quality of the journal (used for validated research, strict publishing rules, each article well referenced by timely articles, etc.)
2. Type of article
   a. Study article—original research study
   b. Review article—summary of previously published studies—not original work
3. Components of article with evaluation questions or issues
   a. Introduction—question is important, appropriate and stated clearly?[19]
   b. Methods[20-22]
      (1) Study population appropriate and adequately described? Suitable sources used to find cases?
      (2) Time period of study relevant?
      (3) Study design applicable to purpose of study?
      (4) Study design described in enough detail?
      (5) Appropriate criteria used to define cases and controls?
      (6) Selection and exclusion criteria described and comparable with other reports?
      (7) Data sources adequate, appropriate and complete?
      (8) Sources of bias in the data? Selection bias? Groups treated equally? Quality of data equal in comparison groups? Outcomes of groups evaluated equally and by persons blinded to treatment/exposures?
      (9) Controls if used are comparable with cases with exposure to risk factors?
      (10) Sources of bias in selection of controls?

(11) Participants if followed in adequate time period? Last to follow-up?
(12) Data quality ensured?
(13) Study variables clearly defined?
(14) Diagnostic, laboratory or statistical methods described in sufficient detail?
(15) Study, if clinical trial, has participants randomized to treatment groups and participants/investigators are blinded to assignment?
(16) Study, if multicenter trial, has adequate procedures for quality assurance?
   c. Results[19,23-26]
      (1) Data values are presented appropriately (means, standard deviations, proportions and differences for paired designs)?
      (2) Statistical tests are appropriate for study design and were performed properly?
      (3) Sample size is adequate? Power of study stated if findings are not statistically significant?
      (4) Confounders are taken into account or should data be reanalyzed to include?
      (5) Adjustments for confounders, if performed, are performed appropriately?
      (6) Data presented provide answers to stated research questions?
      (7) Tables, graphs and charts are appropriate, simple and clear?
   d. Discussion[27]
      (1) Research questions that are stated in the introduction are adequately discussed?
      (2) Conclusions that are drawn are reasonable and justified from the type of study design and the data presented?
      (3) Could other explanations account for the observed results and conclusion?
      (4) Limitations of the study are addressed?
      (5) Suggestions are offered for applications of the findings, which direct future research?
   e. References
      (1) There are adequate references?
      (2) References given are all relevant?

II. Incorporating Research Findings into Practice

A. Performing Research

1. Participate in research to further the field of infection prevention and control

B. Reviewing Research
1. Finding the literature
    a. Peer review journals
    b. Systematic review
    c. Free publications
2. Provide comparisons for your data
3. Use research to guide your infection prevention and control program
4. Consultant
    a. The IP functions as a consultant with expert knowledge and skills; research is a tool that enhances the IP's ability to offer beneficial services to the clients
5. Using research in product review and selection
    a. Participating in product development research
    b. Reviewing research to facilitate decision-making
6. Keep your facility educated
    a. Use recently published studies to educate your infection prevention and control committee
    b. Adapting current practice

Practice Questions for Chapter Six

Chapter Six:

Educations and Research Questions

1. When undergoing the learning process, a leaner proceeds through stages. The stage in which the learner practices new behavior in real situations is known as:
   a. Awareness
   b. Intellectual insight
   c. Emotional insight
   d. New learned behavior

2. There are three major domains in the learning process: cognitive, affective and psychomotor. In the affective learning domain, the individual:
   a. Uses recall application and analytic skills in learning processes
   b. Demonstrates new skills or new ways of acting or doing
   c. Embraces new attitudes, values and beliefs in the learning process
   d. May demonstrate conflict and resistance to the learning

3. According to the education leadership theory, educators should formulate their leadership style based on what quality of the learner
   a. Readiness
   b. Situation
   c. Experience
   d. Education level

4. You are preparing a presentation for a group that is able to learn the material, but is unwilling or insecure about the learning process. Which describes the leadership style that should be used with this group?
   a. Autocratic style, in which the leader provides specific direction about what, when and whom
   b. Democratic style, in which the leader participates as a contributor and facilitator
   c. Encouraging and socializing style, in which the leader promotes collaboration but does not interfere with decision making
   d. Hand-off style where the members determine the direction of the learning

5. The first step in preparation of any educational program is:
   a. Identifying budgetary resources for educational program
   b. Assessing the educational needs of the learning population
   c. Investigating media/projection equipment available
   d. Incorporating the evaluation process in the preparation strategies

6. The main purpose of a needs assessment is:
   a. Identify deficiencies in knowledge, skills or attitude
   b. Provide documentation for regulatory agencies
   c. Assist in developing data collection tools
   d. Assist with the development of instructional objectives

7. Once the purpose of an educational program is established, the instructor must determine the specific actions the learner will perform. These actions are known as:
   a. Course guidelines
   b. Outcomes
   c. Educational goals
   d. Instructional objectives

8. IPs recognizes their audience as adult learners. This is important because adults:
   a. Generally prefer practical rather than academic knowledge, they tend to learn what they can use
   b. May have limited attention spans due to multi-task management
   c. May not provide honest feedback unless encouraged to do so
   d. May feel future education is unnecessary once in a job position of comfort

9. With adult learners, one of the most important roles of the educator is to:
   a. Ensure audiovisual equipment that is consistent with audience profile
   b. Provide an atmosphere of mutual respect, maintain good eye contact and listen to the learners' concerns with little interruption to help validate opinions expressed
   c. Engage the learner in adversarial dialogue if necessary to stress a learning objective
   d. Use role playing in each education session to provide an active role for learner in education process

10. The "train the trainer" method of instruction is often used for wide-scale institutional education programs. For this method to be successful the most important job for the educator is to:
    a. Develop a leader guide in a concise, step-by-step format with curriculum goals and objectives
    b. Spend an appropriate amount of preparation time to cover all topic area and anticipate questions for leaders
    c. Incorporate multilingual chapters as needed
    d. Receive administrative approval before initiation

Questions 11–17 You have recently been hired as an IP at a 250-bed hospital. One of your first duties will be to develop an orientation program for all new employees. This program must be applicable to individuals assigned to nursing and ancillary departments. You realize that these employees will have different educational backgrounds and life experiences.

Questions 11 through 17 refer to the planning, implementation and evaluation of this program. Choose the best answer.

11. Before beginning actual orientation program planning, which of the following should you do?
    a. Become familiar with job requirements in each department
    b. Have an expert from another hospital draft your plan
    c. Survey nursing services for specific infection control needs
    d. Ask all supervisors for their recommendations

12. You know that a plan consists of goals, objectives and resources to meet a particular set of needs. Hospital management has provided you with an adequate budget for education resources, but you must develop goals and objectives. Which of the following is a correctly written program goal?
    a. After completion of the program, the employee will be able to list, with 90% accuracy, 10 infection prevention and control resources in the hospital
    b. After completion of the program, the employee will understand why infection prevention and control is important
    c. To provide information so the employee will feel more secure in the hospital environment
    d. To provide information that will enable the employee to use the infection prevention and control manual

13. Which of the following is a correctly written instructional objective?
    a. After completion of the program, the employee will be able to list, with 90% accuracy, five infection prevention and control resources in the hospital
    b. After completion of the program, the employee will understand why infection prevention and control is important
    c. To provide information so the employee will feel more secure in the hospital environment
    d. To provide information that will enable the employee to use the infection prevention and control manual

14. You will be presenting a monthly, 2-hour orientation program. What teaching strategies could be BEST used?
    a. A 2-hour lecture explaining infection prevention principles
    b. A 2-hour demonstration of how to apply infection control principles
    c. A 1-hour lecture and a 1-hour demonstration of infection prevention principles
    d. A lecture-discussion of infection prevention principles, then break-out into smaller groups for demonstration and return-demonstration of infection prevention principles

15. When designing your teaching plan for general orientation, what subject matter should be included in your outline?
    a. Specific departmental policies; how to use the infection prevention and control manual; handwashing; standard precautions
    b. Specific departmental policies; how to use the infection prevention and control manual; handwashing; specimen collection
    c. Organization's infection prevention and control program; handwashing; standard precautions; specimen collection
    d. Organization's infection prevention and control program; handwashing; standard precautions; individual's role in the prevention of infection

16. When developing your educator role, which of the following SHOULD be used to foster the best learning climate for the adult learner?
    a. Allow the learner to make all decisions for learning goals
    b. Structure class formally so students will not miss important points
    c. Discourage group interaction because time is limited
    d. Relate new information to experiences of the learner

17. To assess learner response and program effectiveness, which of the following is the BEST evaluation tool?
    a. Posttest using open-ended questions, so the adult learner may freely express opinions
    b. Similar pretest and posttest
    c. Pretest with more difficult questions on the posttest
    d. Verbal student response to questions asked at the end of class

Questions 18–20   You are making unit rounds and observe a housekeeper cleaning a blood spill. Although adequate supplies are available, the housekeeper is NOT wearing gloves.

18. Which of the following should be your first response to this situation?
    a. Do nothing at this time; set up an in-service with the environmental services department for next week, because you know that adults learn better in a controlled situation
    b. Review the environmental services department's infection prevention and control policies, and then design an in-service program
    c. Ask the housekeeper to wash his/her hands; then outside the room, review the principles of Standard Precautions with the employee
    d. Call the environmental services supervisor and ask the supervisor to instruct the employee

19. The housekeeper had attended an in-service on cleaning blood spills 1 week earlier. Which of the learning domains is the housekeeper not functioning under?
    a. Cognitive
    b. Affective
    c. Effective
    d. Psychomotor

20. When designing an isolation in-service program for the environmental services department, which of the following teaching strategies is BEST?
    a. A lecture on the use of protective barriers while performing tasks
    b. A simulation of the proper use of protective barriers
    c. A case study of proper cleaning of a patient room
    d. Use the example of the housekeeper not wearing gloves when cleaning the patient's room during a lecture to the department

21. You are giving a learning presentation in an auditorium. Which is true of this setting?
    a. It allows face-to-face participation
    b. It tends to limit active training
    c. It creates closeness of participants and visibility of the educator
    d. It puts the facilitator at the "head" of the table

22. Which of the following is NOT a recommended form of innovation instruction?
    a. Games such as quizzes or word searches
    b. Role play or reenactment
    c. Case studies
    d. Notes written on a blackboard

23. While making surveillance rounds on the surgical unit, you observe a nurse beginning to change a surgical dressing without washing her hands first. Which of the following should be your initial response to this?
    a. Tell the nurse to wash her hands and sign up for next week's in-service
    b. Say nothing because you know learning can take place only in a formal setting
    c. Go immediately to the nurse's supervisor and explain what you observed so she can reprimand her
    d. Ask the nurse, privately, to explain to you the importance of handwashing before a dressing change

24. As part of a program on wound care, you have participants demonstrate how to properly apply an abdominal dressing. In which of the learning domains this exercise reflects change?
    a. Cognitive
    b. Affective
    c. Psychomotor
    d. Objective

25. When designing an in-service program for the engineering department, what should your first step be?
    a. Find out the subject of the last in-service
    b. Ask the manager for his/her suggested topic
    c. Discuss the learning needs of the department members with the manager
    d. Observe the department then develop the educational program you will need to give

26. Which of the following is a correctly written instructional objective?
    a. At the end of the infection prevention and control program, the learner will understand isolation procedures
    b. At the end of the program, the learner will list correctly five infection prevention and control resources
    c. To provide information relating to nosocomial infections
    d. To demonstrate new methods of dressing technique

27. A major goal of the educational process is to:
    a. Enhance the ability of those taught to think in a uniform manner
    b. Decrease anxiety over lack of knowledge and control
    c. Increase competence in identifying and solving problems
    d. Increase tolerance for continuity of ideas

28. Cognitive learning is:
    a. Learning new attitudes, values, beliefs, and ways of learning
    b. Recall or recognition of knowledge involving the acquisition of new abilities
    c. Learning new skills and procedures
    d. A passive form of gaining knowledge or skill

29. A decision to change is necessary before learning can occur. Which of the following is NOT a type of learning that governs change?
    a. Affective learning
    b. Effective learning
    c. Cognitive learning
    d. Psychomotor learning

30. An educational priority of the adult learner is:
    a. Practical knowledge
    b. Abstract concepts
    c. Direction from outside sources
    d. Repetitive tasks

31. The major components of a properly written instructional objective are:
    a. Knowledge, skill and attitude
    b. Relevance, relationship and responsibility
    c. Goals, content and evaluation
    d. Performance, conditions and expected behavior

32. The teaching strategy that provides situational learning experiences close to real situations is:
    a. Self-instruction
    b. Case study
    c. Simulation
    d. Field trips

33. Cognitive learning focuses on:
    a. Reaction time
    b. Basic beliefs
    c. Emotional attitudes
    d. Problem-solving/intellectual abilities

34. The use of pretest and posttest tools allows the instructor to:
    a. Provide learners with test demographics (e.g., mean, range, etc.) within a short time
    b. Get the attention of the learner so that learning may be enhanced
    c. Assess whether learning has occurred
    d. Assess the educational needs of the learner

35. In preparing for an infection prevention and control booth as part of a health fair in a shopping mall, probably the LEAST effective tool to use to present information is:
    a. A black-light handwashing demonstration
    b. Use of a videotape
    c. A straight lecture-type format
    d. A poster board with thought-provoking questions to be answered by the presenter to small groups or individuals

36. You have been asked by a local community center to do a presentation on HIV. Your audience is composed of single adults. When developing your presentation, you should include all BUT which of the following?
    a. Assess learner needs and resources available for presentation
    b. Develop goals and objectives
    c. Identify the domain of learning
    d. Develop a plan for educational experiences and evaluation tool

37. It is important when implementing your teaching plan to establish a climate conducive to adult learning. Which of the following environmental controls WILL NOT maximize adult learning?
    a. Room lighting
    b. Room temperature
    c. Seating arrangements
    d. Music in the background

38. The evaluation of your program is important to assess the effectiveness of your presentation. Which of the following is MOST important to evaluate?
    a. Program design and content
    b. Instructional resources
    c. Quality of the speaker presentation
    d. Whether the learning needs have been met

39. You have been asked to develop an infection prevention and control in-service program for the department of food and nutrition services. You have a copy of the orientation training that is given to all workers in that department. It has a good basic infection prevention and control component, but many of the workers have been in the department for more than 10 years. What is your first action to determine the subjects you need to cover in your lecture?
   a. Develop a lecture based on their basic education program because many employees need a good review
   b. Talk with the department director to find out his major issues with the department workers
   c. Talk with the department's quality improvement coordinator to determine the educational needs of the workers
   d. Make rounds in the department to observe actions that need to be included in your lecture

Questions 40–42 You are an IP at a facility that has had a significant increase in surgical site infections. As part of your surgery department assessment, you need to determine the educational needs of the operating room staff related to infection prevention and control and you plan to implement an educational offering. Based on your knowledge of adult learners, please answer the following questions.

40. In this situation, the most accurate method of assessment that could be conducted quickly would be:
   a. Observation of staff skills
   b. Team meeting to brainstorm knowledge needs
   c. Written test
   d. Request director to conduct a needs assessment

41. In planning the educational offering, you are aware that the primary goal of the teaching/educational process is:
   a. A positive experience for the learner
   b. That learning will take place
   c. Improved work performance
   d. Decreased infections

42. Which of the following methods of teaching would best meet the needs of the operating room staff?
    a. Lecture and slides with some discussion
    b. Self-directed learning modules with some classroom demonstration
    c. Independent videotape review followed by a written examination
    d. Lecture with take-home videotape for review

43. All of the following statements describe adults as learners EXCEPT:
    a. Prefer practical information
    b. Want respect
    c. Use personal experiences
    d. Want a formal structure in the educational process

44. You are conducting a 6-week educational offering. After 2 weeks, you ask each participant to evaluate the learning experience so far. This is a method of:
    a. Summative evaluation
    b. Formative evaluation
    c. Interim evaluation
    d. Median evaluation

45. Which part of a published research study contains a brief summary of the entire research process with interpretation of data, conclusions from the data, limitations of the study and suggestion for future research?
    a. Introduction
    b. Methods
    c. Results
    d. Discussion

46. You are performing a literature review on risk factors for multidrug-resistant *Acinetobacter* during an outbreak situation in your ICU. You are reading an article in your favorite infection prevention journal. You notice that conclusions support a hypothesis you have long considered; however, the methods section is poorly written and hard to follow. What should you do?
    a. Include it in your summary; it supports your concern and will help get you resources to investigate it at your institution
    b. Include it in your summary but note the limitations; it still could be considered for your current cluster
    c. Contact the authors to verify their methodology
    d. Disregard the article you continue your literature review

47. All of the following are features of a well-written methods section EXCEPT:
    a. Time period of the study
    b. Clear criteria for defining cases and controls
    c. Questions the research will answer
    d. Methods of quality assurance

48. Which is not a method of incorporating research findings into practice?
    a. Review and selection of new products
    b. Provide comparisons for CLABSI data in a specialized population
    c. Performing a literature search on UTI risk factors in the elderly
    d. Provide education to the infection control committee regarding MDRO acquisition

49. It has come to your attention that the outpatient surgery department is using a new skin preparation product. What is your first action?
    a. Notify the infection prevention and control committee
    b. Contact the director and insist that the product be discontinued
    c. Look for information about the product and reliable studies
    d. Notify your manager

50. A hospitalist requests to switch to a new central line brand as she has heard that it reduces the incidence of CLABSIs. Your best response would be:
    a. I will present this at the next products committee meeting and will let you know.
    b. Do you have any literature to support this?
    c. Do you know anyone else who is currently using this product?
    d. Let me do a little research and I will get back with you.

Answers for Practice Questions Chapter Six

1.	c	26.	b
2.	c	27.	c
3.	a	28.	b
4.	c	29.	b
5.	b	30.	a
6.	a	31.	d
7.	d	32.	c
8.	a	33.	d
9.	b	34.	c
10.	a	35.	c
11.	a	36.	c
12.	d	37.	d
13.	a	38.	d
14.	d	39.	c
15.	d	40.	c
16.	d	41.	b
17.	b	42.	b
18.	c	43.	d
19.	a	44.	b
20.	b	45.	d
21.	b	46.	b
22.	d	47.	c
23.	d	48.	c
24.	c	49.	c
25.	c	50.	d

References

1. Willyerd KA. Balancing your evaluation act. *Training* 1997;34:53–58.
2. Knowles M. Andragogy. Available online at: http://tip.psychology.org/knowles.html. Accessed November 11, 2010
3. Zemke R, Zemke S. 30 Things we know for sure about adult learning, *Innovation Abstracts* 1984;6:8.
4. Becker R. Taking the misery out of experimental training. *Training* 1998;35:78–79.
5. Hinson P. Education. In: Olmsted RN, ed. *2002 Infection Control and Applied Epidemiology, Principals and Practice*. Washington, DC: Association for Professionals in Infection Control and Epidemiology, 2002.
6. Colthart I, Bagnall G, Evans A, et al. The effectiveness of self-assessment on the identification of learner needs, learning activity, and impact on clinical practice. BEME Guide no. 10. *Med Teach* 2008;30:124–145.
7. Carrico R, Rebmann T, English JF, et al. Infection prevention and control competencies for hospital-based healthcare personnel. *Am J Infect Control* 2008;36:691–701.
8. Bloom's Taxonomy: Learning domains or Bloom's taxonomy. Available online at: http://www.odu.edu/educ/roverbau/Bloom/blooms_taxonomy.htm. Accessed November 11, 2010
9. Hersey P, Blanchard KH. *Management of Organizational Behavior: Utilizing Human Resources*. 5th ed. Englewood Cliffs, NJ: Prentice Hall, 1998.
10. Hersey P, Blanchard KH. Life Cycle Theory of Leadership. *Training and Development Journal* 1969;23:26–34.
11. Dorek PM, Huang S, Chan-Yan C. A lecturing skills course for residents. *Train Learn Med* 1994;6:2.
12. Powers B. Training aids to enhance learning. In: *Instructor Excellence*. San Francisco: Jossey-Bass; 1992.
13. Ryatt A, Lohan K. *Creating Training Miracles*. San Francisco: Pfeiffer & Company, 1997.
14. Cohen N. *Mentoring Adult Learners*. Malabar, FL: Krieger Publishing, 1995

15. Shea G. *Mentoring: A Practical Guide*. Menlo Park, CA: Crisp Publications, 1992.

16. Todd M, Manz JA, Hawkins KS, et al. The development of a quantitative evaluation tool for simulations in nursing education. *Int J Nurs Educ Scholarsh* 2008;5: Article 41.

17. Borella A, Hixon F, Yahl M. TB education on the move [poster], 21st Annual Education Conference, APIC: The next generation, Cincinnati, 1994.

18. Moralejo D, Gaese C. The mock isolation room: a fun way to review infection control. *J Contin Educ Nurs* 1993;24:185–188.

19. Carpenter LM. Is the study worth doing? *Lancet* 1993;342:221–223

20. Sitthi Amorn C, Poshyachinda V. Bias. *Lancet* 1993;342:286–288.

21. Guyatt GH, Sackett DL, Cook DJ. Evidence Based Medicine Working Group: Users' guides to the medical literature. II. How to use an article about therapy or prevention. A. Are the results of the study valid? *JAMA* 1993;270:2598–2601.

22. Jaeschke R, Guyatt G, Sackett DL. Evidence Based Medicine Working Group: Users' guides to the medical literature. III. How to use an article about a diagnostic text. A. Are the results of the study valid? *JAMA* 1994;271:389–391.

23. Munoz A, Townsend TR. Design and analytical issues in studies of infectious diseases. In: Wenzel RP, ed. *Prevention and Control of Nosocomial Infections*. 3rd ed. Baltimore: Williams & Wilkins; 1997:215–229.

24. Victora CG. What's the denominator? *Lancet* 1993;342:97–99.

25. Datta M. You cannot exclude the explanation you have not considered. *Lancet* 1993;342:345–347.

26. Leon DA. Failed or misleading adjustment for confounding. *Lancet* 1993;342:479–481.

27. Glynn JR. A question of attribution. *Lancet* 1993;342:530–532.

CHAPTER SEVEN

THE CERTIFICATION EXAM

CONTENTS

Article	Page
Chapter Seven: The Certification Exam	340
I. Description of the CBIC Exam	340
II. Types of Exam Takers	342
III. Preparation for the Exam	345
IV. Exam-Taking Techniques	346
V. The Computerized Version of the Exam	347
VI. Self-Assessment Recertification Examination	349
VII. Contact Information	350

Chapter Seven: The Certification Exam

I. **Description of the CBIC Exam**

   A. **CBIC—Certification Board of Infection Control and Epidemiology, Inc.**
   1. APIC Certification Association (APICCA) 1981—name changed to CBIC later that year
      a. CBIC—purpose: to improve healthcare by developing a method to demonstrate competency in infection prevention, provide a standard measure of knowledge, encourage individual growth and recognize the infection control professionals who can demonstrate competence in infection control practice
      b. Early testing (began 1983) was 250 questions—shortened to 150 items
      c. Test is accredited by the National Commission on Certifying Agencies (NCCA) which ensures that competency testing is accurate, is of high quality and complies with the standards
      d. Test is available from Applied Measurement Professionals (AMP)
      e. Information is available online about CBIC, including the *Candidate Handbook*, Judicial and Ethics policy, names of board members, etc.
      f. Board members and officers are international and multidisciplinary; board liaisons from APIC and CHICA-Canada are also listed on website
      g. Test is available internationally via computerized method
      h. Exam is available in computerized format Monday through Saturday at over 170 AMP Assessment Centers throughout the United States and selected international sites.
   2. Topics included in the current exam (with number of questions)
      a. Identification of infectious disease processes (18)
      b. Surveillance and epidemiologic investigation (38)
      c. Preventing/controlling the transmission of infectious agents (39)
      d. Employee/occupational health (10)
      e. Management and communication (leadership) (16)
      f. Education and research (14)
   3. Test composed of 150 multiple-choice items (questions or statements)
   4. Content of test items determined by practice (job) analysis surveys; last practice analysis survey done in 2009
   5. All items (the entire question or statement and options) include
      a. Stem—the statement, question, chart or graph; presents the central problem or situation of consideration
      b. Options—all possible options or answers for the stem; this includes "distractors," which are reasonable choices and the "key," which is the correct answer?
   6. Most items have four options: A, B, C, or D

7. Some items are complex multiple-choice—stem (followed by four or five choices, followed by four options composed of the possible choices in combinations)
   1.
   2.
   3.
   4.
      a. 1, 2
      b. 1, 3
      c. 2, 3
      d. 2, 4
8. Exam items are divided into three skill levels
   a. Cognitive level I—the basic recall of information that has been memorized; 25% of the questions or statements will be Cog. I
   b. Cognitive level II—the application level; involves simple application of the facts or interpretation of the data in the stem; 60% of the questions/items will be Cog. II
   c. Cognitive level III—the analysis level; involves evaluation of data, problem-solving or fitting together of a variety of elements into a meaningful whole; 15% of the questions/items will be Cog. III
9. All items have only ONE correct choice
10. There is no penalty for wrong answers; you should guess when you absolutely do not know the answer
11. Passing scores are calculated to compensate for item difficulty and differences between examinations
12. Each test item is evaluated and tested for accuracy, validity and quality of stem and choices by Applied Measurement Professionals (AMP); then approved by the CBIC Test Committee; and finally approved by the CBIC Board
13. Test scores may be cancelled if computer malfunction or misconduct by a candidate is suspected
14. Certification may be revoked by CBIC for falsification of an application, violation of examination procedures or misrepresentation of the certification status
15. Persons needing interpretation of the exam in a language other than English can be provided an interpreter at the candidate's expense. Requests for interpretation must be made in writing to AMP 180 days before the test date and accompany the application. AMP will arrange the interpreter (candidate will not be allowed to arrange the interpreter)
16. Candidates with disabilities will be provided reasonable accommodations. Verification of the disability and a statement of the specific type of assistance needed must be made in writing and sent with the application at least 45 calendar days before

the testing date. AMP must be informed of the need for special accommodations when scheduling the exam time. Wheelchair access is available at all testing centers.
17. Candidate handbook, forms and applications may be obtained by visiting the website: www.cbic.org; or phone: (414) 918-9796 or fax: (414) 276-3349

B. Qualification for Testing

1. Practice must include these components of infection control practice:
    a. Analysis and interpretation of collected infection prevention data
    b. Investigation and surveillance of suspected outbreaks of infection, and three of the following:
        (1) Planning, implementation and evaluation of infection prevention and control measures
        (2) Education of individuals about infection risk, prevention and control
        (3) Development and revision of infection control policies and procedures
        (4) Management of infection prevention and control activities
        (5) Provision of consultation on infection risk assessment, prevention and control strategies
2. First-time candidates, candidates who have not successfully passed the exam and lapsed recertifiers must meet "a" or "b":
    a. Have a current license or registration as a medical technologist, clinical laboratory scientist, physician or registered nurse
    or
    b. Have a minimum of a baccalaureate degree
3. Candidates not meeting the educational requirements may apply for an eligibility waiver, which is available online at www.cbic.org.
4. Self-employed candidates must submit the following with their application: name, address, dates of service, type of service and number of hours for the clients they have worked

II. Types of Exam Takers

A. Know Yourself—Identify the Type of Test Taker You Are and Utilize the Improvement Strategies Suggested

1. Rusher
    a. Characteristics—rushes to complete test before facts are forgotten; arrives early and anxious

      b. Pitfalls
- (1) Unable to read question completely
- (2) High risk for misreading, misinterpreting and mistakes
- (3) Likely to make quick, not well-thought-out guesses

      c. Improvement strategies
- a. Practice progressive relaxation techniques
- b. Develop study plan
- c. Avoid cramming and last-minute studying
- d. Use practice tests to focus on slowing down, answering each question carefully
- e. Read instructions slowly

2. Turtle
   a. Characteristics—moves slowly through each question; repeated rereading; takes 60 to 90 seconds per question versus 45 to 60 seconds
   b. Pitfalls
      (1) Last to finish, often does not complete exam
      (2) Has to quickly complete last questions, increasing chance of errors
   c. Improvement strategies
      (1) Take practice tests focusing on time spent per item
      (2) Place watch in front of you
      (3) Mark answer sheet for halfway point

3. Personalizer
   a. Characteristics—mature person who has personal knowledge and insight from life experiences
   b. Pitfalls
      (1) Runs risk of relying on experience, may develop false understandings and stereotypes
      (2) Personal beliefs and experiences may not be norm or standard
   c. Improvement strategies
      (1) Focus on principles and standards that support nursing practice
      (2) Avoid making connections between patients in exam clinical situations and personal clinical experience
      (3) Focus on generalities, not on experiences

4. Squish
   a. Characteristics—views exams as threats; preoccupied with grades and personal accomplishment

b. Pitfalls
   (1) Procrastinates studying for exams
   (2) Unable to study effectively because waits until last minute
   (3) Increased anxiety over test because of late studying of poor quality
c. Improvement strategies
   (1) Establish a plan of disciplined study
   (2) Use defined time frames for studying content and taking practice exams
   (3) Use relaxation techniques
   (4) Read carefully
   (5) Return to difficult items

5. Philosopher
   a. Characteristics—academically successful person who is well disciplined and structured in study habits; displays great intensity and concentration during exam; searches questions for hidden or unintended meaning; experiences anxiety over not knowing everything
   b. Pitfalls
      (1) Overanalysis causes loss of sight of actual intent of question
      (2) Reads information into questions, answering with own added information rather than answering the actual intent of question
   c. Improvement strategies
      (1) Focus on questions as they are written
      (2) Work on self-confidence and not on question; initial response is usually correct
      (3) Avoid multiple rereadings of questions
      (4) Practice with sample tests

6. Second guesser
   a. Characteristics—answers questions twice, first as an examinee, second as an examiner; believes second look will allow one to find and correct errors; frequently changes initial responses (grades own test)
   b. Pitfalls
      (1) Altering an initial response frequently results in an incorrect answer
      (2) Frequently changes answers because the pattern of response appears incorrect (e.g., too many "true" responses)
   c. Improvement strategies
      (1) Reread only the few items of which one is unsure
      (2) Avoid changing initial responses
      (3) Take exam carefully and progressively first time, allowing little or no time for rereading
      (4) Study facts
      (5) Avoid reading into the questions

7. Lawyer
   a. Characteristics—attempts to place words or ideas into the question (leads the witness); occurs most frequently with psychosocial or communication questions, which ask for the most appropriate response
   b. Pitfalls
      (1) Veers from the obvious answer and provides response from own point of view
      (2) Reads a question, jumps to a conclusion
   c. Improvement strategies
      (1) Focus on what patient is saying in question, not what is read into the question
      (2) Choose response that allows patient to express feelings that encourage hope, a response that clarifies, identifies feelings or avoids negating or confronting patient feelings

III. Preparation for the Exam

A. Decide When You Wish to Take the Exam

1. Decide what date you can be ready to take the test—allow 3 months study time for the first time test-taker
2. Make a "contract" with yourself to take the test on that date

B. Develop Your Thinking Skills

1. Understand thought processes related to Cog. I, Cog. II and Cog. III items in the test
2. Build your thinking skills
   a. Concentrate on learning the subject well, not just memorizing a lot of facts; quality—not quantity
   b. Develop memory skills that trigger retrieval of needed facts: Acronyms (PERRL), acrostics (**E**very **G**ood **B**oy **D**oes **F**ine), ABCs (each letter stands for a term), imaging (visualize picture), rhymes, music and links
   c. Improve higher level thinking skills by exercising the analysis of memorized facts; small group reviews are good for this

C. Know the Content

1. Prepare well for studying, be organized
   a. Create your own study area or space
   b. Define and organize the content to be studied
   c. Do a content assessment of material:
      (1) No review required
      (2) Minimal review will be necessary

(3) Intensive review will be necessary
(4) Start from the beginning
d. Develop a study plan of the content
e. Use study time wisely
2. Actual study suggestions (suggested source: *APIC Text* 2009)
a. Study in short intervals during your peak time
b. Quick review of material on exam day
c. Study the correct content, not details
d. Fit your studying into the same type as test type
e. Use your study plan, keep to a schedule
f. Actively study, take notes as you study
g. Use study aids, study guides, review courses, study groups
h. Know when to quit, when your energy and attention wanes
i. Allow extra time to study chapters that have complex information
j. Study 2 to 3 hours each night/day, at least 3 days a week and then again on the weekend
k. After you have covered most sections of the *APIC Text*, begin reviewing the sections of this *Review Guide*
l. Take the questions at the end of each chapter. This will tell you what areas you need to review and those on which to spend more time. Do not be upset if you do not agree with all of the answers. Research the topic. The more work you do to find out the answer, the more likely the answer will be imprinted in your memory. (If you truly feel the answer indicated is wrong, contact APIC headquarters)
m. Do not forget to schedule and pay for your test on the date you selected.
n. Study in groups if you have friends and APIC chapter members who can get together with you to test each other; many people schedule study group meetings weekly

IV. Exam-Taking Techniques

A. Before the Exam

1. Know the actual test type (e.g., multiple choice)
2. Be aware of the purpose of the test and type of questions
3. Recognize the components of the test questions—background statement, stem and list of options (distractors)
4. Take practice tests
5. Be prepared on the day of exam—know the site, building, travel route, timing
6. Get plenty of rest the night before the test—do not cram

B. Taking the Exam

1. Identify key words in the test question
2. Recognize item types—selection of one best answer or multiple answers
3. Read directions carefully
4. Follow basic test-taking rules—read questions carefully, time yourself, do not change answers, etc.
5. Use muscle relation techniques during the test to keep your stress down

C. Psych Yourself Up for Taking the Exam, Work on Stress Reduction

1. Good attitude
2. Keep your goals in mind
3. Think positively
4. Use positive self-talk, expect success
5. Feel good about yourself
6. Know yourself
7. Realize that failure is possible
8. Persevere, endurance
9. Develop strategies to reduce fear and anxiety

V. The Computerized Version of the Exam

A. Application for Exam

NOTE: These instructions were taken from the *CBIC Candidate Handbook* (2010) edition. Candidates should obtain their own copy of the *Candidate Handbook* and follow the instructions in the handbook to be sure they are accurate in preparing for the course

1. Administered via computer at over 170 AMP Assessment Centers and selected international sites (typically at H & R Block offices)
2. There are NO application deadlines
3. U.S. citizens may take the test online at www.goAMP.com. Eligibility will be confirmed online. If eligibility is confirmed, the candidate may schedule an examination appointment and make payment by credit card.
4. Candidates may submit a paper application (from the CBIC handbook or website: www.cbic.org). Application must contain all information, appropriate documents and fees and be legible. Notice of eligibility is sent within approximately 2 weeks. If eligibility is confirmed, an examination appointment can be made. Confirmation notice contains toll-free number to contact AMP for scheduling test date and location or the candidate can schedule the exam online at www.goAMP.com
5. The eligibility and acceptance of the application is good for 90 days. A candidate who fails to schedule an appointment for examination within the 90-day eligibility period

must submit a complete application and examination fee to reschedule an examination appointment
6. Candidate must arrive on time (unscheduled candidates or late by 15 minutes will not be admitted)
7. The candidate may reschedule ONE exam appointment at no charge. Cancellation of an appointment must be done at least 2 business days before the exam to prevent forfeiture of application fees (888) 519-9901
8. To be admitted to the testing center, candidate must present 2 forms of identification (one with a current, acceptable photograph)
9. Candidate will be instructed to enter his/her Social Security number and capture his/her own photograph (which will remain on screen and will print on your score report)
10. Before attempting the exam, candidate will be given a practice test
11. Three hours are allowed for completing the 150 test items
12. Anyone with a disability can describe his/her needs on a form located in the *Candidate Handbook*. It includes a section for "Professional documentation" to validate the disability
13. For the cost of the exam or SARE, please refer to the website: www.cbic.org or the *Candidate Handbook*

B. Rules for the Exam

1. Report on the date and at the time scheduled (candidates arriving more than 15 minutes late will not be admitted and will forfeit their fees and registration)
2. No books, papers or reference materials are allowed to be brought into the testing center. Pencils will be provided
3. Scratch paper will be provided to use during the exam but must be turned in before leaving
4. No questions may be asked during the test
5. During the examination, comments may be provided for any questions by clicking on the exclamation point (!) button.
6. Eating, drinking or smoking is not permitted in the testing center
7. A break may be taken during the test, but extra time is not allotted
8. The supervisor may dismiss a candidate from the exam for any of the following reasons:
    a. Candidate's admission is not authorized
    b. Candidate creates a disturbance
    c. Candidate receives or gives help to another candidate
    d. Candidate attempts to write down questions or make notes
    e. Candidate attempts to take the exam for someone else
    f. Candidate is seen using notes
9. No electronic devices, including cell phones, pagers, cameras, tape recorders or personal digital assistants (PDAs) are allowed in the testing center

10. Programmable calculators are not permitted but silent, hand-held, solar or battery-operated calculators without paper tape or alphabetic keypads may be used.
11. The exam time allowed is 3 hours; computer screen will have remaining time on screen (if distracting, can be turned off)
12. Answer each question; do not leave any blank
13. No guests, visitors or family members are allowed in the exam room or reception area.
14. No personal items or belongings will be allowed in the assessment center. Only keys and wallets may be taken into the test room.

Anyone creating a disturbance, getting help during the test or violating one of the above rules of conduct will be reported (their score will not be recorded), and the cost of the exam will not be refunded.

C. Following the Exam

1. Candidate is requested to fill out a short evaluation of the exam
2. Obtain the score report from the testing supervisor
3. Score will contain
   a. "Pass" or "fail" indication
   b. Raw score for each major category is indicated
   c. Total score is based on 135 questions (15 items are pretest items)
   d. Minimum passing score is determined by Angoff method, which estimates the passing probability for each exam item

VI. Self-Assessment Recertification Examination (SARE)

A. Facts about the SARE Exam

1. SARE is a 150-question, multiple-choice, web-based exam
2. SARE questions are different from questions used on standard certification exam but are based on the current CBIC Job Analysis
3. Anyone may purchase the SARE for personal self-assessment or to provide an alternative recertification method for currently certified persons
4. For recertification, the SARE must be completed and mailed by December 31 of the year of recertification
5. Applications for the SARE are included in the *CBIC Certification Handbook*
6. The SARE is geared toward the advanced professional, at a minimum seventh year of practice, and the computerized CBIC exam is geared toward a 2-year practitioner. Many of the questions on the SARE are more difficult than those on the CIC exam
7. If a candidate fails the SARE test when attempting to recertify, the computer test must be taken for any attempts during the next 5 years

VII. Contact Information

CBIC Executive Office
555 East Wells Street
Suite 1100
Milwaukee, WI 53202-3823
Phone: (414) 918-9796
Fax: (414) 276-3349
www.cbic.org info@cbic.org

Applied Measurement Professionals (AMP)
Examination Services
18000 West 105th Street
Phone: (913) 895-4600
Fax: (913) 895-4651
www.goAMP.com; info@goAMP.com

2010 Infection Prevention Competency Review Guide

Evaluation

Please complete and return this evaluation when you have finished using the *Infection Prevention Competency Review Guide*. Your feedback is important as APIC strives to continuously improve educational products. Thank you!

I. Sections used:

- ☐ I. Identification of Infectious Disease Processes
- ☐ II. Surveillance and Epidemiological Investigation
- ☐ III. Preventing/Controlling the Transmission of Infectious Agents
- ☐ IV. Employee/Occupational Health
- ☐ V. Management and Communication
- ☐ VI. Education and Research
- ☐ VII. The Certification Exam

II. Please check the appropriate response:

	Excellent	Good	Fair	Poor
Content	☐	☐	☐	☐
Method of presentation	☐	☐	☐	☐
Usefulness for self-study	☐	☐	☐	☐
Relevance to practice	☐	☐	☐	☐
Met personal goals	☐	☐	☐	☐

	Very High	Moderate	Low	Very Low
Degree of difficulty	☐	☐	☐	☐
Cost of materials	☐	☐	☐	☐

III. Comments:

IV. I plan to take the certification exam next:
☐ Spring ☐ Summer ☐ Fall ☐ N/A

Please return to:
APIC Products Department, 1275 K Street, NW, Suite 1000, Washington, DC 20005–4006

About the Author

Carol M. McLay

Dr. Carol M. McLay received her nursing diploma from Algonquin College in Ottawa, Canada and her Bachelor of Science in Nursing from the University of Ottawa.

She has a Master of Public Health degree in epidemiology from Rollins School of Public Health at Emory University and completed her Doctor of Public Health degree in epidemiology at the University of Kentucky.

Dr. McLay worked for 12 years as an RN in a variety of hospital settings before finding her passion in Infection Prevention and Control. She considers herself fortunate to have been employed in the Hospital Infections Program (now the Division of Healthcare Quality Promotion) at the Centers for Disease Control and Prevention, Atlanta, Georgia while she was completing her MPH degree.

She spent several years as the Director of an Infection Prevention and Control department and has been certified in infection control (CIC) since 2000. In 2006, Dr. McLay was a co-founder of Bluegrass Public Health Consultants and has been working throughout the United States as a consultant in the fields of epidemiology, infection prevention and control and public health. She is also a public health clinical instructor at the University of Kentucky College of Nursing in Lexington, Kentucky.

Her publications and presentations have largely been in the areas of patient safety and infection prevention and control. She was awarded APIC's Blue Ribbon Award in 2001 and has won several awards for Best Oral Presentation. She enjoys traveling to speak at both regional and national lectures. She was a contributing author to the 2002 *APIC Ready Reference to Microbes*.

Dr. McLay currently resides in Lexington, Kentucky with her devoted husband, three precocious young children, two hyperactive dogs and two wily cats.